THE HERBAL APOTHECARY

100 Medicinal Herbs and How to Use Them

JJ PURSELL

with photos by Shawn Linehan

Timber Press
Portland, Oregon

Photo credits begin on page 277.

Published in 2015 by Timber Press, Inc.

Timber Press
The Haseltine Building
133 S.W. Second Avenue, Suite 450
Portland, Oregon 97204-3527

Printed in China

Text design by Kristi Pfeffer
Cover design by Laken Wright

Library of Congress Cataloging-in-Publication Data

Pursell, J. J., 1973– author.
    The herbal apothecary: 100 medicinal herbs and how to use them/JJ Pursell; with photos by Shawn Linehan.—First edition.
        pages cm
    Includes bibliographical references and index.
    ISBN 978-1-60469-662-2 (hardcover)—ISBN 978-1-60469-567-0 (pbk.)
    1. Herbs—Therapeutic use—Handbooks, manuals, etc. 2. Materia medica, Vegetable—Handbooks, manuals, etc. I. Title. II. Title: One hundred medicinal herbs and how to use them.
    RM666.H33P872 2016
    615.3'21—dc23
                                        2015009786

A catalog record for this book is also available from the British Library.

THE HERBAL APOTHECARY

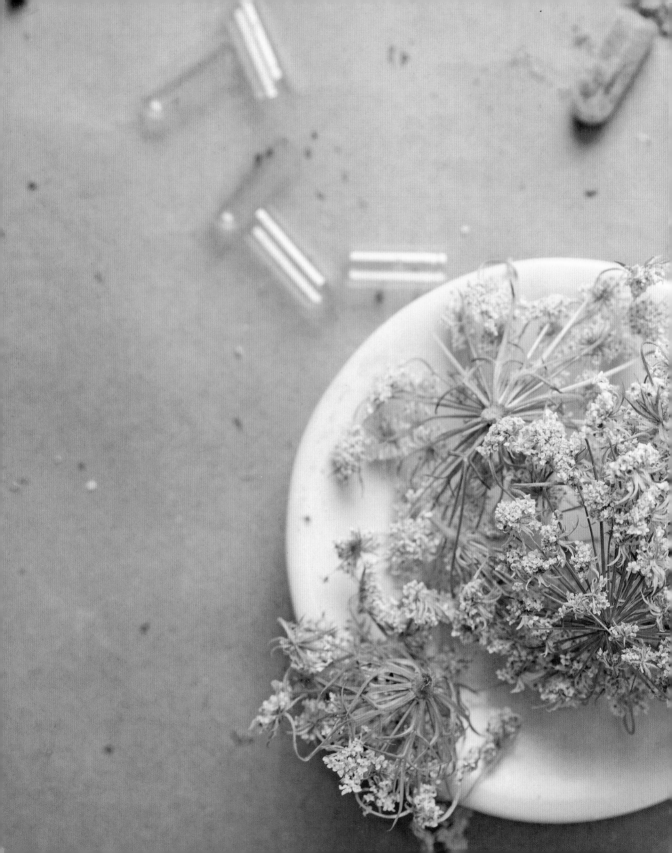

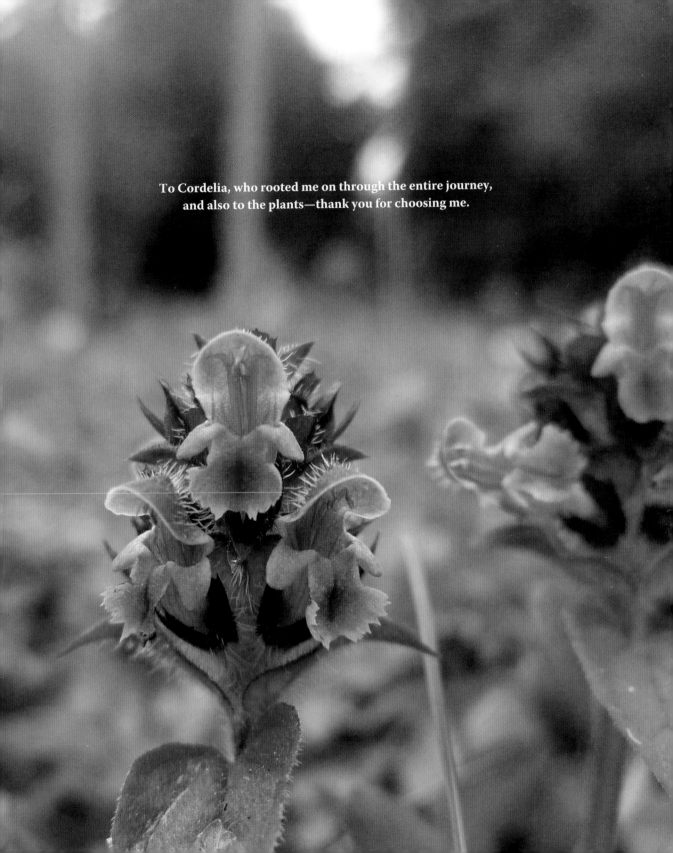

To Cordelia, who rooted me on through the entire journey,
and also to the plants—thank you for choosing me.

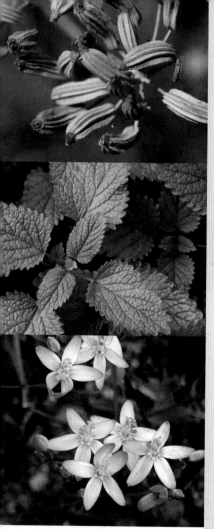

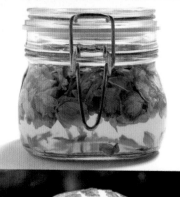

Contents

Preface 8

FROM HERBAL TRADITIONS TO MODERN PRACTICE: AN INTRODUCTION 10

The Way of the Herbalist 16

An Ancient Medicine 20

Plots to Pharmaceuticals 23

BASIC HUMAN ANATOMY 27

The Cardiovascular System 28

The Respiratory System 31

The Gastrointestinal System 34

The Endocrine System 37

PLANTS FROM THE TRADITIONAL WAYS: A DIRECTORY OF MEDICINAL HERBS 40

Getting to Know the Plants: How to read the plant directory 44

Agrimony 54

Angelica 55

Balsam fir 56

Balsam poplar 57

Bayberry 59

Bearberry 60

Bistort 62

Blackberry 63

Black cohosh 64

Black haw 66

Black walnut 67

Blessed thistle 69

Bloodroot 70

Blue flag 72

Blue vervain 73

Bogbean 74

Boneset 76

Borage 77

Buckthorn 78

Bugleweed 79

Burdock 80

Calamus 82

Cedar 83

Centaury 85

Chaga 86

Chaparral 87

Chickweed 88

Chicory 90

Cleavers 91
Couch grass 92
Cowslip 93
Cranesbill 95
Culver's root 96
Echinacea 97
Elder 98
Elecampane 100
False unicorn 101
Fennel 102
Gentian 104
Goat's rue 106
Goldenrod 107
Grand cactus 108
Gravel root 109
Greater celandine 110
Hawthorn 111
Hops 112
Horehound 114
Horny goat weed 115
Horse chestnut 116
Hydrangea 117
Jamaican dogwood 118
Juniper 119
Lady's slipper 121
Larch 122
Lemon balm 123
Licorice 124
Linden 126
Lobelia 127
Lovage 129
Lungwort 130
Maitake 131
Mistletoe 132
Motherwort 133
Mullein 135

Nettle 136
Oatstraw 138
Oregon grape 140
Pennyroyal 141
Plantain 142
Poplar 144
Purple loosestrife 146
Queen of the meadow 147
Raspberry 149
Rauwolfia 150
Red clover 152
Red root 153
Reishi 154
Rosemary 155
Sage 156
Schizandra 157
Self heal 159
Shiitake 160
Skunk cabbage 161
Solomon's seal 162
Sorrel 163
Squaw vine 164
St. John's wort 165
Sumach 167
Sweet violet 168
Thyme 169
Tormentil 170
Usnea 171
White oak 173
Wild carrot 174
Wild cherry 175
Wild yam 177
Wood betony 178
Wormwood 179
Yarrow 181
Yellow dock 182

AN HERBALIST'S LABORATORY 184
Creating an Herbalist's Kitchen 187
Formulating Herbal Blends 189
Delivering the Herbs: Herbal Applications 193

HERBAL TREATMENT PLANS 236
Acne 239
Bumps, Bruises, and Other Childhood Conditions 242
Fatigue and Brain Function 244
Female Complaints 246
Inflammation and Pain 250
Insomnia 253
Menopause 256
Respiratory Ailments 258
Skin Conditions 262
Stress and Adrenal Problems 264
Tummy Complaints and Irritable Bowels 266
Wounds 268

Metric Conversions 272
Herbal Suppliers 273
References 274
Acknowledgments 276
Photo Credits 277
Index 280

Preface

As a child I was always drawn to plants, leaves, flowers, and such. I used to collect acorns as prized possessions, and my imaginary friends were talking trees. Although many of us grow up and often get distracted from our true callings in life, I was fortunate to have the plants persistently remind me of the work I was meant to do. For me, herbalism is a way of life. It is walking with intention every day and giving thanks to the bounty that is all around us, sustaining us. While modern medicine has propelled us into drastic healing measures, herbs continue to create opportunities to return to a gentler approach to health and wellness.

A long time ago, I heard a story about how plants came to help people. A few years later I was walking in the woods and suddenly realized I'd become quite lost. After wandering for hours, I sat down to calm myself and noticed the most beautiful grove of trees. Looking up at them, I felt the warm sun on my face and then felt what seemed like a mother's embrace. As the trees comforted me, I remembered the story and took out my notebook to write it down. This is the story I remembered.

A long, long time ago, we used to be all one—the humans, the animals, the rock people, the water, the wind, the plants, and everything else that was on the Earth. Together we formed one tribe and shared the same language. We were able to communicate and keep the balances of nature in check through a relationship of mutual respect and boundaries.

Then a man killed a bear, and everything changed drastically. This direct act of taking a life upset the balance of the world and great grief settled over the land.

The bear clan came together to discuss what needed to be done. Because such an act had never before happened, most of the bears were unsure of how to proceed. The young warrior bears wanted to take immediate action and get revenge. They wanted to use the force they had never used in battle to kill man and wipe him from existence. They thought that such swift action would result in a return of balance and harmony. The elders listened and finally agreed to let the warrior bears do as they wished.

The warrior bears set out to make a bow and arrow, just as man had done. They asked a young birch tree for an offering to make a strong and sturdy bow. And after they had stripped the bark and shaped the bow, they went looking for the right bowstring to complete it. They tried many things, all of which were not strong enough and quickly broke. They approached the elders and asked, "What did man use for his bowstring?" The elders' gentle eyes looked upon them lovingly, for even though they agreed to let the warrior bears proceed, they knew this path was not the way to peace. Despite this, they said, "The man used dead bear intestine as the string for his bow, because it is strong and filled with tension." At this, the warrior bears all looked frightened and confused about what to do next.

Then one of the eldest bears offered up his body so the warrior bears could continue on this path. It was his time, he said, to go with the setting sun. And he did. And the warrior bears gave thanks and used his intestines to make bowstrings. After all the bows were finished, the warrior bears wanted to practice using them. What happened next was more disappointment. As the bears pulled back the bowstrings, each one snapped under the sharpness of their claws.

What were they to do? One bear suggested they cut off all their claws so that they might use their bows. But at this notion, the elders asked everyone to gather together for another meeting. For this meeting, they called upon every creature of the Earth—the other animals, the plant people, the water people, the creepy crawlies, the wind, grandmother moon, grandfather sky, and Mother Earth herself.

They asked for everyone to think about what was the best course of action. The warrior bears continued to argue that by eliminating man, the world would be returned to peace and balance. They asked for everyone to join them to accomplish this task. Surprisingly, everyone was in agreement—everyone, that is, but the plant people. The plants asked the wise old ginseng for his advice. The old ginseng pondered a moment and then said that he would meditate for three days in a cave in the mountains. After the three days he would know what was best for the world.

So up went the wise old ginseng to meditate in the cave in the mountains. And although this was a quiet place, each day the mosquito would buzz up to the ginseng and ask, "What are you going to do? How are we going to help? What is your decision?" And each day, ginseng would reply, "When I am done with my meditation, I will know what is best for the world." Those mosquitos can be so annoying.

After three days, the wise old ginseng descended from the cave. Once again, everyone gathered, anxiously awaiting his thoughts. After a slow, deep breath, the old ginseng said, "Although we are one with the world, we cannot be one with this decision. We the plant people must help man, for they are naïve and, like children, need healing and guidance. From this day forth, plants will offer themselves to man in hopes of creating balance in their health by healing them."

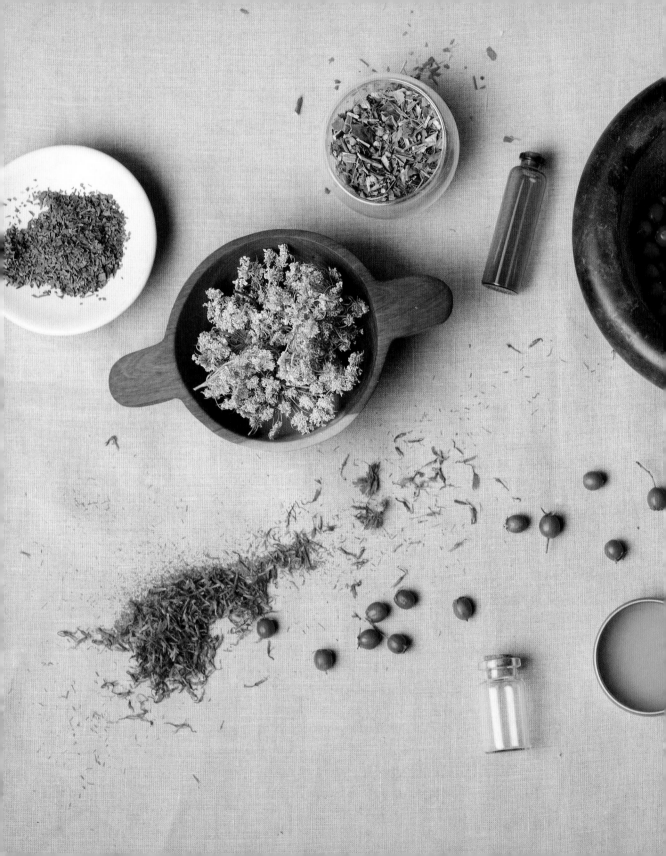

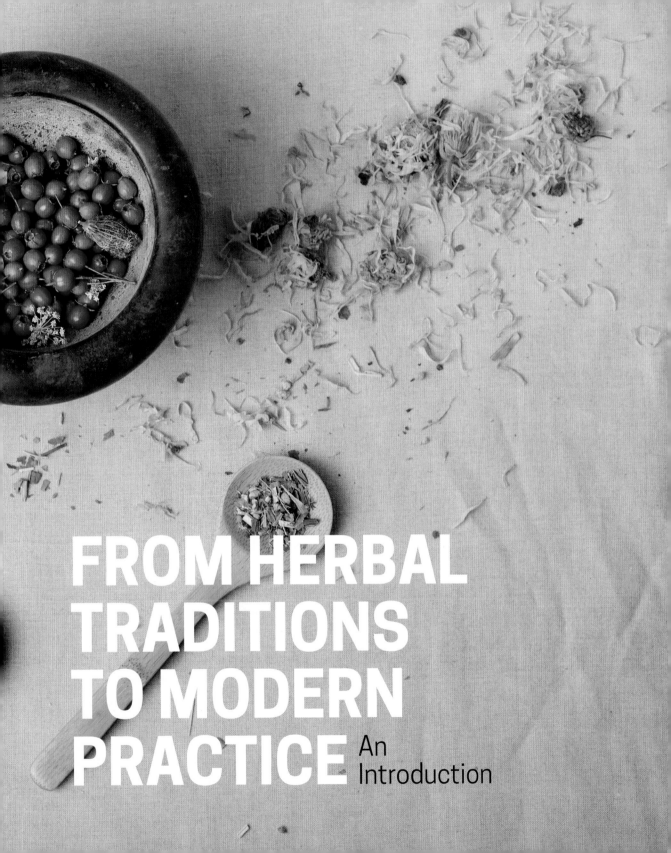

FROM HERBAL TRADITIONS TO MODERN PRACTICE

An Introduction

What is it about plants that draws us in and creates a strong desire to learn their secret ways of healing? Perhaps it is a remembrance of a time long ago, when we all knew how to use them as medicine. Or it may be a desire to deepen our connection to nature and to study its healing bounty. Some of us are driven by the simple curiosity of learning an approach to medicine that differs from that of the established mainstream. However you discovered your interest in herbal medicine, you should know that herbalism and herbal medicine are time-honored traditions with a lot to offer you, your family, and your community.

Herbs are used for healing by much of the world's population, yet herbalism has often been considered folk healing and some herbs have been deemed unsafe for general consumption. Some may say that we don't need to use herbs, because today we have modern medical techniques and a pill for every situation. Some believe that we should leave behind the old ways because they are ineffective, and we should adopt new ways because they are superior. As a result of such beliefs, the herbal knowledge that was once common in every household is now a rare commodity. But times are changing, and the call to return to our roots is being heard by more and more of us.

You can learn about herbs in many ways. One of the best ways to learn is from teachers who share stories and valuable knowledge. They can offer keen insights into herbs and their uses. Find teachers within your community who practice the traditional ways of herbal medicine. Take a class or workshop, or work on an herb farm. Form a mentoring relationship to gain perspectives on how to use the plants.

It is also important that you spend time with the plants. Find an herb growing in your yard, or sit outside with a cup of herbal tea. What do you see? What does it smell like? When you drink tea made from the herb, how does it make you feel? Until you've spent time touching, seeing, smelling, and tasting the plant, your knowledge is incomplete.

And then, of course, you can consult the many available books on herbs and herbalism. We are fortunate to have access to books written long ago and to the generations of books written since. They include many aspects and influences (such as astrology) of herbal medicine, and most agree on which plant should be used when and how each is used. This information was drawn from years of study, research, and experience. Once in a while, however, you will find information in one source that differs from what you have learned elsewhere. I continue to find humor in my students' despair with the differing opinions they sometimes find as they research herbs. But this is a good thing! Each herbalist provides a detailed account of his or her own experience with the herb and how it works.

This information results from the time the herbalist has spent with the plant. You may have a completely different experience with the same herb, and that is fine.

One thing most herbal professionals do agree about is that herbs serve particular functions when they are consumed.

- Herbs help the body eliminate waste. If the body experiences poor digestion or sluggish detoxification, herbs move out the old to make way for the new.
- Herbs promote healing. Their mineral and vitamin content help the body heal and reestablish proper form and function.
- Herbs increase overall energy in the body. Herbs provide a boost that helps the body heal and detoxify, which increases day-to-day energy levels.

This book is for the beginning herbal enthusiast who is looking for a lot of information in one place. Many books on herbs focus on specific plants, medicine-making, or the history of herbs, but I wanted to write a book with a bit of everything, from both the traditional and scientific perspectives. As an herbalist turned biochemist, turned naturopathic physician, I am a gatherer of information. This book is my attempt to share some of what I've learned about herbs. I think its components will help you understand herbal medicine in a philosophical, scientific, and traditional way. By weaving in anatomy, plant descriptions, and herbal treatment ideas, I have provided information that I hope will help you view this dynamic system from a holistic perspective to gain a clear understanding of how and when to use plants as medicine.

As you begin your herbal studies, remember that traditional herbalism is far more complex than what is presented in this book. Herbalism focuses on a deeper level that involves the concepts of tissue states (excitation, depression, atrophy, stagnation, tension, relaxation), the four qualities or natures (hot, cold, dry, damp), the patient's temperament, and the energetics (the subtle energies) of the plant. If you want to know more about these subjects, read *The Practice of Traditional Western Herbalism* by Matthew Wood (2004).

Although there are many philosophies, we don't really know how herbs actually work as medicine. We do know, however, that they work in a holistic way to treat entire bodily systems rather than a single symptom, and they nourish and restore balance in the body so that organs in disharmony can return to optimal function. When a plant is taken into the body, it is recognized on a cellular level. Not only does the body identify the plant's constituents, but it also seems to know how to break them down and put them to work where they are needed. Although herbs can be effective on many physiological aspects and levels, they work with the body to recognize and attend to the area in greatest need first. We can

also get creative with formulation, blending various herbs into combinations that focus with even greater intention.

Many herbs are high in minerals that feed the body with the healing components needed to improve cellular regeneration, circulation, elimination, and organ function. We can scientifically test physiological function after herbs are administered to show their effectiveness. Consider several examples. Ginger contains very potent anti-inflammatory compounds called gingerols. Several clinical studies involving arthritis patients found that ginger extracts affected the inflammatory process at a cellular level to reduce pain and inflammation. Blood cell counts measured after administration of immune-stimulating herbs show increased white cell counts. Biopsies taken after herbal administration have shown positive changes in cellular structure.

Modern medicine has done an excellent job of isolating plants and body parts, but it is severely lacking in the dynamic principles of holism and systemic unity. Whether you are considering a plant or your body, be mindful of the complete system rather than the individual parts or symptoms. When you use herbs, think about the entire plant and how it will affect the body in a holistic manner. For example, meadowsweet tea is often used to treat stomach problems and can be particularly helpful for children with diarrhea. One constituent (a scientifically active component within the herb) of meadowsweet is salicylic acid, which is an important ingredient in aspirin. When salicylic acid is taken in an isolated form, it can cause irritation to the stomach wall. But in addition to salicylic acid, meadowsweet contains antioxidants called polyphenols, which protect the stomach wall. This means that meadowsweet offers the desired action of pain relief without the side effect of stomach irritation.

In my practice, I rarely see a patient who experiences an issue in isolation. When one system or organ is struggling, it is likely that other systems or organs are suffering as well. When we use herbs, we must consider several important points as we integrate this way of thinking to treat the body from a holistic perspective.

- Identify and treat the cause. Although acute situations, such as burns, can often be quickly soothed with herbs, long-standing disharmony requires investigation and the promotion of balance within all bodily systems.
- Look at the whole body. What bodily discomforts do you view as normal? What symptoms have you experienced for so long that you almost don't feel them anymore? In the hustle and bustle of our busy lives, we can become disconnected to what is happening in our bodies and the signs and signals of distress.
- Trust the power of nature. Take a look around, and you will see that healing plants are everywhere. Many plants that grow in particular climates are specific to treating the illnesses

of that region. Where I live in the Pacific Northwest, for example, rosemary and cedar grow in abundance. Both are excellent for our ever-present damp conditions that can affect the respiratory tract and joints.
- Prevention is key. Don't kid yourself that you can live a long and healthy life and do nothing to sustain it. Be an advocate for your body. Treat it well, know its signs and symptoms of distress, and learn how to assist it when it speaks to you.

Wherever you are on your herbal journey, I'm happy to be a part of it. Speaking from experience, I know it can be life changing to recognize a healing plant and use it to help you feel better. Go slowly through the book to absorb all that is contained within and reread it several times to cement certain concepts for forever learning. Most of all, get out among the plants. They are the best teachers. I hope that you will use this book as an everyday tool and view it as a bridge toward living and healing in a more holistic way. Teach yourself and share with others. Reclaim the knowledge that was once exchanged freely by all.

The Way of the Herbalist

At one time, throughout the Americas and elsewhere, plant medicine was commonly taught in households and shared within communities. Although the popularity of modern medicine has resulted in a decrease of these practices, in North America at least, the use of herbal medicine is making a mass resurgence, and herbal practitioners are guiding others through the mystery and practicality of the power of herbs.

It is difficult to pinpoint the beginnings of herbal medicine, but we do know that tribal cultures have used healing plants for many generations. Herbs were originally eaten as simple foods, but human curiosity being what it is, some devoted time and energy to experiment with plants and began recognizing their value in health and healing. Since prehistory, herbs have been used for illness and fever, broken bones, blood diseases, and many other conditions. People eventually recognized that using herbs preventatively seemed to promote some of their strongest effects, strengthening the body to fight off illness. One such example is the vinegar of the four thieves, consumed by robbers from Marseilles, France, during the bubonic plague epidemic. After plundering the homes of those who had fallen ill, none of the thieves who took daily doses of the vinegar succumbed to the plague.

At one time, medicinal herbs were often grown in home gardens, including simple herbs known for their ability to relieve fever, heal wounds, and treat bites. Herbal remedies were commonplace, and if a person didn't know the appropriate herb to treat an illness, he could go to a house where rosemary grew, knowing this would be the place to get herbal information. Much like the telling of any good story, herbal remedies were shared when knowledge was passed from generation to generation. Many of our grandmothers, in fact, cooked up herbal concoctions and stored them in the cupboard. At some point, as the era of modern medicine ascended, herbal remedies began to be mistrusted as inferior medicine—not because they were harmful or dangerous, but because they were considered inferior to the new synthetic medications.

As a budding herbalist, you have a lot to consider and much to be excited about. I've spoken with countless people about their interest in herbs and when it began. For many, it was a simple realization that what was being presented about using herbs medicinally seemed to make a lot of sense. Unlike the often overwhelming and confusing American model of modern medicine, herbal medicine presented something familiar and comforting. I like to think that understanding the basics of herbs and how they work gives us confidence that if we or our family members experience a cold or the flu, an upset tummy, or a muscle strain, for example, we can responsibly care for ourselves and our loved ones. One aspect of herbs that I particularly enjoy is the relationship built between the person and the plants. Every journey is different, and plant medicine encourages that, offering endless resources and building bonds from knowledge and experience.

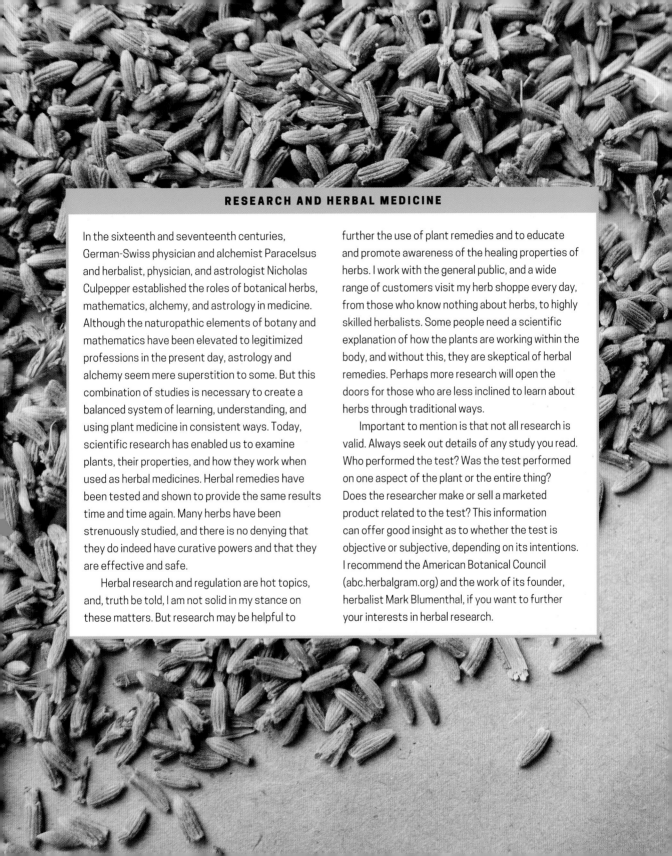

RESEARCH AND HERBAL MEDICINE

In the sixteenth and seventeenth centuries, German-Swiss physician and alchemist Paracelsus and herbalist, physician, and astrologist Nicholas Culpepper established the roles of botanical herbs, mathematics, alchemy, and astrology in medicine. Although the naturopathic elements of botany and mathematics have been elevated to legitimized professions in the present day, astrology and alchemy seem mere superstition to some. But this combination of studies is necessary to create a balanced system of learning, understanding, and using plant medicine in consistent ways. Today, scientific research has enabled us to examine plants, their properties, and how they work when used as herbal medicines. Herbal remedies have been tested and shown to provide the same results time and time again. Many herbs have been strenuously studied, and there is no denying that they do indeed have curative powers and that they are effective and safe.

Herbal research and regulation are hot topics, and, truth be told, I am not solid in my stance on these matters. But research may be helpful to further the use of plant remedies and to educate and promote awareness of the healing properties of herbs. I work with the general public, and a wide range of customers visit my herb shoppe every day, from those who know nothing about herbs, to highly skilled herbalists. Some people need a scientific explanation of how the plants are working within the body, and without this, they are skeptical of herbal remedies. Perhaps more research will open the doors for those who are less inclined to learn about herbs through traditional ways.

Important to mention is that not all research is valid. Always seek out details of any study you read. Who performed the test? Was the test performed on one aspect of the plant or the entire thing? Does the researcher make or sell a marketed product related to the test? This information can offer good insight as to whether the test is objective or subjective, depending on its intentions. I recommend the American Botanical Council (abc.herbalgram.org) and the work of its founder, herbalist Mark Blumenthal, if you want to further your interests in herbal research.

Herbalists are doing amazing things all around us. Consider, for example, author, healer, and teacher Rosemary Gladstar, and her work as a founder of United Plant Savers. The work of United Plant Savers involves research, education, and conservation of native medicinal plants and their habitats. Through her passion, Rosemary has become a visionary beyond the normal constructs of her career. She began blending medicinal herbs for teas in the 1970s, because she believed in the medicine and felt called to share it with others.

Mark Blumenthal is another dedicated herbalist who has truly devoted himself to the study, trade, and research of herbal medicine in North America. As the founder of the American Botanical Counsel, he encourages the public to make educated, responsible choices about herbal medicine as an accepted part of healthcare. The counsel's mission is to provide education using science-based and traditional information to promote responsible use of herbal medicine to serve the public, researchers, educators, healthcare professionals, industry, and media. Mark started his herbal journey as a hobbyist. As a young adult in the 1960s, he began picking up herb books at natural grocery stores and visiting the woods to identify the plants he was studying. His first real business venture, selling herbs to small, local grocers, eventually grew into a company that created and distributed Mark's own herbal products. Since then, he has become a leader in herbal product regulation. Through years of work, Mark came to realize that herbal education was the missing link in North America and decided to dedicate his life to this endeavor.

Health consultant Donnie Yance, founder of the Mederi Centre for Natural Healing in southern Oregon, is a great example of an herbalist and visionary. After he read the book *Back to Eden* by Jethro Kloss, his life was never the same. Inspired by herbs and their potential, he dove in headfirst and sought out herbal education through the Sequoyah College of Herbology. Eventually he opened the Centre for Natural Healing, which specializes in herbal formulation and compounding, especially for treating cancer.

Margi Flint owns and operates EarthSong Herbals, a busy family practice and herb school in Marblehead, Massachusetts. She has more than 35 years of herbal practice experience. She sees clients for consultations and offers many classes throughout the year. She is also the author of a textbook for herbalists, *The Practicing Herbalist: Meeting with Clients, Reading the Body*, a valuable resource for anyone interested in practicing herbalism.

Wanting to offer more opportunities for herbal education and clinical experience, Paul Berger created the North American Institute of Medical Herbalism and subsequently the Colorado School of Clinical Herbalism. His work has led the way to provide herbalists with the confidence to pursue their interests in positive and successful consulting careers.

Phyllis Hogan, Linda Quintana, Mimi Kamp, Matthew Wood, Sean Donahue, Jill Stansbury, David Hoffman, Sarah Holmes, David Winston, Karyn Sanders—the list of inspiring herbalists goes on and on, but all have a common thread: their spark was ignited by a passion for herbal medicine. If you are still reading this, my guess is that your spark has also been ignited.

As interest in herbal medicine continues to grow, you'll find more opportunities to get involved, and perhaps you'll decide to devote your professional life to the study of herbal medicines, as I have done. I went to naturopathic school to obtain my doctorate in medicine so that I could be licensed to do what I wanted with herbs. I was afraid that without a credentialed degree that provided legitimacy, I would be limited in continuing my profession as an herbalist. Although school was definitely an important part of my journey as a person, my original concerns about getting the degree proved to be unwarranted. I do believe in education, particularly when it comes to using herbs, but focusing on herbs, if that is what you want to do, is the best course of action. Go into the woods, be with yourself and the plants, find teachers, take classes, and sign up for internships. Surround yourself with herbs and devote your time and study to them.

You can find teachers and herb schools in many communities, but if you want something more academically structured, Maryland University of Integrative Health, Bastyr University, and the California Institute of Herbal Studies are options to consider. If you love herbs and want to help others, study the herbs and become the herbalist you want to be. Although herbalists are not doctors allowed to practice medicine in North America, we can provide information to others about improving their health using herbs. Share what you learn so that others can benefit. I often hear students and herbal enthusiasts deny themselves the title of "herbalist." If you love herbs and are studying them, I'm here to inform you that you are indeed an herbalist.

What does the future hold? These are exciting times for herbalists. We are witnessing the art of herbalism rapidly regaining its rightful place as a modality for health and healing. However, as herbalism flourishes and winds its way back into the mainstream, it is eliciting a unique set of problems and concerns. Be aware of such issues to protect the future of herbalism. Understand the practice of sustainable harvesting and wildcrafting, know where your herbs come from, protect habitats from destruction, educate yourself thoroughly on how herbs work within the body before using them, and support herbalist guilds and communities through membership. Most importantly, live in kindness and at peace, and enjoy yourself in whatever herbal relationship you choose, whether as a hobbyist, an enthusiast, or a professional.

An Ancient Medicine

The story of medicinal plants is an ancient one that threads many cultures from around the world into a common tapestry. The first medicinal drugs were in the form of herbs, plants, roots, flowers, and fungi. Archaeologists have uncovered evidence, including symbolic depictions and fossilized sediments of the plants depicted, which suggests that medicinal herbs were used in the Paleolithic Era, some 60,000 years ago. The first legitimized documentation of herbal remedies begins with the Sumerians in ancient Mesopotamia (present-day Iraq), who lived more than 5000 years ago. They carved recipes on clay slabs, or tablets, that included drug preparations referring to more than 250 plants. Imagine the plant life utopia at that time! Some of these writings suggest advanced understanding of plant constituents, such as the alkaloid principles of poppy, henbane, and mandrake. These herbs must have been tried through experimentation, as no one during that time would have known the full effects of the plants. I'm sure that, for some of them, some lessons were tough to learn. The Sumerians, considered one of the world's first urban civilizations, were originally recorded as a matriarchal society that viewed everything from a natural perspective, understanding that nature controlled all and was bountiful. Similar to Daoists, the Sumerians watched nature and its cycles to correlate similar cycles within the human body for healing practices.

In China, people were experimenting with plant medicine as well. Around 2500 BC, the first Chinese herbal, *Shen Nung Pen T'sao ching*, was written by Emperor Shen Nung. It focused on grasses and roots, documenting 365 herbs. An interesting and dedicated herbalist, Shen Nung personally tasted each of these herbs and—you guessed it—unfortunately died due to a toxic overdose, all in the name of plant medicine. He came from an agricultural background and was often referred to as the Yan Emperor, or divine farmer. His work is considered the basis for Chinese herbalism, which is universally accepted in China and practiced throughout the world. Many of the herbs he mentioned are still widely used today, including camphor, podophyllum, jimson weed, cinnamon bark, ginseng, gentian, and ma huang. (The ma huang shrub first brought the drug ephedrine to modern medicine.)

The East Indian traditions of Ayurveda (science of life) and the *Vedas* scriptures are filled with abundant references to medical treatments using plants. Ayurvedic herbalists Charaka (*circa* 800 BC) and Sushruta (*circa* 500 BC) were two of the first to write preparations from plant, mineral, and animal sources. These were the first formulations, or herbal blends, for creating healing prescriptions. Sushruta categorized plants into subdivisions according to diseases and plant treatments. Ayurvedic practices are some of the most practical when it comes to using herbs with foods, understanding the simple knowledge that food is medicine. Healing spices such as nutmeg, pepper, clove, caraway, and turmeric all descend from Ayurvedic culture and are often used today.

In another part of the world, Egyptians were no strangers to the use of plant medicine, particularly because of their close relationship with Babylonia and Assyria. They shared similar plant medicine and theurgist (supernatural) philosophies, but there is no question that Egyptians were much less fond of the metaphysics of medicine. Most of our knowledge of Egyptian plant medicine comes from the writings of historians, especially Manetho (*circa* 300 BC). Another valuable resource are the wall depictions of monuments and tombs. The *Papyrus Ebers*, written around 1550 BC, includes 700 plant, mineral, and animal species and more than 800 prescription entries. Upon discovery and translation, this was the largest materia medica (a body of collected knowledge about the therapeutic properties of a substance used for healing) and prescription document found from this time period. Many of the prescriptions include herbs such as pomegranate, senna, castor oil, centaury, garlic, coriander, juniper, and willow. Despite Egypt's inhospitable growing terrain and the surrounding desert, the Egyptians cultivated many indigenous plants for medicinal use.

Moving forward, although many herbalists have made significant contributions in the field of plant medicine, a few have devoted their lives to the study of herbal medicine. Here is an abbreviated history.

It is difficult to think of the roots of plant medicine without including Greek botanist Theophrastus (371–287 BC), considered the father of botany. At an early age, he began his studies under Plato. After Plato's death, he attached himself to Aristotle. Needless to say, his interests were wide-ranging, extending from biology and physics, to ethics and metaphysics. But his love of plants resulted in his authoring two books, *De Causis Plantarum* and *De Historia Plantarum*, which generated a classification system of more than 500 medicinal plants. This was the first document of its kind to include the importance of gradual dosing to acclimate the body to treatment. This was extremely important information at the time regarding the proper use of herbs, especially those with a high toxicity content; knowing how to use them could be the difference between life and death.

Pedanius Dioscorides (AD 40–90), from current-day Turkey, was a physician, pharmacologist, and botanist who is most remembered as the first to consider plant medicine as an applied science. As a physician, he traveled extensively with Roman militaries and studied the plants in-depth wherever he went. His work *De Materia Medica* has been translated many times over as the primary herbal encyclopedia from the Middle Ages to the Renaissance. His book offered not only plant descriptions, but also the names of each plant and foraging information. He also mentions such preparations as extracts by the maceration method followed by evaporation, and how to express the fresh juice of plants and concentrate it in the sun. *De Materia Medica* was also one of the first books to document how to store plants, providing the basis for modern storage.

Along this historical journey is Roman physician Aelius Galenus, or Galen of Pergamon, who escalated the teachings of Hippocrates to become the foundations of western medicine. Galen promoted and wrote often about Hippocrates's system of the four humors (blood, yellow bile, black bile, and phlegm), healing modalities, and herbs. He believed that humors were formed in the body, rather than ingested, and suggested that the body reacted to consumed foods by producing different humors. Warm foods, for example, tended to produce yellow bile, while cold foods tended to produce phlegm. Other factors could affect the production of humors as well, including the time of year, a person's age, where they lived, their profession, and even their life circumstances. Using this system, Galen was able to blend herbs to balance out deficiencies or excesses depending on a patient's condition. His work also led to the creation of a book that compiled the first list of plant drugs with similar actions. He classified plants into simples (herbs with only one quality), composites (herbs with more than one quality), and entities (herbs with specific qualities, such as purgatives, emetics, and poisons). This classification was particularly helpful to herbalists of the time, because it provided a cross-reference for similar herbs based on treatment and condition. For 1500 years, Galen's book was in popular use, until 1858, when his work and theories were decisively displaced by Rudolf Virchow's newly published theories of cellular pathology.

But before Virchow, a select few had significant impacts on the field of plant medicine, including Hildegard von Bingen (1098–1165), who was sent to live with Benedictine nuns at age 8 because of her gifts as a visionary. Her experience in the monastery gardens and helping to heal the sick allowed her to accumulate extensive knowledge of plants and herbal healing techniques. She composed various books that focused on the scientific and medicinal properties of plants, stones, fish, reptiles, and animals, including *Causae et Curae*, which examined human healing through the lens of nature and its cycles. Her approach was similar to the theories of Chinese Daoism, blending a holistic approach with Hippocrates's humors.

From the fifteenth through eighteenth centuries, plant medicine was researched, documented, and shared around the world through translation. Prior to this, traditional plant medicines were consumed as simple preparations, such as teas, drops, poultices, and salves. But with new knowledge and texts becoming available, herbalists began to compound plants and ingredients, and these blends were in high demand. Herbalists had an opportunity to work empirically (based on experience) rather than experimentally, which was probably a great relief. This was the time of John Gerard, Nicholas Culpepper, and Carl Linnaeus. Despite being discounted by physicians of the time, Culpepper's work in the healing and herbal field was still extremely popular with the masses and continues to be used today. The consensus was that the new compounded medicine was stronger, and stronger was better. Because of the value placed on these medicines, they were sold at a high price and not available to all. Sound familiar?

Plants to Pharmaceuticals

The nineteenth century provided an important turning point for herbal medicine. With the high demand for more sophisticated drugs, scientists began looking at the active constituents of plants, which led to the first experiments that isolated plant components, including alkaloids from poppies, ipecacuanha, strychnos, and quinine. With these advancements, scientific pharmacy was born, and remedies were filled with plant derivatives.

- Asiaticoside, derived from gotu kola, helps heal wounds.
- Berberine, derived from barberry, has antimicrobial and antibiotic properties.
- Camphor, derived from the camphor tree, causes dilation of the capillaries and increases blood circulation.
- Codeine, derived from the opium poppy, helps relieve pain and reduce coughs.
- Etoposide, derived from the may apple, is an antitumor agent.
- Scopolamine, derived from jimson weed, has strong sedative effects.
- Taxol, derived from the Pacific yew, is used to treat a variety of cancers.

Unfortunately, this practice led to herbal medicine being taken from the people and given to those who wanted to control it.

Currently, plant-derived pharmaceuticals make up one-fourth of the drugs available in American pharmacies. Almost all pharmacies prescribe medicines derived from plants. Many countries, including the United States, have both pharmaceutical and herbal pharmacies, and in some countries they are considered of equal importance in treating illness. In Russia, Germany, and the United Kingdom, for example, herbal medicines are a part of the mainstay medical experience. Knowledge about how and when to use them is offered at each pharmacy.

Despite this, most American allopathic (mainstream) doctors are neither trained nor offered continuing education on the history of plant medicine, herbal knowledge, or herbal pharmaceutical contraindications. Many suggest that plant medicine is ineffectual and dangerous, but herbalists know that education is key, and any good practitioner will include education in each treatment plan.

Pharmaceutical drugs typically consist of one chemical, whereas plants can contain hundreds. It is usually easy to determine the side effects of one chemical component, but grasping the potential side effects of the endless components in a plant is difficult. Interestingly, the multitude of components in a plant also explain why some herbs have contradicting qualities—an herb may be both stimulating and relaxing or both astringent and dilating. In addition, two or more of a plant's constituents often work together to achieve a physiological effect. The bark of cat's claw is a good example. Research on extracts of the whole cat's claw plant demonstrated its ability to boost the human immune system. In efforts to understand the aspects that accomplish this, scientists isolated and extracted several alkaloids, hoping to identify the single component that provided this benefit, so that it could be replicated and marketed. As it turned out, the isolated alkaloids were actually much weaker in action when they were separated from the rest of the plant. In cat's claw, alkaloids and tannins synergistically work together to optimize the body's immune system.

Those developing new pharmaceuticals may also encounter a variety of problems. In particular, they cannot patent crude plant preparations—in other words, they cannot patent nature. Therefore, drug developers are constantly on the lookout for single plant components that they can isolate and change slightly so they can patent it. Consider coumarin, for example, which is found in red clover, aniseed, fenugreek, and other herbs. Coumarin increases blood flow in the veins and decreases capillary permeability. After isolating coumarin from a plant, biotechnicians added a small salt molecule. This did not alter the action of coumarin, yet it produced a new substance that was patentable.

The biological activity of a newly produced pharmaceutical drug is of little importance to its manufacturer, because the drug can be controlled through increasing or decreasing dosage and application. After they've identified and extracted the chemical compounds and created the drug, they can manipulate it by adding other chemical elements to change the way it performs. In an alchemic context, this is quite amazing. Dosing is

key, but it doesn't necessarily guarantee that a drug is safe. Prescribed drugs have very specific dosing requirements, but even if a patient takes the appropriate amount, the drug can be toxic and can even lead to death.

In 2004 I attended the Medicines of the Earth conference in Black Mountain, North Carolina. This is one of my favorite conferences because of the wide range of speakers and topics, and it tends to be research- and science-heavy. That year, a panel of leading herbalists, including David Hoffman, Donnie Yance, and Jill Stansbury, cited several statistics that left an impression on me. The topic was herbal safety, and during the discussion, someone mentioned the staggering number of hospitalizations and deaths related to pharmaceutical drugs, a number that grows each year. Melody Peterson, author of *Our Daily Meds* (2008), states that approximately 100,000 Americans die each year from properly prescribed medications as a result of known side effects. What this means is that the doctor prescribed the medication correctly, the pharmacist filled it correctly, but the medication simply failed the patients, leading to their deaths.

Since 1983, the American Association of Poison Control Centers has recorded every type of poisoning that has occurred in the United States, including those caused by dietary and herbal supplements. Keep in mind that most herbal medicine poisonings are caused by someone taking too much of something and not necessarily the prescribed or proper dose. Even with that consideration, the numbers of annual deaths resulting from herbs is still less than 1 percent of the total annual deaths resulting from prescription drugs.

Many pharmaceutical compounds include inorganic components that the body either struggles to break down or cannot break down, and this can cause cellular communication issues and toxicity within the body. In addition, most pharmaceuticals lead to acidity in the body, which inhibits proper digestion of nutrients. By nature, plants contain many of the same compounds found in the human body, which enables cellular recognition and the body's innate ability to break down the components.

Finally, pharmaceutical drugs are prescribed to mask the symptoms a patient is experiencing. Here's an (oversimplified) example. You have chronic heartburn, so you take acid-blockers. Although these drugs may change your day-to-day digestive state for a while, most of them eventually become ineffective, and their long-term use can cause other health issues. Herbs certainly can be used to treat acute symptoms, but the herbal medicine philosophy is to treat the underlying cause to improve overall health and be rid of the need for medications.

We are in the midst of an era in which synthetic drugs and antibiotics are failing to keep us healthy, and this makes plant medicine even more important.

Herbal supplementation costs less than a typical pharmaceutical prescription. The beauty of herbs is that they are often readily available in nature, and if you are qualified and trained to identify the herb in the wild, and the plant is not protected in some way, it is free for the taking. And the various application options—from tea, to poultices, to washes, to liquid extracts—give us a wide cost variable that makes one form or another available for every economic class.

Why else do we use herbs? They enable us to be proactive in our health so that in our later years, we can hope to have fewer health compromises. You have only one body, so treat it like a temple. Give thanks every day. How you do so is your choice.

BASIC HUMAN ANATOMY

Knowing how your body functions is powerful knowledge that you can apply directly to how you use herbs. For example, perhaps you suffer from acid reflux, which occurs at the top of the gastrointestinal system, or maybe flatulence is the issue, which is farther along. When you understand how the gastrointestinal processes work, you'll be able to choose the best herbs to deal with each particular belly complaint.

All bodily processes are controlled by organs that are part of several systems that work together to keep us alive and well. Herbalists believe that disease is caused by system imbalance. If one bodily system is unbalanced or unhealthy, others may be affected as well. For this reason, herbalists treat the acute situation and support the underlying causes to create sustained change and health. This is fundamental to holistic healing.

The following pages offer information on the cardiovascular, respiratory, gastrointestinal, and endocrine systems of the body. Although I have separated them to help you understand their physiological functions, they are most truly interconnected, as are all bodily systems.

The Cardiovascular System

At one time or another, we've all listened to a heartbeat—the steady thump, thump of a continuous pulsation in the chambers inside the largest muscle in the body, equal in size to a large turnip at 8 to 10 ounces. The heart's chambers and passageways pump blood to every living cell in the body. In classical Chinese medicine, the heart is referred to as the empress. Empress heart governs both the flow of blood and distribution of oxygen, water, nutrients, waste materials, immune cells, and hormones. As the ruler, the heart is where everything begins, and as with any good leader, the heart should be calm in spirit, gracefully guiding peace throughout the body to create balance in all physical functions.

I love being human. Each of us is a big body of thoughts, functions, and feelings, with an advanced brain that connects all these sensations. No one can deny that humans have a highly functioning limbic brain system that deals specifically with emotions. Although our emotions can at times be overwhelming, they are some of the unique and beautiful aspects of living as a human being. And which organ feels and responds to each and every emotion we experience? The heart.

Although the brain sends messages to the heart, the heart sends far more signals to the brain, and these signals significantly affect cognitive function such as attention, perception, memory, and problem-solving. In reality, emotions are an important aspect to health and particularly to the heart. Studies have shown that anger, stress, or grief can affect a person's ability to think clearly and remember things correctly as a result of erratic signals sent from the heart to the brain. Studies with a heart rate monitor have shown that emotional states also affect the heart's rhythm. During times of stress and negative emotions, heart rate patterns become erratic and disordered, with increased or abnormal rates. These studies also monitored the hearts of people who were experiencing a sense of calm or positive emotions, revealing an ordered and stable heart rate.

Extreme emotion or heartbreak, sadness, and depression physically affect our hearts. Countless studies have shown how depression and feelings of isolation and loneliness affect the heart. Heartbreak can cause people to become sick, or even die, following the death of a loved one. Modern technology has made it easier for us to have limited physical contact with others, yet most of us still feel the physical need to share friendship, deep love, gratitude, values, or simple contact through a smile. Without such contact, the heart and cardiovascular system can undergo physical changes, such as irregular functioning or hardening of the arteries. The repetitive experience of negative emotions also leads to atherosclerosis (hardening of the arteries) and inflammation in the heart. Atherosclerosis, of course, is one of the leading causes of heart attacks and strokes.

Although heart disease is considered a congenital or genetic disease, many people develop heart disease without these predispositions. By looking beyond the symptoms that arise from heart disease to take a closer look at the causes of heart pathologies, we may save our lives or, at the very least, help ourselves lead more joyful lives.

So what does all of this have to do with herbs? As a naturopathic physician, acupuncturist, and herbalist, I am always returning to the concept of wholeness and to how herbs can affect the physical functioning of the heart and other organs. Although herbs may not directly address the cause of a heart illness, they can often be helpful in improving day-to-day health.

Herbs for the cardiovascular system

A broad range of herbs support the heart and cardiovascular system. Some increase the efficiency of the heart function, while others increase the strength of the heartbeat or normalize the heart rate. Herbal remedies nurture the heart in deeper ways as well. Because cardiac well-being depends on spiritual as well as physical attributes, you can drink cordials (tonics taken in small amounts to strengthen the body, mind, and spirit) or take nervines (tonics used to help calm the body, mind, and spirit) to support the heart.

Cardiac herbal remedies are typically divided into two main groups: cardiotonics and cardioactives. Cardiotonic herbs restore tone and function to heart. They do not usually produce a dramatic effect, but they are nourishing and tonifying to the whole system, improving overall function and health. Cardiotonics should be taken long-term to create sustained positive physical change and improve heart rate and rhythm, decrease

BASIC HEART FUNCTION

The cardiovascular system comprises the heart muscle itself, and the arteries, veins, and capillaries that transport blood and other materials throughout the body. The heart is divided down the middle, with two chambers per side: a left atrium and ventricle on one side, and a right atrium and ventricle on the other. Normally, valves between each heart chamber ensure that blood flows in one direction only. Veins carry blood into the heart and arteries carry blood out. After being pumped through the heart, oxygenated blood is sent throughout the body via the aorta (the largest artery in the body), and the pulmonary artery carries deoxygenated blood (blood depleted of oxygen) to the lungs to be refortified with oxygen.

palpitations, decrease blood pressure, and potentiate a calm heart. Cardiotonic herbs include hawthorn berry, garlic, linden, yarrow, motherwort, ginkgo, grand cactus, coleus forskohlii, and guggul.

Cardioactive herbs can have a dramatic effect on the heart, often increasing the efficiency of heart muscles without increasing their need for oxygen. As heart disease worsens, the heart's ability to maintain normal circulation decreases. Cardioactive herbs help circulation and stimulate urine production, which lowers blood volume, lessening the load on the heart. The presence of glycosides in these herbs enables the heart to increase contractibility and pump more blood throughout the body. The downside to cardiac glycosides, however, is that they are often toxic, and because of this, foxglove and some other herbs are no longer available for general consumption. Cardioactive herbs include lily of the valley, purple foxglove, Scotch broom, and squill.

Cardiovascular stimulants increase the movement of blood and stimulate the cardiovascular system using heating herbs such as cayenne, ginger, and cinnamon.

Vasodilators such as prickly ash and ginkgo widen the blood vessels to decrease constriction and restriction.

Hypertensives work to decrease overall blood pressure but seem to focus on diastolic pressure, reducing the heavy burden on heart and vessels.

Effective herbs include garlic, linden, mistletoe, olive leaf, and rauwolfia.

Diuretics such as corn silk, dandelion leaf, and parsley leaf increase kidney action to flush fluids that can reduce total blood volume, easing a heavy heart load.

Vascular tonics tone and support vascular health and are helpful for treating varicose or spider veins. Effective herbs include butcher's broom, collinsonia, ginkgo, and horse chestnut.

Nervines may be helpful if heart disease worsens as a result of negative emotions. Several herbs, such as motherwort, skullcap, oatstraw, and linden, have an affinity for, or association with, the heart and often calm stress and reduce heart palpitations.

The Respiratory System

I often sit in my living room, looking out the window, watching the giant cedars and firs sway in the breeze. I particularly love windy days, as the air circulates around and through these magnificent beings. I can almost see them breathing fully and freely, as the forceful air fortifies them and causes old leaves and limbs to drop, perhaps all for the best. In Chinese medicine, we always look at nature as a reflection of the human condition, and to me, these trees present a great image of the human respiratory system—like giant lungs that breathe in and out the life breath of our world.

Many of us are unconscious of breathing in and out, yet we do it twelve to twenty times per minute, depending on our age. Our lungs oxygenate our bodies, moving vital oxygen into the bloodstream as we breathe in and removing carbon dioxide waste as we breathe out—just as trees and other organisms take in what they need and discard the rest. Our breath also resonates at an emotional and spiritual level for each of us, as we breathe in what is pure and necessary and release all that is not in our best interest. Have you noticed that your breathing feels restricted when you feel stress? Would it not be better to release each breath fully and not hold on to what you don't need?

Over time and as we age, we tend to use less and less of our lung potential to breathe, and our breath becomes shallower. I often ask patients to take a deep inhalation, and I see their bellies go in and their chests puff up. This is a clear sign that I need to initiate breath retraining. When they are breathing only from the top lobes of their lungs, they are not reaching the full potential of oxygenation. Such shallow breathing can affect cells, nerve functions, muscle action, circulation, digestion, and their body's long-term physical and emotional condition.

Returning your awareness to the simple rise and fall of your breath can have dramatic positive effects on your overall well-being. When was the last time you sat and checked in with your breath? Try it now. Place both feet on the ground and rest your hands in your lap. Begin by observing your breath, in and out. Do nothing to change it. What do you notice? Now take a deep breath, noticing how you breathe in. Do you feel any constriction? Now take another deep breath in, and begin the breath at the root of your belly. Fill your abdomen, making it big and round. Draw the breath to completion by reaching the tops of your lungs, and then slowly exhale. Do this five times. How do you feel now?

With every breath, oxygen travels through the lungs and to the heart, and is then distributed throughout the body in the bloodstream. Within the lungs are little air sacs, where oxygen hitches a ride onto red blood cells. When oxygen and blood cells bind together, carbon dioxide is released into the bloodstream as a by-product, carried back to the lungs, and expelled when we breathe out. The spongy, elastic tissue of the lungs stretches and constricts with each breath. The upper parts of the lungs can contract strongly (which enables us to cough) because cartilage is present. The lower parts have very little cartilage and therefore are not able to contract as strongly, which is often why a respiratory infection in the lower lung area can be difficult to heal.

The respiratory system also includes the upper respiratory tract, including the nose, mouth, and throat. In addition to detecting odors, the nose moistens, filters, and warms the air we breathe in. Cilia and goblet cells are the two most prominent features of the upper respiratory tract. The tiny hairs of cilia wave around and block foreign particles from entering the respiratory system. They are the first line of defense in keeping the upper respiratory system free of foreign material. I often imagine them as go-go dancers, waving wildly and making it difficult for others to weave through the crowd. Goblet cells produce and secrete mucus to create a protective barrier from irritants such as allergens and polluted matter. Cilia can be damaged and paralyzed through smoking, inhalation of harmful chemicals, and inflammation caused by food, bacteria, or viruses. As a result, more goblet cells are produced, which increases mucus in the nasal cavity, creating chronic congestion and post-nasal drip. If you suffer constant nasal congestion, don't blame the goblet cells, because they are just trying to protect you. But correcting the imbalance is important.

Herbs for the respiratory system

With the many categories of respiratory herbs, you can customize your needs by mixing and matching, depending on your constitution and symptoms. Many herbs can be used to reduce irritation, congestion, and asthma, and some can relax or stimulate the entire respiratory system.

Respiratory tonics heal, repair, and strengthen the overall respiratory tract and its components. I often recommend that my patients use respiratory tonics that include thyme, elecampane, rosemary, or mullein for a month each year as a lung wellness program. As a culture, we are increasingly focused on detoxing, cleansing, and purging. As an herbalist, I focus on fortifying, toning, and improving. If we strengthen our bodies, they will purge toxic materials on their own. Tonics are great to use before cold, flu, or allergy season begins, to fortify the body's overall function and bolster the entire respiratory system. Anyone with a history of smoking would do well to use tonics, because they can heal cellular damage and improve respiration. Good respiratory tonics include elecampane, mullein, and coltsfoot.

Anticatarrhals help with stuck phlegm accompanied by inflamed mucous membranes in the airways or body cavities, which often occurs in response to an infection. By reducing the inflammation, the phlegm is more likely to decrease as well. Effective anticatarrhals include cayenne, coltsfoot, elder flower, elecampane, eyebright, ginger, goldenrod, goldenseal, mullein, and plantain.

Mucolytics generally break up phlegm and work well when combined with anticatarrhals. Some dissolve mucus, some move it out by thinning it, and some draw it out of passageways. By the time you need a mucolytic, you want it to work quickly, so that the cold causing your spouse to snore in seismic magnitudes will be silenced.

Effective mucolytics include angelica, aniseed, cayenne, cinnamon, fennel, garlic, and ginger.

Respiratory stimulants (expectorants) quicken or enliven respiratory function. These herbs jump-start the respiratory system and are helpful for moving gunk up and out and mobilizing respiratory circulation. Effective respiratory stimulants include cedar, coltsfoot, horehound, hyssop, and thyme.

Lymphatic herbs support the lymphatic system and swollen glands throughout the body. Using lymphatic herbs for a day or so not only mobilizes white blood cell circulation, but helps to flush away the waste overload accumulating in the lymph glands. Effective lymphatics include echinacea, blue flag, poke root, red clover, and wild indigo.

Demulcent herbs are soothing and protective to irritated or inflamed tissues. They release soothing fluids that calm such tissues. These herbs can help soothe the respiratory tract any time there is repetitive coughing or pain with breath. Cooling by nature, they can lower the heat level that is often caused by accumulated phlegm in the lungs. Effective demulcents include fennel, licorice, marshmallow, and slippery elm.

Respiratory relaxants also assist in calming irritated tissues of the respiratory tract, but unlike demulcents that secrete soothing fluids, relaxants cause restricted tissues to relax. Think about a full day of coughing when you are sick, when your lungs have had the workout of a lifetime and are tender and sensitive. Taking just a bit of an herbal respiratory relaxant is like slipping into a warm bath. In fact, go ahead and get into that bath and sip herbal tea at the same time. Effective respiratory relaxants include coltsfoot, mullein, pleurisy root, and thyme.

Bronchodilators are masters at opening the respiratory pathways to assist with breathing, whether resulting from asthma, bronchitis, pleurisy, COPD (chronic obstructive pulmonary disease), or smoker's cough. In my opinion, Mormon tea is the best herbal remedy for opening the airways. Unfortunately, the herb ma huang, the active component of Mormon tea and the source of ephedra, is difficult to find because of past abuse of ephedra in weight-loss products. Nevertheless, ma huang is one of the best herbs for opening airways quickly when breath is restricted. Effective bronchodilators include coleus forskohlii, grindelia, lobelia, ma huang, and red clover.

Antimicrobial herbs specialize in attacking the body's invaders by stimulating positive cellular forces such as white blood cell defenders. Bacterial and viral elements can be prevalent particularly in closed spaces such as offices and schools. Using antimicrobial tinctures regularly in small doses (3 drops) will sustain the defensive barrier and help rid the body of potential illness. Effective antimicrobials include lavender, red root, rosemary, usnea, and yarrow.

The Gastrointestinal System

I love food, but food doesn't always love me back. As I tell my 3-year-old, our taste buds can be tricksters, and they love to trick us into eating all sorts of things that our body doesn't really like. Habits are hard to break, and some of the hardest are dietary related.

In some cultures, people's lives revolve around mealtime and food preparation. I wish I could spend hours every day cooking and eating and taking herbs to stimulate digestive juices and ensure digestive success. To create sustained change, we need to be mindful of what and how we eat. Unfortunately, we grab food on the go, skip meals, and often work while we eat. I'd like to say that herbs can heal any gastrointestinal complaint, but they are only one part of the equation. Nevertheless, when you know how the gastrointestinal system works and you use bitter, demulcent, carminative, laxative, and antispasmodic herbs appropriately, you can heal most gastrointestinal upsets.

In many cultures around the world, aperitifs and digestifs are included as part of the meal. Aperitifs and digestifs are herb-based infusions or extracts made with or without alcohol. Tradition shows the benefits of both on digestive functions. Aperitifs eaten before a meal prepare the body to receive food and jump-start digestive juices. They can also help stimulate an absent appetite. Digestifs are taken after a meal to help reduce gas and bloating and to aid in successful digestion. Some take digestifs directly prior to the main course of a meal, as it is often the richest part. I encourage you to try both aperitifs and digestifs. After consuming them with meals, check in with your body. Does your digestion change, and if so, how? Are you more comfortable after a big meal?

As you work in the kitchen preparing a meal, you may pull items out of the cupboards and the refrigerator, and then perhaps cut up meat and vegetables before turning on the stove. These actions provide the necessary visual and olfactory cues to your brain. The stimulated brain sends messages to your central nervous system to switch to the parasympathetic (rest-and-digest) mode, which dilates all the blood vessels in the body, particularly those in the gastrointestinal tract. This stimulates the secretion of stomach acid, or hydrochloric acid (HCl). You'll know you are on track when you begin to salivate.

After all the preparation is completed and the food is cooked, you sit down and begin slowly chewing your food (the key here is slowly). Again you'll notice the increased saliva in your mouth. Within your saliva is the first phase of digestion, a little enzyme called amylase. As you chew your food, amylase coats it and begins breaking it down. As the swallowed food travels to your stomach, stomach acids are waiting for it. Your stomach turns on like a washing machine and heats up like an oven, tumbling the food with the acid to break it down to a recognizable molecule: a protein, a carbohydrate, a sugar, and so on. Then the stomach sends cues to your pancreas to release the appropriate pancreatic enzymes to break up the molecules into nutrients or waste. And that's how it should reach your small intestine. Ideally, everything that enters your small intestine is either useable energy (nutrients) or waste. Its main job is to return the nutrients to your body and send the waste out to the large intestine (colon).

Many of us fail to eat slowly enough to digest our food properly. Or, perhaps by the time we remember to eat, we simply grab whatever is close by and gobble it down. When we don't slow down, we never transition to that rest-and-digest phase and we remain in a tightly sympathetic (go-go-go) state. After we swallow, no stomach acids are awaiting the food in our stomach, because it hasn't had time to prepare. As the stomach tries to secrete enough acids to begin breaking down the food, the body works hard to catch up, but instead of the pancreas getting involved, the food arrives at the small intestine in a rather whole form. The small intestine therefore has to take on a second job and attempts to break down nutrients and waste. Incredibly, this can take up to three days, as the small intestine tries to salvage any nutrients it can. At some point, everything left is condemned to waste and is sent to the large intestine. As a result, intestinal irritation and malabsorption issues arise. This process also takes an exorbitant amount of energy, leaving us feeling tired and worn down.

Herbs for the gastrointestinal system

The good news is that herbs can help at each point along the gastrointestinal journey, and if our bodies can absorb food nutrients and successfully eliminate wastes, we have more energy, leading to a positive sense of well-being. If you don't have the luxury of being able to cook every meal and of stimulating the digestive process before a meal, herbs can help.

Bitter is one of the five flavors recognized by our taste buds (along with sweet, sour, salty, and umami, or savory). Unfortunately, bitters are lacking in many diets, and this may be a contributing factor to the indigestion epidemic. When bitter-tasting compounds touch their taste receptors on the tongue, a signal is sent to trigger the entire gastrointestinal system to get ready to eat. Bitter flavor says to the body, "Hey! Wake up! Food is on the way!" The positive effects of bitter herbs and foods are endless. They help the stomach secrete hydrochloric acid, and when sufficient acid is present, the stomach can break down food more efficiently and signal the pancreas to start its job. This improves the digestion and metabolism of dietary fats and increases the peristalsis (the movement action) of the small intestine. As a result, less burden is placed on the liver and gallbladder, so fewer toxins build up in the system, and acidity decreases throughout the body. Effective herbal bitters include dandelion, gentian, goldenseal, hops, horehound, wormwood, and yarrow.

Carminatives relieve gas and can be consumed preventatively before meals or consumed after eating to relieve discomfort. Carminatives are sweet in flavor and highly aromatic. One of my favorite examples is the small bowl of mukhwas often served at Indian restaurants. This after-meal snack or digestive aid is created primarily of fennel seeds, aniseeds, coconut, sesame seeds, and peppermint essential oil. Take a pinch next time you go out for Indian food and chew it up after the meal. Carminatives combat flatulence in two ways: by suppressing the formation of gas in the intestines, which reduces the amount that needs to be expelled, and by promoting gas expulsion, essentially clearing out the intestines to help stop the flatulence. Effective carminatives include angelica, aniseed, basil, catnip, cinnamon, cumin, fennel, gentian, oregano, peppermint, spearmint, wintergreen, and wormwood.

Digestive demulcents soothe and reduce irritation of the gastrointestinal tract. Anyone who experiences chronic heartburn or intestinal cramping most likely has inflamed gastrointestinal tissues. These herbs can soothe and heal damaged tissue. Effective demulcents include comfrey, goldenseal, Irish moss, oats, marshmallow, and slippery elm.

Purgatives and laxatives are used to eliminate waste from the large intestine. A purgative's main job is to begin intestinal contraction quickly to get out whatever is inside—think food poisoning. Laxatives, on the other hand, offer a gentler approach to moving the bowels and help to expel stool. Laxatives are perhaps a good choice after you eat a heavy meal that causes slight constipation. Effective purgatives include cascara sagrada, rhubarb, and senna. Effective laxatives include barberry, buckthorn, dandelion root, and yellow dock.

Astringent herbs help knit tissues together. When chronic inflammation occurs in the bowels, tissues begin to pull apart, which can lead to leaky gut syndrome, irritable bowel disease, and diverticulosis. Astringent herbs can help reduce and stop this destruction. Effective astringents include agrimony, bayberry, nettles, plantain, raspberry, white oak bark, and yarrow.

Antispasmodics can quickly provide relief for pain and spasms in the large or small intestinal tract. They can also reduce nervous tension held in the abdomen that may be causing pain. Effective antispasmodics include black cohosh, chamomile, crampbark, fennel, hops, lobelia, skullcap, and valerian.

The Endocrine System

The endocrine system includes a number of glands that secrete hormones that communicate with the body to regulate bodily functions. As the body's chemical messengers, hormones transfer information and instructions from one set of cells to another. Many different hormones move through the bloodstream, but each type of hormone is designed to affect only certain cells.

Using herbs to bring health to the endocrine system can balance the body and ease symptoms. Insomnia is a good example of an issue that results from disharmony in the body, when long-term stress is the true cause of sleepless nights. Although you can take many herbs for acute sleep issues, such as hops, valerian, and kava, to balance the entire body, you need to treat the root cause of the issue. Alleviating and healing the underlying stress response by supporting the endocrine system through herbal medicine can cure insomnia and other stress-related issues.

The top complaints I hear at The Herb Shoppe and in my private practice regard stress and fatigue. The most common symptoms that accompany it are anxiety, insomnia, inflammation, blood sugar issues, and digestive upsets. Many of these problems result from an under-functioning endocrine system. Fortunately, an abundance of herbs is available to help with such complaints, whether they are experienced acutely or constitutionally.

If someone has been on the go for a long time or experiences recurring stress, the adrenal glands can be overworked. These two little endocrine glands, about the size of almonds, sit right above your kidneys. One of the adrenal glands' main functions is to secrete and balance hormones within the body, including cortisol, which is largely responsible for regulating blood sugar, reducing inflammation, and moderating stress. When blood sugar is low, cortisol helps you maintain physical function, so you don't get lightheaded and pass out. Cortisol

THE SYMPATHETIC AND PARASYMPATHETIC STATES

The central nervous system, which controls many functions of body and mind, is always in one of two states: the sympathetic or the parasympathetic. The sympathetic nervous system is the fight-or-flight state that prepares us for action, when surges of adrenaline direct the body's energy toward survival. Although we all need our sympathetic system, some people thrive on it—they like the buzz. They continuously push themselves, fueling up with caffeine and sugar to maintain a constant sympathetic state, or what I refer to as sympathetic dominance.

On the flip side, the parasympathetic state is known as the rest-and-digest state, and when the body is functioning properly, the parasympathetic balances the sympathetic state. In this state, the body relaxes, and blood and oxygen flow increases. This is the best state for mealtimes and sleep.

GLANDS OF THE ENDOCRINE SYSTEM

The endocrine system includes the hypothalamus, pituitary gland, thyroid, parathyroids, adrenal glands, pineal gland, reproductive glands, and pancreas, which all secrete hormones at various rates.

■ The hypothalamus is a small but powerful gland in the brain that secretes hormones to maintain homeostasis (equilibrium) in the body. It is responsible for regulating body temperature, thirst, hunger, sleep cycles, and mood.

■ The pituitary is regulated by the hypothalamus but is considered the master gland of the endocrine system. Located at the base of the brain, this gland probably produces more hormones than any other gland in the body, acting as prime minister, constantly evaluating what is occurring in the body and responding to it. It regulates growth, blood pressure, body temperature, and pain relief. It also controls some functions of the sexual organs.

■ The thyroid gland is situated in the neck by the Adam's apple. The thyroid regulates the metabolism and controls how quickly the body uses energy. It also creates proteins and controls the body's sensitivity to other hormones. In the clinic, I have often noticed thyroid dysfunction caused by digestive imbalances.

■ The parathyroid glands regulate blood calcium levels in the body.

■ The adrenal glands produce cortisol and adrenalin. They also support the thyroid and reproductive glands. Underfunctioning adrenal glands pull energy from the thyroid and reproductive glands, reducing their function.

■ The pineal gland secretes melatonin, which aids sleep patterns. It also converts important nervous system messages into endocrine system responses.

■ The reproductive glands include the ovaries, uterus, and testes. They secrete myriad hormones, all focusing on the varying elements of reproduction and reproductive cycles.

■ The pancreas is considered a glandular organ and resides in the upper cavity of the abdomen. It has two main functions: it secretes enzymes that break down food into components such as proteins, lipids, carbohydrates, and nucleic acids; it also secretes hormones that help control blood sugar levels.

is also released when acute or chronic inflammation is present in the body—whether it's a sprained ankle or an old football injury that flares up. Cortisol acts to keep the inflammatory fires from rising too high. Another trigger for cortisol release is emotional stress, such as that which occurs with performance anxiety or during a difficult conversation with a co-worker or loved one.

If any of these symptoms continues for too long, cortisol is constantly being released. At this point, two things occur. First the body stops releasing cortisol as it senses that you are trying to establish a new order. For example, if you continue skipping meals, disregarding inflammation and stress, your body will stop trying to compensate. Second, the body reaches a critically low level of cortisol, because you've used so much of it. When this happens, all cortisol is retained in case a physical trauma were to occur and cortisol would be necessary to keep you alive during shock. When you are no longer releasing cortisol in response to daily needs, you are no longer compensating. This often leads to a rise in day-to-day complaints of dizziness, insomnia, blood sugar disorders, inflammation, anxiety, and pain.

Herbs for the endocrine system

Fortunately, many wonderful herbs can be used to tone the endocrine system. The four best types of herbs for treating the endocrine system are the adaptogens, bitters, alteratives, and nervines.

Adaptogen herbs can be viewed as tonics. They are the best class of herbs for treating the endocrine system and stress. Plants contain amazing mechanisms to help them deal with stress, whether it involves a soil disturbance or an environmental or pathogen attack. Plants release hormones, much like humans, to adapt to the issue. When we take adaptogens, they modulate and rewire our response to cortisol needs, increase our endurance for stress, and help us respond to it. Effective adaptogens include ashwagandha, borage, eleuthero, holy basil, rhodiola, and schizandra.

Bitters get everything moving by producing a generalized force of motivation that improves the functions of the entire endocrine system. Bitters help the body increase production of hormones when underproduction is the problem, and they decrease production when overproduction occurs. Hypothyroidism, for example, is the underfunctioning of the thyroid gland. Gentian, a strong bitter herb, is a good herb for treating underactive thyroid and helps increase its hormone production. Bugleweed, another strong bitter, is used for hyperactive, or overactive, thyroid function, helping to decrease the overproduction. Effective bitters include barberry, boneset, bugleweed, gentian, goldenseal, hops, horehound, and yarrow.

Alterative herbs cleanse and promote proper blood functioning. They assist the hormones to travel more easily through the bloodstream by increasing the assimilation of nutrients and fortifying eliminative functions. They are best when used long-term, because they work slowly and gradually. Effective alteratives include burdock, cleavers, dandelion root, Oregon grape, red clover, sarsaparilla, and yellow dock.

Nervine herbs help to calm the body, mind, and spirit. They also fortify frayed nerve endings that result from chronic stress and unrest. Whether your monkey mind is keeping you awake at night or you're jumping from fright at the slightest sound, nervines can help. In my opinion, everyone needs nervines, and I recommend them often. Effective nervines include chamomile, lemon balm, lavender, linden, oatstraw, passionflower, wood betony, skullcap, St. John's wort, and vervain.

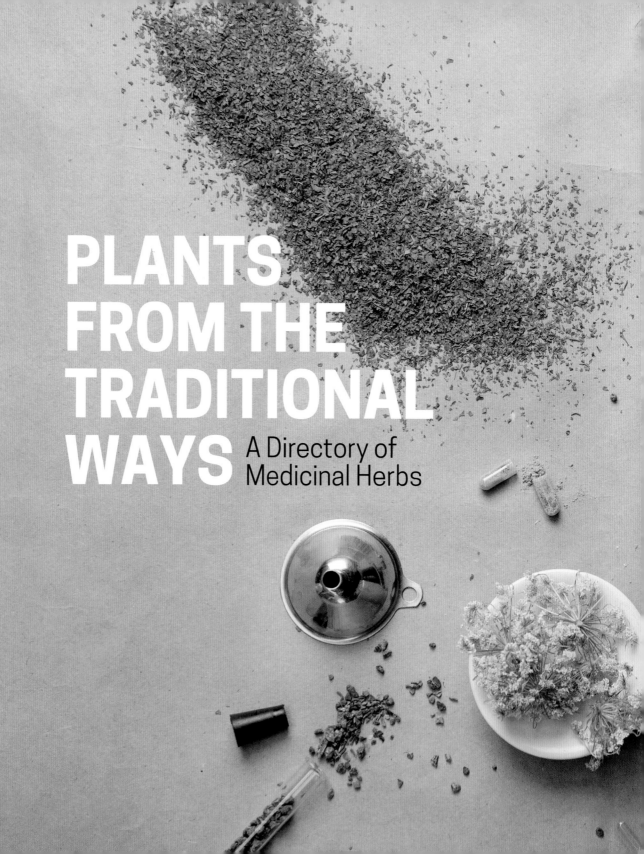

PLANTS FROM THE TRADITIONAL WAYS

A Directory of Medicinal Herbs

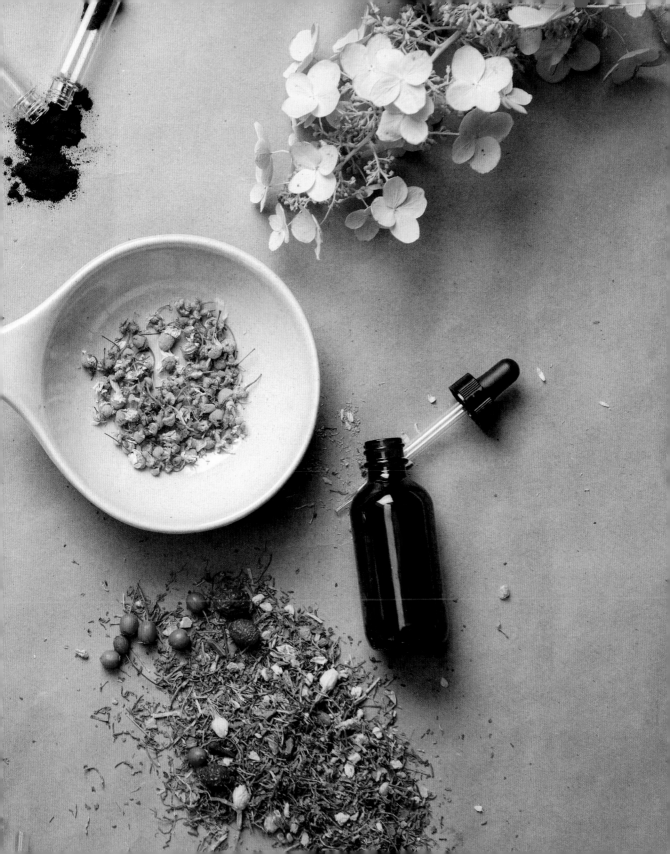

Every fall I commence my annual herbal certification class. Once a month when we come together, I provide information-packed lectures on plants, their healing qualities, and the anatomical systems they affect. Because there is so much information to absorb, I often see my students' heads swimming by the end of each lecture, but I hope they swim happily away with new and exciting knowledge. After years of teaching this class, I know one thing for sure: you can read about plants all day long, but until you go out and find them and sit with them, you really don't know anything. True learning begins when you interact with these fascinating plants.

In their 1973 book *The Secret Life of Plants*, authors Peter Tompkins and Christopher Bird explored the physical, emotional, and spiritual relationships between plants and people. They discussed numerous researchers who have dedicated their lives to the study of plants and the outcome of their research. For example, in the 1950s, Dr. T. C. Singh studied the relationship between music and plants by playing traditional Indian music over a loudspeaker in several villages where several varieties of rice were growing. During the experiment, rice production in those villages was 25 to 60 percent higher than the regional average. Another researcher, Marcel Vogel, found that plants responded to

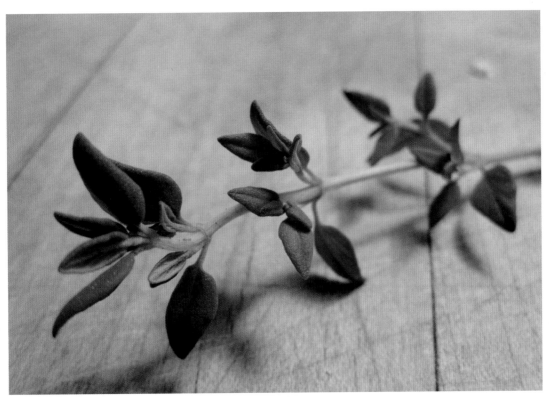
Thyme leaves

the thoughts of people in their presence. Vogel was the first to perform experiments that connected plants and human intentions, when a person willed a freshly picked leaf to survive weeks after it had been plucked. And then there is Cleve Backster, a polygraph examiner in the late 1960s. One night, he decided he would attach the polygraph electrodes to the plant on his desk to see what would happen. When he watered the plant, the polygraph responded similarly to how it would respond to a human experiencing emotional stimulus. Then he took it up a notch, knowing that the most effective way to trigger humans into a strong emotional reaction, to cause the polygraph to jump, was to threaten their well-being. He dunked one of the plant's leaves in hot coffee. When this resulted in no polygraph reaction, he conceived an idea of more intensity: he would burn the plant.

The moment the idea came to his mind and he imagined the flame touching the leaf, a dramatic change in movement occurred on the polygraph. Backster had not moved, had not struck the match, but had simply thought of the leaf burning, which caused a reaction in the plant.

Although I do not encourage you to try to evoke such reactions from plants, I do encourage you to get out into the wild or into your garden and simply sit with the plants. As you read through these plant entries, some will almost jump off the page, almost willing you to get to know them. I suggest you study these plants first. Even if you think you know everything about a particular herb, take a look with fresh eyes to allow the plant to share its secrets with you. If you know ten plants, and know them well, you have all the medicine you need. Who are your plant allies?

Getting to Know the Plants
How to Read the Plant Directory

Each of the listings in the plant directory starts with the plant's common name, followed by its botanical Latin name. I believe that learning the botanical names will serve you far better than learning the common names. Latin is the universal language of horticulture, and if you know a plant's Latin name, no matter where you are in the world, you can ask for a plant by its true botanical name. This is extremely helpful if you are trying to find medicinal herbs in a foreign country. Common names can also be helpful in locating herbs, but common names can be regionally oriented, meaning that a plant name in one region may not be the same name used in another. For that reason, I've also included alternative common names for each plant.

The plant family is also included, along with the parts of the plants used in herbal medicine. Understanding groupings of characteristics within a plant family can help you identify plants as you search for them in the wild. For example, plants in the mint family, Lamiaceae, can often be identified by their square stems.

Organs or systems affected

Some herbs have an affinity for certain organs or bodily systems—that is, they are specifically aligned to improve the overall function of a bodily tissue, organ, or system. By providing the supporting elements for the tissues, organs, or functions, these herbs help the targeted system operate more proficiently. When you know the specific organs and bodily systems that are best served by an herb, you can choose the most appropriate herbs for treatment. This knowledge helps you begin to categorize herbs in a new and informed way and provides a foundation for formulating herbal remedies and blends.

Therapeutic actions

Therapeutic actions are the primary healing characteristics of an herbal medicine. Knowing the terms used for therapeutic actions will improve your understanding of how herbs work and interact with the body.

DEFINITIONS OF
THERAPEUTIC ACTIONS

---

adaptogen increases resistance and resilience to stress; as a tonic, it increases the overall sense of well-being.

alterative gradually restores proper functioning of the body, increasing health and vitality; sometimes referred to as a blood cleanser.

analgesic relieves pain.

anti-asthmatic treats or prevents asthma.

antibacterial destroys or stops the growth of bacteria.

antibilious helps the body remove excess bile.

anticatarrhal reduces inflamed mucous membranes of the head and throat, and often reduces phlegm.

antidepressant helps to prevent, cure, or alleviate mental depression.

antiemetic stops vomiting.

antifungal destroys or inhibits fungal growth.

antihemorrhagic helps control hemorrhaging or bleeding.

anti-inflammatory helps control inflammation.

antimicrobial helps destroy microbes (germs).

antioxidant protects cells from damage.

antipruritic prevents or relieves itching.

antirheumatic helps ease pain of rheumatism and inflammation of joints and muscles.

antiseptic removes toxins from the body and waste accumulations such as pus.

antispasmodic calms nervous and muscular spasms or convulsions.

antitussive relieves coughs.

antiviral opposes the action of a virus.

aperient helps promote bowel movements; a very mild laxative.

aperitive stimulates the appetite.

aphrodisiac increases the capacity for sexual arousal.

aromatic presents strong aromas, often because of the presence of volatile oils.

astringent constricts and pulls tissues together and helps decrease secretions.

bitter stimulates appetite or gastrointestinal function.

cardiotonic increases the strength and tone of the heart.

carminative soothes digestion and helps to expel gas and relieve bloating.

cathartic active purgative that produces bowel movements.

cholagogue increases bile flow from the gallbladder.

counterirritant produces an inflammatory response.

decongestant removes mucus congestion.

demulcent soothes inflammation of mucous membranes.

deobstruent removes obstructions from the alimentary canal (the digestive organs).

depurative removes impurities and cleanses the blood.

diaphoretic increases perspiration and opens the pores of the skin.

diuretic increases urine flow.

emetic produces vomiting.

emmenagogue regulates and at times induces normal menstruation.

emollient softens and soothes the skin.

expectorant facilitates removal of secretions and phlegm.

febrifuge reduces or relieves fever.

galactagogue promotes the flow of breast milk.

hemostatic controls or stops the flow of blood.

hepatic supports the liver.

laxative helps loosen the bowel contents for easier elimination.

mucolytic helps break down thick mucus.

nervine calms the body, mind, and spirit.

nutritive provides nutrition, and is often high in vitamins and minerals.

pectoral helps heal the lungs.

purgative causes fast evacuation of the bowels.

relaxant induces relaxation.

restorative brings balance to a particular organ or system.

rubefacient reddens skin, dilates blood vessels, and increases local blood supply.

secretolytic increases the production of mucus in the respiratory tract.

sedative exerts a soothing, tranquilizing effect on the body.

stimulant temporarily increases body or organ function.

stomachic supports the stomach.

styptic stops bleeding.

tonic increases systemic strength and tone.

vulnerary treats wounds.

Nature

Knowing the plant's nature helps you understand its effect on bodily tissues. For example, if an herb has a cool nature, it provides a cooling effect on tissues. An herb with a dry nature helps dry tissues when that is required. This eclectic herbal wisdom is one of the oldest and most traditional ways of classifying herbs.

Plant constituents

Plants are made up of various and plentiful constituents, or components. Learning an herb's constituent parts provides direct clues as to what actions the plant will perform in the body. When you learn about the constituents of a plant, you are learning how the plant functions as a healing agent. You can use that knowledge to predict what will happen when you apply or ingest it. What part of the plant creates a positive resolution to wounds, dysfunctions, or dismays?

Often, we can identify some of a plant's constituents using our senses. A plant's appearance, taste, and smell can offer clues about which constituents are present. Highly aromatic plants almost always contain volatile oils (concentrated aromatic oils). A sweet taste is an indication that carbohydrates are present, and a sour flavor tells us that the plant probably contains tannins. Just as we learn to identify flavors in foods or notes in wine, we can learn to identify herbal constituents with a little practice. For example, if you put a small piece of gentian root into your mouth and chew, you will quickly taste its bitter constituent. Chew a bit of marshmallow root, and you can quickly identify the demulcent (soothing and mucilaginous) constituent. Drink some raspberry leaf tea, and you'll notice the astringent or tannin constituent. As you move through this aspect of your learning, always engage the plants.

Although we may prefer to learn about herbs and the medicine they possess from the Earth-centered traditions of sensing, using, growing, and wildcrafting, we can also know the plants from a scientific perspective. Knowing the constituent properties of herbs can give you keen insight into how they may function with some predictability.

When a scientist analyzes a plant in a lab, she can extract its individual constituents and study each part separately. She can then classify the constituents by their actions and reactions to certain stimuli, and in the process, determine how each constituent performs in the body. For example, a volatile oil typically creates a disinfectant action in the body because of its ability to penetrate barrier surfaces. When a plant's volatile oil constituent performs consistently in the body, it can be isolated from the plant and re-created in a lab as a medication that can move through cell walls (or penetrate barrier surfaces) into a cell to begin healing.

Although scientists separate the plants into their constituents in a lab, you don't have to do it this way. Herbalist Peter Holmes, who works to integrate Chinese medicine theory and western herbalism, believes that science alone is ineffectual in herbal medicine, because it cannot accurately describe a thing that is alive, ever-changing, and persistently interacting with its surroundings. Although we are able to separate and identify each of a plant's constituents, remember that separating a plant into individual parts reduces it to a mere specimen, and this reduces the plant's full potential. Rosemary Gladstar, renowned herbalist and founder of Sage Mountain Retreat Center & Native Plant Preserve, points out that some plants have identified constituents that serve no organic function for the plant itself, yet they seem to benefit everything around them, such as the soil and other plants. These plants seem to be growing simply to heal the Earth—and, perhaps, us.

PLANT CONSTITUENTS AND THEIR BASIC FUNCTIONS

*Several common plant constituents act and function in specific ways within the body.
This information provides some perspective into the scientific side of herbal medicine.*

CONSTITUENT	ACTION	SOLUBILITY	DESCRIPTION
Acid	Antimicrobial, heals wounds and inflammation	Water, alcohol	Most often associated with phenolic acids. Can bond with other plant materials. Rebuilds muscle fibers and heals nerve endings. Serves an important role in digestive health. Sour flavor causes the mouth to pucker. Generally considered safe.
Alkaloid	Varied	Water, alcohol (some)	Although thousands have been identified, their specific function is unclear. Appear to affect both body and mind (such as with psilocybins and morphine). Tend to act on the liver, nerves, lungs, and gastrointestinal system. Odorless and colorless (except Oregon grape and goldenseal's berberine). Considered mildly safe to highly toxic.
Anthraquinone	Stimulates gastro-intestinal system, quickens intestinal transit time	Insoluble in water or boiling alcohol	Prevalent in most plants and herbs, especially senna and rhubarb. Often identified by yellow color and bitter taste. Best known as a purgative that gently stimulates the bowels, 8–10 hours after ingestion. Add bile salt production herbs (dandelion root, milk thistle, turmeric) in conjunction; they are needed to bind with waste for proper elimination. Although not water soluble, senna and buckthorn teas help with constipation because other constituents in these herbs stimulate the bowels. For the full anthraquinone action, use a tincture (alcohol). Generally considered safe, though overdosing can cause intestinal gripping, especially with diarrhea or irritable bowel.
Bitters	Increases gastric secretions, improves digestion	Water, alcohol, vinegar (slightly)	Important for gastrointestinal physiological function. Once tasted, triggers response in the digestive process, increasing appetite, stomach acids, pancreatic enzymes, and detoxification by the liver. When mixed with another herb, can stimulate the herb into action. For example, blending bitter horehound, a respiratory expectorant, with mullein, a broad respiratory agent, stimulates an overall healing effect for the lungs. Generally considered safe.

CONSTITUENT	ACTION	SOLUBILITY	DESCRIPTION
Carbohydrates	Provides systemic energy, reduces tissue inflammation and irritation	Water, glycerin, alcohol (slightly)	Plentiful in the plant kingdom, provides a direct energy source as simple sugars (pure energy) or as more complex forms that secrete a protective film to soothe and heal irritated tissues (via demulcent herbs, such as comfrey leaf, marshmallow root, slippery elm bark). Stimulates relaxation and secretions in mucous membranes (such as lungs and bladder) to soothe, calm, and heal. Generally considered safe.
Coumarin	Reduces inflammation, anticoagulant, antispasmodic	Water, alcohol	Aromatic by nature (think fresh mown grass) and prevalent in the plant world. Within the plant, helps limit growth and prevent infections and parasites. In the body, increases blood flow and decreases capillary permeability. Use with caution because of mild toxicity.
Flavonoid	Antioxidant	Water, alcohol	Plant acid that turns chemical responses on or off in the body. Stimulates immune function, regulates secretory functions, affects genetic expression, and regulates cellular functions. Necessary for complete absorption of vitamin C. Inhibits formation of free radicals from cellular damage (especially oregano and rosemary). Generally considered safe.
Glycoside	Supports cellular absorption	Water, alcohol	Comprises a non-carbohydrate molecule bound to a sugar molecule, such as a plant acid, flavonoid, or anthraquinone combined with a sugar molecule. The sugar bond increases absorption rate in the body, beneficial if plant contains something you need, such as salicylic acid for quick headache relief, but is not such a good thing when the plant contains a poison, such as cyanide, that is easily released when damaged and then readily absorbed. Know what type of glycoside is in the plant you are using to determine how to use it safely. All work with cellular absorption and seem to be activated when the plant is crushed, mashed, or damaged. Use with caution.

CONSTITUENT	ACTION	SOLUBILITY	DESCRIPTION
Saponin	Heals skin	Water, vinegar, alcohol	When mixed with water, saponins (such as soapwort) create a foamy, bubbly reaction. When you make tea, if you see foam at the top of your mug, you can bet saponins are present. Saponins such as sassafras are used in the body to create cortisol and sex hormones. Taken as tea or capsules, they are nonsystemic—they react in the intestinal tract, leaving little by-product for the liver to detox. Studies show they can also bind cholesterol, minimizing its absorption through the gut—good to know for anyone on cholesterol-lowering medications. Generally considered safe.
Tannin	Astringent	Water, vinegar, glycerin, alcohol	A phenol that, when eaten, causes lips to pucker and pulls moisture from the mouth. As an astringent, binds tissues together, often helping reduce inflammation or irritation. Can create a protective layer to reduce damage to internal membranes and skin and can help stop internal or external bleeding by constricting blood vessels and releasing cellular components that harden certain tissues. This action is protective by nature, but not appropriate for women who are menstruating or those who need to avoid constriction of blood vessels, such as those with atherosclerosis or migraines. Generally considered safe.
Volatile oils	Antiseptic	Distillation (best), alcohol (some), water (poorly)	Volatile and flammable liquids, typically colorless, that tend to oxidize (and evaporate) rapidly when exposed to air. Break down readily, and soon after consumption, trace elements can be found in breath, saliva, tears, urine, and breast milk. Can act systemically or locally when externally applied. Many affect central nervous system and stimulate white blood cell production. Use with caution because they readily permeate tissues.

Flower essence

Herbal medicine is typically physical medicine—that is, consuming medicinal herbs creates a physical change in the body. When we use herbs as medicine, we want to create a sustained change within the body to promote health or healing. Flower essences are used to affect the emotional or psychological aspects of healing. The first flower essences were formulated in the 1930s by Edward Bach, who created the popular Rescue Remedy. Organizations such as the Flower Essence Society have conducted research and training in the use of flower essences for more than 30 years. To understand flower essences, you must recognize that a human is more than just a physical body, and that the body is actually a combination of matter and consciousness intertwined. This consciousness can be identified as the spiritual essence, or self. Flower essences are energetic imprints of the life force of plants that interact with our spiritual essences, helping to evoke specific qualities within us. Whenever possible, I've included each herb's flower essence, or its energetic attributes, to provide the full picture of the plant's potential in health and healing.

Medicinal uses

Every medicinal herb has particular affinities for healing in the human body. I describe each herb's particular usefulness in healing along with the specifics regarding how the herbal healing occurs.

Contraindications

Contraindications are difficult to document, because many of them are not scientifically founded or clinically experienced first-hand. Some herbs have been condemned as a result of a single study, and others are labeled dangerous because an isolated extracted constituent is considered toxic, without consideration of the plant's entirety and its unique ability to work as a whole. In addition, some people use herbs without having a solid knowledge about how and when to use certain plants, which can cause ill effects. As my mentor, teacher, wise woman, and dear friend Linda Quintana always used to say, plants have been used for generations to heal, but they need to be used wisely, with respect. That said, take the contraindications listed here seriously, and carefully heed the instructions regarding dosages, particularly for children, people with compromised health, and pregnant women. And never, ever consume or use any plant that you do not clearly recognize as edible and safe.

Medicine cabinet

I describe the most common applications and dosing for each particular herb. You can also refer to the standard medicinal dosing in the "Adult Dosing Basics" table, unless a dose is specifically indicated. Refer to "An Herbalist's Laboratory" for clear descriptions of each application type.

DEFINITIONS OF MEDICINE CABINET TERMS

decoction The process of simmering roots or bark to create a tea for drinking.

fomentation A topical application of a cotton cloth soaked in a strong herbal infusion or decoction and placed onto an affected area as needed.

infusion A brew that pulls the active principles of the herbs into water, typically created by pouring hot water over the herbs and letting the mixture steep.

liniment A topical application that can increase blood circulation and stimulate healing.

menstruum A substance, or solvent, that pulls medicinal constituents from solid plant matter into a liquid, such as with herbal tinctures.

poultice Direct application of the plant (fresh, dried, or powdered) onto the body.

tincture A liquid, often alcohol and water, into which the fresh or dried herb's medicinal constituents have been extracted.

Identification and cultivation

Knowing how to identify a plant serves as an advantage when you're looking for a plant in the wild, or in the garden, but it also helps you understand characteristics within a plant family and shared features such as actions and uses. In addition, basic cultivation information helps you grow the herb in your own garden.

HARDINESS ZONES

Each plant description includes key characteristics of the plant as well as its USDA hardiness zone ratings. These zones are based on average annual minimum temperatures. Knowing a plant's hardiness zone will help you determine whether the plant will survive in your climate. The lower the zone number, the colder the winter temperatures.

To learn which zone you garden in, see the US Department of Agriculture Hardiness Zone Map at at usna.usda.gov/Hardzone/ushzmap.html.

For Canada, go to planthardiness.gc.ca/ or atlas.agr.gc.ca/agmaf/index_eng.html. For Europe, go to uk.gardenweb.com/forums/zones/hze.html. For the UK, search for "hardiness" at rhs.org.uk.

Wildcrafting

Some foraging and wildcrafting information is provided if the plant is found in North America. Wildcrafting herbs, or harvesting wild plants, is an ancient tradition that today involves ethically harvesting herbs in their natural environment. It doesn't necessarily involve traipsing through the deep woods. If you've gone into your backyard to gather dandelion leaves for tea, you've wildcrafted.

Although historically herbalists have collected their own herbs for medicinal use, not all of us live in wilderness-rich areas and can easily find or grow all the medicines we need, so we depend on wildcrafters to bring us what we cannot find. Today, in fact, wildcrafting can be a quite lucrative profession. If you want to forage for yourself, however, this book provides information regarding when and where to find the herbs you seek. It also provides information about when not to gather wild plants, particularly when they are considered endangered or threatened. Remember that when you harvest a plant, you enter into a relationship with it. It is your responsibility to prepare the plant for wildcrafting before you begin your work removing any of its parts or its entirety. Acknowledge your intentions and ask for permission—from the landowner and from the plant—before you remove anything. Be considerate of the wildcrafting site and leave no trace of your having been there.

You must also respect the laws of wildcrafting. Overharvesting has been a problem for decades and has led to plants becoming endangered or threatened. For this reason, you should always know the endangered and threatened status of the plants in your area before you collect anything, and never harvest any plant considered endangered or threatened.

Harvest mindfully to ensure the future growth and health of any plants you disturb. In general, harvest only a third of what is available, or a third of any single plant, to enable it to continue to survive and grow. Always leave most of the strongest plants at the harvesting site to ensure continuation of the species.

While gathering roots and rhizomes, replant root crowns and rhizome pieces directly in the ground, especially if a bud is present, to help the plant regrow. If you need to strip bark, do not remove it from a living part of the plant. Instead, look for freshly fallen branches and remove bark from those parts. If you must remove bark from a healthy part of a plant, remove only very small, vertical strips, and never, ever girdle a tree (remove bark horizontally around the entire trunk) or you will kill it entirely. If you cut too much, the wound you create opens a path for bacterial and fungal infections, which can kill the tree.

Study your plants and have someone guide you before you begin harvesting—in other words, know your plants before you collect! Whether you are wildcrafting for personal use or professionally, you can gain a lot from the experience. If you are just beginning, you may experience moments of exhilaration or frustration as you search for a particular plant.

Be prepared by gathering items you might need before you head out to collect herbs in the wild.

SUPPLIES FOR WILD HARVESTING

Gloves

Sturdy all-terrain shoes

Hat

Compass, so you don't get lost in the woods

Sharp pocket knife with a 2- or 3-inch blade

Sharp scissors or pruners

Hand trowel

Harvesting basket or paper bag—not plastic, which does not allow air circulation

Herbal bug repellant

Patience

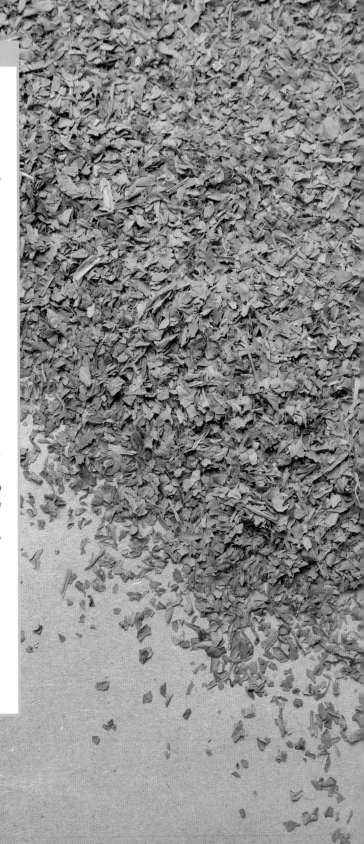

HOW TO DRY HERBS

Unless the herbs required are clearly indicated as fresh, you'll use dried herbs for most recipes in herbal medicine, including those in this book. You can dry your own herbs after harvesting them if you process them correctly to ensure that you capture all the benefits of the medicine. Some plants, such as hops, need very particular drying procedures that are beyond the scope of this book, but most herbs can be easily harvested and dried for future use to maintain their medicinal value. If you are processing roots, wash them thoroughly and cut them into small, useable pieces before drying. Leaves and flowers can be processed whole or cut into smaller pieces.

After collecting herbs, place them on a dry bed sheet or on an old, clean window screen in the shade. A warmer day is best to ensure that all the moisture is extracted. Never place herbs in the direct sun, because direct sunlight is damaging and diminishes their potency. A warm, shaded spot is best. Situate the sheet or screen off the ground to achieve airflow around the herbs. I often tie the four corners of the sheet to four chairs, which allows for 2 or 3 feet of airflow underneath. Drying can take 1 to 3 days, but hopefully not much longer. The herbs need to dry relatively quickly to avoid mold formation.

Store dried herbs in sealed glass containers unless you live in an extremely humid climate. In humid areas, glass tends to collect heat and sometimes moisture, leading to mold growth. If you live in a humid area, store dried herbs in brown paper bags instead. Keep them in a cool, dark place to help them stay viable for many months, or longer.

Agrimony

Agrimonia eupatoria

Also called church steeples, cocklebur, sticklewort, philanthropos **Family** Rosaceae **Parts used** Aerial parts, roots

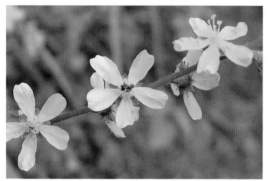

Agrimony flowers

> *Agrimony is delicately scented but powerful in cleansing the liver, giving tone where needed and supporting the kidneys and bladder.*

Organs or systems affected Bladder, kidneys, liver, central nervous system, respiratory system **Therapeutic actions** Astringent, tonic, diuretic, cholagogue, relaxant **Nature** Mildly sweet, sour, bitter, cool, dry **Plant constituents** Bitter, flavonoids, tannins, vitamin C, volatile oils **Flower essence** Helps those who are inwardly troubled by fear and anxiety, and who may worry excessively about illness, finances, or problems with work or life, yet present a cheerful, carefree face

Medicinal uses

Resolves kidney and bladder ailments Agrimony eases the pain and helps pass kidney stones. Because of its astringent qualities, it is used for bladder incontinence and bedwetting. It helps tone weak bladder tissues and relaxes bladder tension, enabling more control over bladder function. Its astringent nature is helpful throughout the body where tone is lacking (such as stretched ligaments that do not properly hold bones in place).

Relieves liver congestion Agrimony is used to support overall liver function, specifically jaundice. In Chinese medicine, the liver houses the emotion of anger. Agrimony helps release emotions and tension held in the liver that cause physical congestion, which manifests as skin complaints, gastrointestinal and gallbladder malfunction, and changes in vision. It also helps correct the imbalance of other organ systems.

Reduces sympathetic dominance Agrimony can help those who hold emotions in their tummies or who habitually hold their breath when dealing with extreme stress or pain. Holding your breath during pain causes the release of natural endorphins that help suppress the pain; however, the repetitive patterning of such behavior results in a cascade of negative physical effects, including the inability to oxygenate the body fully, leading to more tension. Agrimony relaxes the appropriate areas to enable your central nervous system to switch from a sympathetic dominant state to a parasympathetic state, or the rest-and-digest phase, which increases blood flow to restricted areas.

Contraindications Because agrimony opens elimination pathways in the body and relaxes the sympathetic nervous system, taking it orally may increase the efficacy of prescribed medication. Consult with your doctor before using agrimony.

MEDICINE CABINET

Infusion 1 or 2 teaspoons per cup, steep 8 to 10 minutes, 1 to 3 cups per day
Tincture 1 dropperful 3 times per day

Identification and cultivation

Numerous pinnate leaves, with larger 6- to 8-inch leaves close to the ground, growing smaller at the top, to 3 inches. Small, bright yellow flowers are borne on slender spikes, approximately ⅓ inch across, with five narrow and oval shaped petals. Flowers face up and out toward the sun until withered, and then face down. Plants thrive in hedges and fields and along ditches. Perennial. Grow in calcareous soils lightened with a little sand, full sun. Zones 5–9.

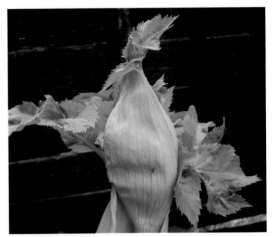
Emerging angelica

Angelica

Angelica archangelica

Also called garden angelica, Norwegian angelica, holy ghost **Family** Apiaceae **Parts used** Roots

> *Angelica is the perfect convalescent cure.*

Organs or systems affected Intestines, stomach, uterus, cardiovascular system **Therapeutic actions** Tonic, stimulant, relaxant **Nature** Sweet, bitter, warm **Plant constituents** Volatile oils, flavonoids, phytosterols, bitters, tannins, furanocoumarins **Flower essence** Enhances protection and guidance from spiritual beings, especially during threshold experiences such as birth, death, or other life passages

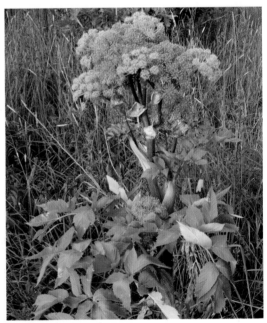
Angelica going to seed

Medicinal uses

Helps the body recover from illness Angelica helps return proper functioning to bodily systems after they have been off track, such as after one has been ill for a while, and the appetite is suppressed, circulation is sluggish, and hormones are not properly regulated. It can also help balance the central nervous system by regulating overstimulation or sluggishness.

Restores reproductive wellness Angelica has long been used to warm the uterus and its surrounding blood vessels. It also appears to affect hormones directly and helps balance the endocrine system. Some research indicates that it has an estrogen-increasing effect, making it useful in some cases of amenorrhea (the absence of menstruation) or premenstrual syndrome (PMS).

Restores digestive wellness As a stimulant, angelica can provide positive effects on the entire gastrointestinal system, aiding proper gastrointestinal secretions, absorption, and elimination.
Contraindications Angelica contains furanocoumarins, which increase skin photosensitivity and may cause dermatitis with long-term use.

MEDICINE CABINET

Decoction 1 or 2 teaspoons per cup, simmer 10 to 15 minutes covered, 1 to 3 cups per day
Tincture 10 to 30 drops, 1 to 3 times per day

Identification and cultivation

Stalks are hollow, short, and thick. Small leaflets are bright green and toothed. Yellow-green flowers are borne on umbels (in which short flower stalks spread from a common point). Spindlelike, fleshy roots are best harvested in the fall. Grows in damp places in lowland and mountainous areas, especially along streams, rivers, and seashores. Biennial. Grow in most soils, full sun to part shade. Zones 4–9.

Balsam fir

Abies balsamea

Also called Canada balsam, Christmas tree, fir pine, sapin, silver fir **Family** Pinaceae **Parts used** Outer and inner bark, shoots

> *All parts of the balsam fir can be used as medicine to heal the lungs and skin.*

Organs or systems affected Bladder, lungs, skin
Therapeutic actions Stimulant, antiseptic, analgesic **Nature** Sweet, moist **Plant constituents** Resin, terpene acids, bitters, essential oils, vitamin A, calcium, iron, fluorine

Medicinal uses

Heals respiratory and throat ailments Balsam resin is a strong choice for healing the respiratory tract and eliminating a sore throat. It helps soothe persistent coughs and heals all types of pulmonary infections. Balsam shoots are best for this.
Clears cystitis and intestinal inflammation The inner bark is used to clear out cystitis and gastrointestinal inflammation.
Helps one give up smoking Balsam can help alleviate side effects such as irritability, constipation, and insomnia as one gives up the smoking habit.
Relieves external pain Balsam salve or liniment can be applied topically to help allay discomfort with conditions such as burns, wounds, hemorrhoids, sore nipples, strained muscles, and toothaches.

MEDICINE CABINET

Infusion 1 teaspoon per cup, steep 8 to 10 minutes covered, 1 to 3 cups per day
Tincture 1 dropperful, 1 to 3 times per day
Salve or liniment Use as needed

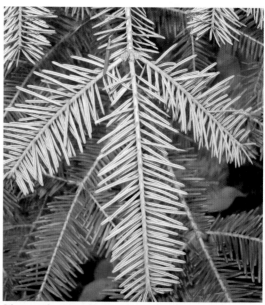

Silvery undersides of balsam fir needles

Identification and cultivation

Evergreen conifer with blunt needles, ¾ to 1½ inches long, dark green on top with silvery undersides. Smooth, scaly bark is covered in pitch. Oblong, purplish cones grow upright along the branches, break open when mature, and are never intact when they hit the ground. When foraging, remove tips from limbs only where your permit authorizes you to do so. Trees must be taller than 10 feet, and no more than 14 inches can be cut. Do not remove tips from the top third of the tree and do not remove more than a third of the tips. Do not disturb the main stem or leader. Can be propagated from seed in a greenhouse in early spring. Grow in well-drained soil, full sun to part shade. Zones 3–6.

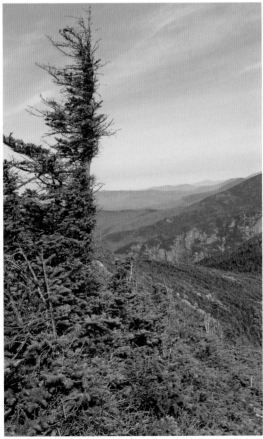

Balsam fir

Balsam poplar

Populus balsamifera

Also called balm of Gilead, tacamahac **Family** Salicaceae **Parts used** Bark, buds

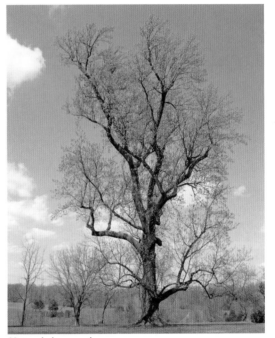

Mature balsam poplar

This tree produces much medicine from buds and bark to heal the skin, kidneys, and respiratory tract.

Organs or systems affected Intestines, kidneys, lungs, skin **Therapeutic actions** Buds: stimulant, tonic, diuretic, demulcent, expectorant. Bark: expectorant, cathartic, tonic, stimulant **Nature** Bitter, aromatic, cool, moist **Plant constituents** Phenolic glycosides, salicin, essential oils, resins, tannins, acids, mannitol, fatty oils **Flower essence** Assists those who are inconsistent or are unable to react appropriately with emotion

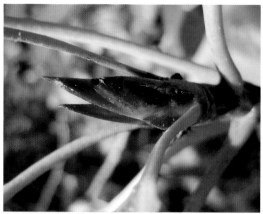
Emerging balsam poplar bud

Medicinal uses

Treats skin conditions Balm made from buds make an excellent treatment for skin troubles. Use as a muscle rub or chest congestion balm, or for more complex skin issues such as eczema, psoriasis, and folliculitis. It can reduce pain, cool the skin, and relieve itching. Used internally and externally.

Moistens respiratory system and lower intestines The bark has a particular affinity for the lungs and gastrointestinal system, where it moisturizes dry and damaged tissues. In the lungs, it helps with dry coughs and to expectorate hot phlegm. The healing stimulates movement where movement is needed, such as in the bowels when constipation is present. Poplar is a simple laxative that stimulates peristalsis activity (the movement of the colon to push along waste, in contrast to a purgative action that intentionally irritates the lower bowel to rid the body of matter quickly).

Supports kidney and bladder elimination Bark and buds help support the kidneys and bladder in elimination with or without infection. The kidneys do an extreme amount of filtration each day, particularly with bodily infection, fever, or both. Balsam poplar helps the kidneys eliminate toxins.

Relieves rheumatism and gout Because of its anti-inflammatory and pain-relieving effects, balsam poplar has traditionally been used to ease the pain of rheumatism and gout.

Contraindications Those with cottonwood allergies should avoid balsam poplar.

MEDICINE CABINET

Infusion Bud infusion, 1 teaspoon per cup, steep 8 to 10 minutes, 1 to 3 cups per day
Decoction Bark decoction, 1 teaspoon per cup, simmer 10 to 12 minutes covered, 2 to 4 cups per day
Oleic resin 1 tablespoon in lemon juice and honey, 3 or 4 times per day (resins are soluble in alcohol and oil, but not water)
Tincture 1 dropperful, 3 or 4 times per day
Salve Massage ointment into desired area for 5 to 10 minutes

Identification and cultivation

Mature trees reach 50 to 70 feet. Deep brown stems are smooth and round. Smooth bark is white to dark gray. On mature trees, bark may be rough and uneven or may crack. Buds are conical, pointed, with closely overlapping scales, and very fragrant. Smooth leaves are ovate or heart shaped. Collect buds in late winter and early spring before they open. Wear gloves to protect hands from sticky resin. Never harvest buds that are partially open; they are susceptible to mold and could already contain spores. Remove bark only from fallen branches; taking bark from a live tree can kill the tree in its entirety, something we plant lovers want to avoid. Thrives in moist forest sites. Live seeds have short survival time and must be sowed within a few days of ripening. Grow in deep and rich soil, or damp soil, full sun to part shade. Zones 2–5.

Bayberry

Morella cerifera (also *Myrica cerifera*)

Also called wax myrtle, waxberry, candleberry, tallow bush, vegetable tallow **Family** Myricaceae **Parts used** Bark

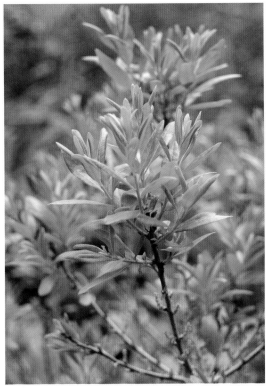
Bayberry

> *Bayberry makes its way into congested spaces in the body, breaks up the congestion, and releases it.*

Organs or systems affected Liver, lungs, cardiovascular, respiratory, and gastrointestinal systems **Therapeutic actions** Astringent, stimulant, alterative, tonic **Nature** Pungent, bitter, warm, dry **Plant constituents** Triterpenes, flavonoids, resins, phenols, myricinic acids, tannic and gallic acids, gum, wax

Medicinal uses

Frees system from obstructions and toxins Bayberry has a particular affinity for the cardiovascular, respiratory, and gastrointestinal systems when they are overburdened by hardened mucus. Within the heart and cardiovascular system, bayberry works as an astringent and vessel toner, steadily increasing circulation and creating a positive outward flow of blood. Within the gastrointestinal system, bayberry works as a tonic to resolve damp conditions and promote healthy breakdown and absorption. It pulls together excessive fluids and stimulates the release of toxins.

Warms the body Bayberry warms the body, enabling bodily systems to work efficiently. It is a good choice at the beginning of a cold, when a slight increase in body temperature is needed to create an inhospitable environment for most bacteria and viruses. As the bayberry's warmth creates a gentle perspiration, the attacking threat is pushed out.

Improves reproductive health Bayberry has plenty to offer women's health. It has antispasmodic abilities and acts on both the sympathetic and parasympathetic nervous systems. It is often combined with motherwort for suppressed or late menses, particularly when the condition is caused by what Chinese medicine calls a cold uterus, when vessels to the uterus are constricted and the blood is not flowing properly to maintain a healthy hormone or nutrient balance. Some consider bayberry a valuable asset in childbirth.

Stimulates lymphatic system Bayberry is useful when glands feel swollen or tender, which is often the cause of lymphatic congestion, when the body works overtime to rid itself of problems such as viral or bacterial infections.

Treats canker sores Bayberry can be helpful in treating sores in the mouth and throat.

Contraindications Extremely large doses may cause vomiting.

MEDICINE CABINET

Decoction 1 or 2 teaspoons per cup, simmer 10 to 12 minutes covered, 2 to 4 cups per day

Oil ½ teaspoon to swollen lymph glands or canker sores, 1 or 2 times per day

Tincture 1 dropperful, 1 to 3 times per day

Identification and cultivation

Dense evergreen shrub, 2 to 5 feet. Outer bark layer is grayish and peeling, covering a hard, red-brown fibrous inner layer. Shiny, dark green, lanceolate leaves release fragrance when bruised. Catkins bear tiny yellow flowers. Small globular berries grow in groups, at first green and turning greenish white with a hard, waxy surface. Grows in dry woods and fields or in thickets near swamps and marshes. Gather in late fall or early spring. When planting, dig holes two to three times wider and deeper than the rootstock, and surround the root ball with about 5 gallons of compost. Grow in well-drained, slightly acidic soil, full sun to part shade. Zones 7–11.

Bearberry

Arctostaphylos uva-ursi

Also called uva-ursi, upland cranberry, kinnikinn-ick, foxberry **Family** Ericaceae **Parts used** Leaves

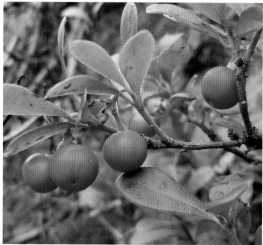

Bearberry

This ground cover's antiseptic and toning attributes are particularly helpful to the kidneys and bladder.

Organs or systems affected Bladder, kidneys
Therapeutic actions Diuretic, astringent, soothing tonic, antiseptic **Nature** Pungent, cold, dry
Plant constituents Flavonoids, tannins, acids, triterpenoids, essential oils, resin, allantoin, trace minerals including iron, calcium, chromium, selenium, magnesium **Flower essence** Heals the feminine aspect within us all and helps us better connect with and understand the healing powers of nature; also aids in pathologies of the ovaries

Medicinal uses

Creates antiseptic and diuretic action One of bearberry's main constituents is a glycoside called arbutin. When ingested, arbutin travels through the body largely unchanged until it reaches the kidneys, where it creates both diuretic and antiseptic actions. This stimulates a flushing reaction that cleanses the mucous membranes of the bladder, which is particularly helpful with bladder infections. The plant's tannins aid to balance the pH of urine, lowering acidic bladder environments.

Tones the bladder and helps dissolve kidney stones As an astringent, bearberry helps tone the tissues of the bladder, particularly when there is enuresis (uncontrolled urination), kidney infection, prostate constriction, and incontinence. It has the triple action of calming and toning the tissues and serves as an astringent for excessive discharges. With incontinence, it seems to impart tone specifically to the sphincter of the bladder, which holds the urine in. For people who worry about needing a bathroom everywhere they go, bearberry can provide comfort. It has often been used to help dissolve kidney stones.

Regulates labor contractions Peter Holmes (2007) and others clearly state bearberry's ability to help regulate contractions during active labor as well as to encourage labor to progress.

Contraindications Bearberry should be used for 7 to 10 days; it should not be used long-term for fear of exhausting eliminatory organs. It should not be used with children, because it overstimulates the bladder. It can also turn the urine green.

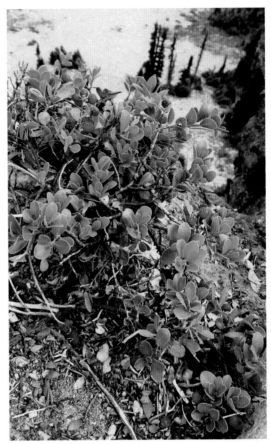
Bearberry plants

Identification and cultivation

Low evergreen shrub with shiny, small, leathery, dark green leaves rounded at the apex, arranged alternately on smooth, woody stems. Racemes of three to fifteen pink-white flowers. Bright red berries ripen in autumn. Harvest leaves in late spring and summer. After drying, store leaves immediately to prevent their reabsorbing water from the air. These slow growers can be difficult to transplant and establish. Tolerates drought. Grow in well-drained, acidic, sandy soil, full sun. Zones 2–6.

MEDICINE CABINET

Infusion 1 teaspoon per cup, steep 8 to 10 minutes, 1 to 4 cups per day. For acute problems, drink 4 ounces at a time, as needed.
Tincture 10 drops or 3 dropperfuls, 1 to 3 times per day

Bistort

Persicaria bistorta

Also called snakeweed **Family** Polygonaceae
Parts used Roots

> *This herb is used to stop bleeding through its strong astringent action.*

Organs or systems affected Uterus, gastrointestinal system, respiratory system **Therapeutic actions** Astringent, alterative **Nature** Pungent **Plant constituents** Tannins, resin, saccharides, mucilage, acids **Flower essence** Provides loving support at times of major life changes

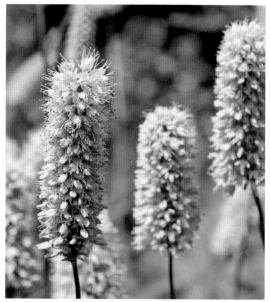

Bistort flowers

Medicinal uses

Stops bleeding through astringent action Bistort can be used wherever an astringent is needed in the body. For example, in an overflow of menses, bistort can help taper off the bleeding. Also useful for nosebleeds, lung hemorrhages, diarrhea, and bleeding hemorrhoids.

Alleviates toxins from the body Bistort gives us an opportunity to study the doctrine of signatures, because its root resembles a snake moving in action. Traditional herbalists say it is superior at protecting the body and eliminating poisons as it snakes its way through the gastrointestinal tract.

Contraindications Generally regarded as safe.

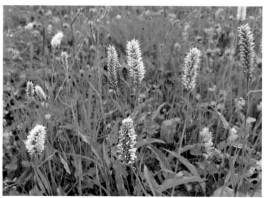

Bistort

Identification and cultivation

Single, erect, simple stems, 12 to 24 inches. Upper side of large ovate leaves are blue-green. Multiple white flowers appear early summer to midsummer on a terminal cylindrical spike. Grows in the lower parts of mountain ranges. Harvest roots in early autumn. Divide clumps in early spring for transplanting. Grow in moist soil that does not dry out, full sun to part shade. Zones 3–9.

MEDICINE CABINET

Fomentation For nosebleeds, saturate cotton ball and insert into nose, or take internally using decoction or tincture.
Decoction 1 or 2 teaspoons per cup, simmer 10 to 12 minutes covered, drink as needed
Sitz bath 6 tablespoons per quart, steep 1 hour
Tincture 10 to 30 drops, as needed

Blackberry

Rubus fruticosus

Also called bramble, dewberry, goutberry, thimbleberry **Family** Rosaceae **Parts used** Leaves, roots

> *Some of the finest syrup to ease throat pain can be made with the simple blackberry.*

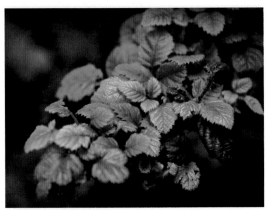

Blackberry leaves

Organs or systems affected Gastrointestinal system, respiratory system **Therapeutic action** Astringent **Nature** Sweet, sour, cool, dry **Plant constituents** Tannins, gallic acid, villosin, starch, calcium oxalate **Flower essence** Helps to create competent manifestation in the world; affects clearly directed forces of will, and intentional and decisive actions

Medicinal uses

Aids digestion Blackberry is specific for damp stomach and intestinal conditions with increased mucus, food stagnation, and often loose bowels. It is an astringent and tones the body. Blackberry was once considered one of the most beneficial herbs for the stomach. Unfortunately, its use has declined due to its commonness, which I find silly. We are funny creatures, quickly abandoning those things that work for us. Traditionally, the Oneida people of the American Great Lakes region used blackberry to protect themselves from the various diseases of the white man, suggesting its ability to keep the gastrointestinal tone intact, strong, and able to pass whatever is foreign or harmful from the body.

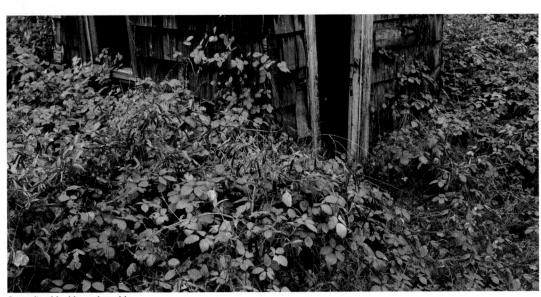

Sprawling blackberry brambles

Soothes sore throats Blackberry cordial or syrup is an excellent treatment for sore throats.
Contraindications Although effective as an herbal astringent to control bleeding, blackberry leaf should not be used for an extended period because its high astringency may inhibit menstrual bleeding and may cause constipation or diarrhea. Although that seems like contradicting information, herbs affect people with different physical constitutions in different ways.

```
┌────────── MEDICINE CABINET ──────────┐
     Infusion 1 or 2 teaspoons per cup, steep 8 to
           10 minutes, 1 to 3 cups per day
          Syrup 2 to 4 teaspoons per day
   Tincture 1 to 3 dropperfuls, 3 times per day
└───────────────────────────────────────┘
```

Identification and cultivation

Stems are heavily toothed, prickly, and bright green, 3 to 6 inches tall. Compound leaves arranged alternately, with three to five leaflets. Blooming in late spring to early summer, flowers are up to 1 inch across, with numerous stamens and yellow anthers, five white petals, and five green sepals with pointed tips. Petals are longer than sepals, rounded, and often wrinkly. Grows in natural meadows, at river and pond margins, in overgrown farm fields or recent burns, along country roads and lanes, and under power line rights-of-way. The guides recommend disturbed ground or abandoned places where trees and undergrowth have been removed, providing several decades of sunny ground for fast-growing berry bushes to colonize. Perennial shrub. Plant in spring. Grow in sandy, acidic soils, full sun. Zones 3–10.

Black cohosh

Actaea racemosa (also *Cimicifuga racemosa*)

Also called black snakeroot, squaw root, rattle root, bugbane, macrotys, tall bugbane, bugwort, rattleweed **Family** Ranunculaceae **Parts used** Rhizomes, roots

> *Black cohosh is a key herb in balancing estrogen within the body and treating overexertion of mind and muscle.*

Organs or systems affected Heart, lungs, stomach, uterus, cardiovascular system, musculoskeletal system **Therapeutic actions** Antispasmodic, stimulant, diaphoretic, astringent, diuretic, expectorant, alterative, emmenagogue **Nature** Bitter, pungent, sweet, cool, dry **Plant constituents** Resin, aromatic acids, essential oils, glycosides, alkaloids, triterpenoids, salicylic acid, isoflavonoids, saponins, tannins, mucilage, sulfur, potassium, magnesium, potassium phosphate **Flower essence** Helps one heal from addictive or abusive relationships and supports the ability to confront rather than retreat from situations as necessary

Medicinal uses

Supports hormone function in menopause Traditionally black cohosh has been used as a women's herb to support and balance hormone function and uterine health. In modern times, black cohosh has been put to the test—or lab, I should say. Studies show that black cohosh has an estrogenic effect and is supportive to certain conditions that are driven by estrogen deficiency, including menopause, hot flashes, vaginal dryness, and reduction in the ability to climax with sexual interaction. Anything estrogenic raises red flags these days, and one concern has

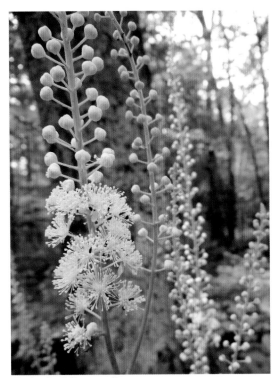
Black cohosh flower stalks

Relieves anxiety and muscle tension Research supports the traditional use of black cohosh as a relaxant and antispasmodic. I often prescribe it to patients who have muscle tension combined with an overactive nervous system, making them anxious or leading to insomnia. This same reaction can also have specific relaxing effects on the heart, slowing the rate yet strengthening the force of the pulse.

Relieves rheumatism and inflammatory pain Because of its salicylic aspect (nature's aspirin), black cohosh is often used for aches and pains. It seems particularly good for lower back discomfort.

Provides emunctory system support Black cohosh is used for breaking up mucus in the lungs and aiding eliminatory secretions of the kidneys, liver, and lymphatic system.

Contraindications Should not be used during the first trimester of pregnancy. Extremely large doses can create mild cramping and nausea. Those with liver disease should avoid this herb.

been the increase of estrogen stimulating breast cancer growth. Again, we return to the lab and find that black cohosh does not exert estrogenic effects on breast tissue. One particular test used a standardized black cohosh tincture and found, as many others do, that the herb offered relief of menopausal symptoms without systemic or breast-specific estrogenic effects. Given at full-term pregnancy time, black cohosh can be helpful to initiate and regulate labor contractions.

Enhances sense of well-being Serotonin contributes to a general feeling of happiness and well-being. Recent reports indicate that the extract of black cohosh binds and activates serotonin (5-HT) receptors. Receptors are located throughout the body, but many are concentrated in the gastrointestinal system, platelets, and central nervous system.

MEDICINE CABINET

Decoction 1 or 2 teaspoons per cup, simmer 10 to 12 minutes, 1 to 3 cups per day

Fomentation 3 tablespoons per pint, apply to affected area

Tincture 3 to 60 drops, 1 to 3 times per day

Identification and cultivation

Leaves are arranged alternately with long petioles, on unbranched, slender, smooth stems, 3 to 8 feet long. Wandlike racemes bear flowers on 8- to 20-inch stems. Knotty roots spread horizontally, 4 to 6 inches. Grows in shady and rocky places. Perennial. Listed as endangered in some areas. Propagate in early spring, just as the soil warms up; plants tend to emerge very early. Grow in humus-rich, moist, well-drained soil, full to part shade. Zones 3–8.

Black haw

Viburnum prunifolium

Also called stage bush, sweet viburnum, American sloe, king's crown, sheepberry, snowball tree
Family Adoxaceae **Parts used** Bark, root bark

Black haw supports, nourishes, and relaxes the female reproductive system.

Organs or systems affected Uterus, central nervous system, gastrointestinal system **Therapeutic actions** Astringent, relaxant **Nature** Sweet **Plant constituents** Triterpenoids, coumarin, bitter, valerianic acid, salicosides, tannins

Medicinal uses

Promotes and calms tension Black haw is considered a nutrient tonic that builds the blood where it is deficient, making more nutrients available in the body and calming the gastrointestinal system. It's also a good choice for anyone who holds tension in the stomach, which causes dysfunction in the gastrointestinal system.

Eases menstrual symptoms Native Americans used black haw for almost all complaints of the female reproductive cycle. Similar to its cousin, crampbark, black haw is not only antispasmodic, but it can work as a tonic rather than symptomatically—that is, it can be used preventatively rather than in acute situations only. Depending on the length of PMS symptoms, it is a good choice to take during the latter half of the menstrual cycle, from ovulation until end of menses, as well as premenstrually, one to five days before bleeding, to relieve nervous irritation. If used acutely it is an ideal choice for dysmenorrhea, or spasm cramping, before or with menses.

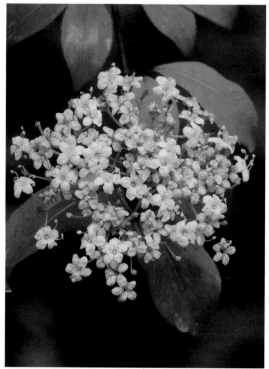
Black haw flowers

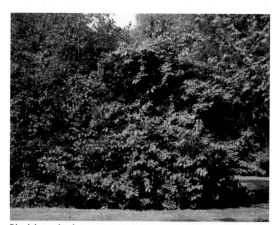
Black haw shrub

Relaxes the nervous system Black haw relaxes the nervous system, particularly during pregnancy and premenstrually, when digestion and the nervous system are not balanced. It helps to improve overall digestive function and ease the stress that sometimes accompanies pregnancy. It is valuable in assisting in uncomplicated labor. It can also arrest and prevent miscarriage.

Contraindications Generally regarded as safe.

MEDICINE CABINET

Decoction 1 tablespoon per cup, 2 to 4 cups per day
Tincture 1 or 2 dropperfuls, 3 or 4 times per day, or every hour as needed until symptoms subside

---

Identification and cultivation

Shrub, 12 to 15 feet, with dark green, ovate leaves, 1 to 4 inches long. White flowers are borne on cymes. Because the root bark is the usable part of the plant, you must uproot the entire shrub, therefore killing the plant. In some areas, native black haw has been overharvested, and this is a concern. For this reason, you should use a homeopathic preparation of root bark unless you grow the plant yourself. You can, however, wild harvest bark from fallen branches in the spring after flowering. Deciduous shrub. Grow in well-drained soil, full to part shade. Zones 3–9.

Black walnut

Juglans nigra

Also called carya, walnoot, Jupiter's nuts
Family Juglandaceae **Parts used** Leaves, hulls

Black walnut is a great choice for clearing the bowels, toning the colon, and ridding the body of unwanted invaders.

Organs or systems affected Intestines, pancreas, stomach, thyroid **Therapeutic actions** Alterative, laxative, astringent **Nature** Bitter, pungent, cool, dry **Plant constituents** Flavonoids, tannins, acids, bitters, essential oils, alkaloids, protein, calcium phosphate, oxalate, trace minerals **Flower essence** Assists with change, including changing patterns, behaviors, habits, or lifestyle

Medicinal uses

Detoxifies colon and body Black walnut has long been used to support the cleansing of the lower bowels and to help to rid the body of built-up toxins. When the colon is inflamed, weak, and

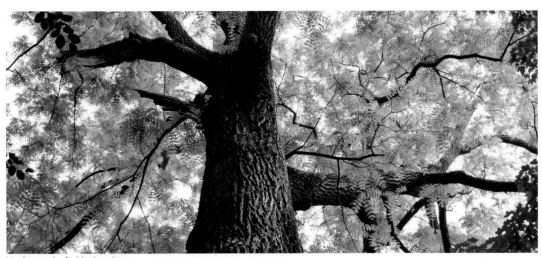

Up the trunk of a black walnut

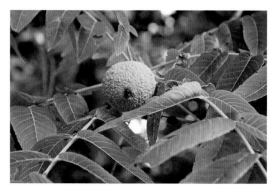
Black walnut fruit and leaves

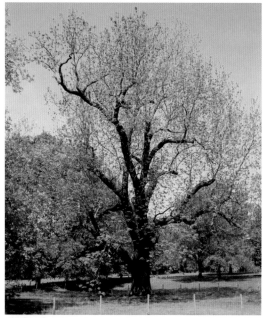
Black walnut tree

Fights bacterial, parasitic, and fungal infections
Black walnut tincture is not only high in a plant form of iodine, but it also has antibacterial, anti-parasitic, and fungicidal properties. The amount of iodine in black walnut tincture is so high that it can be used as a substitute for iodine antiseptics. As an oxidizing agent, black walnut upsets the cellular balance of any bacteria or other microbial entity it meets. A little goes a long way for external applications as well as internally for traveler's diarrhea. Because of its ability to disrupt and remove bacteria and fungus, I often recommend it to be added with salt to the neti pot to help clear a sinus infection and congestion.

Treats hypothyroidism and goiter Contemporary herbalists Phyllis Light and Matthew Wood use black walnut in the treatment of hypothyroidism and goiter.

Contraindications Can cause ringing in the ears. Some believe this to be caused by the die-off of a parasitic infection.

MEDICINE CABINET

Fomentation 3 tablespoons per pint, steep 1 hour, strain. Soak cotton cloth in infusion, apply to affected area.
Infusion 1 or 2 teaspoons per cup, steep 15 minutes, 1 to 3 cups per day
Tincture 3 to 30 drops, 3 times per day. In a neti pot, use 1 dropperful of tincture combined with salt and water.

---

allowing malabsorption to occur, black walnut is a trusted ally to tone the tissues and help the colon better assimilate nutrients, especially fats and proteins. When the colon is back on track, the liver is less burdened by the toxins that a sick colon releases into the bloodstream (also known as bad blood). When one has bad blood, faulty metabolism, and insufficient liver detoxification pathways, the skin is often affected, and this shows up as eczema, acne, rosacea, boils, and similar afflictions.

Identification and cultivation

Stout, gray-green twigs have a chambered pith. Compound leaves arranged alternately, with fifteen to twenty-three finely toothed leaflets. Round nuts with a hard, corrugated shell are 1½ to 2 inches in diameter. Grows in moist woodlands. Harvest leaves in spring and hulls at time of fruiting. Deciduous tree. Grow in moist, well-drained soil, full sun. Zones 4–9.

Blessed thistle

Cnicus benedictus (also *Centaurea benedicta*)

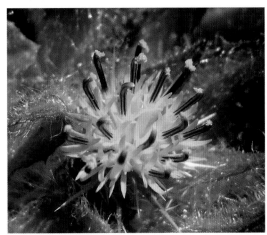
Blessed thistle flower

Also called holy thistle, lady's thistle, carduus, cardin, St. Benedict's thistle **Family** Asteraceae **Parts used** Aerial parts

> *This potent bitter purifies the gastrointestinal system, liver, kidneys, and skin.*

Organs or systems affected Intestines, kidneys, liver, skin, stomach **Therapeutic actions** Alterative, carminative, cholagogue, diaphoretic, diuretic, febrifuge, nervine, stimulant **Nature** Bitter, cool, dry **Plant constituents** Bitter glycosides, alkaloids, flavonoids, essential oil, tannins, resin, acids, mucilage, potassium, calcium, magnesium, iodine **Flower essence** Assists those who need comfort in the natural ways of giving and receiving

Medicinal uses

Assists in breast milk production Blessed thistle has been used for centuries to activate the mammary glands to increase breast milk supply. Research indicates it is still one of the most commonly chosen herbs for this use. Galactagogues, or herbs that increase breast milk supply, work by increasing the hormone prolactin in the body, therefore increasing milk production. In my practice I often combine blessed thistle with other herbs such as goat's rue, shatavari, nettle, hops, and fenugreek. This balanced blend increases the prolactins and provides trace minerals and B vitamins. It also helps the new mom relax, which can help the let down of breast milk occur more easily.

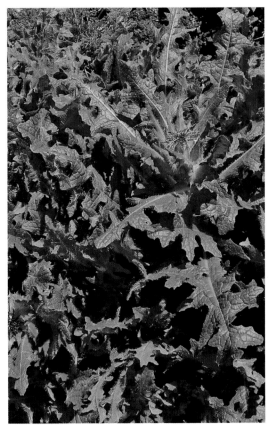
Blessed thistle

Tonifies liver and cleanses the blood Blessed thistle works to tonify the liver and in turn cleanse the blood. It appears to stimulate overall circulation, which is helpful for purification. When the body experiences a combination of decreased circulation and waste buildup, headaches can result. In *The Complete Herbal* (1653), Culpepper often recommends blessed thistle for the treatment of simple headaches and to increase circulation to help with brain stimulation and decrease foggy thinking. Blessed thistle is also used for headaches that accompany menopause. Perhaps the binding of excess estrogens and androgens may alleviate hormone-driven headaches.

Detoxifies skin It can be used topically to calm skin problems such as chicken pox, acne, and boils that result from internal issues. Apply fomentation to pull out toxic elements gently and soothe the skin.

Contraindications Generally regarded as safe.

MEDICINE CABINET

Fomentation 3 tablespoons per pint, steep 1 hour, strain. Soak cotton cloth in infusion and apply to affected area.
Infusion 1 or 2 teaspoons per cup, steep 10 minutes, 1 to 3 cups per day
Tincture 10 to 30 drops, 1 to 3 times per day

Identification and cultivation

Round stems are straight, branched, and wooly. Thin, lanceolate, hairy leaves are 2 to 3 inches long. Yellow flowers are borne on branch ends. Collect the leaves on a hot and dry midsummer afternoon, just before flowers bloom. Grows in open, sunlit pastures, especially around livestock; it thrives around manure. Blessed thistle is considered a noxious, invasive weed, so do not plant it in your garden. Perennial. Birds enjoy the seed, so try to gather seed before the birds do. Zones 5–9.

Bloodroot

Sanguinaria canadensis

Also called Indian paint, tetterwort, red paucoon, coon root, snakebite, sweet slumber
Family Papaveraceae **Parts used** Rhizomes

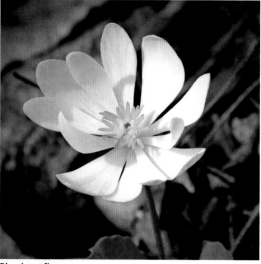

Bloodroot flower

> *Bloodroot is an essential aspect of the escharotic (scab-forming) treatment for cervical dysplasia.*

Organs or systems affected Heart, liver, lungs, uterus **Therapeutic actions** Stimulant, emetic, expectorant, restorative **Nature** Pungent, bitter, hot, dry **Plant constituents** Alkaloids, resin, sanguinaric acid, acids, starch **Flower essence** Helps those who have deep feelings of unworthiness and who tend to exclude themselves from groups or community

Medicinal uses

Treats cervical dysplasia During an annual gynecological exam, women's health physicians focus on the health and wellness of the cervix

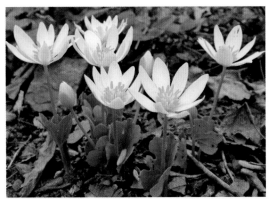
Bloodroot

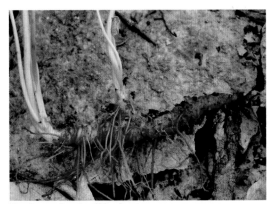
The deep red roots of bloodroot

and vaginal canal. By collecting a sample of cells from these areas, we can detect whether cervical dysplasia is present and if estrogen is at a healthy level. Cervical dysplasia refers to abnormal pre-cancerous and cancerous tissue on the surface of the cervix. It is measured in grades of severity. CIN I (cancer in situ) represent mild cervical dysplasia and can have a low rate of progression to cancer. In contrast, CIN II and III, moderate to severe cervical dysplasia, is more likely to progress to invasive cervical cancer if not treated. Bloodroot is an essential part of the escharotic treatment for cervical dysplasia. It is typically combined with zinc chloride and applied directly onto the face of the cervix. Many studies document the effectiveness of this treatment. Blood-root is a viable option in place of such procedures as conical biopsy or loop electrosurgical excision (LEEP) procedures.

Stimulates and warms organs As a stimulator, bloodroot speeds up the central nervous and cardiovascular systems. Because of this action and its innate warming quality, it produces warmth in its organ affinities. It is a good choice for warming the lungs, gastrointestinal tract, or uterus to improve function. Used in larger doses, it helps expel phlegm from the lungs, and lower doses relieve bronchial irritation, aid in digestion, and mildly increase peripheral circulation. It can also stimulate menstruation.

Contraindications Bloodroot should be avoided by pregnant women and by those who are breast-feeding. It should not be used for children. It should not to be taken long-term due to the alkaloids present and the potential for toxic buildup.

MEDICINE CABINET

Decoction 1 teaspoon per cup, simmer 10 to 12 minutes covered, once per day

Salve Apply small amounts, 1 or 2 times per day

Snuff A pinch for sinus infections or headaches

Syrup 1 teaspoon, 1 to 3 times per day, best when combined with other herbs

Tincture 5 to 10 drops, 1 to 3 times per day

Identification and cultivation

Bloodroot's sheathlike leaf is wrapped around the flower and increases in size after flowering. Palmate leaves are gray-green, lobed, and covered with hairs. Waxy white flowers bloom in early to midspring. Rhizomes are thick, round, and fleshy, and produce a red-orange juice. Grows in open woods. Perennial. Listed as endangered in some areas, plants are easily propagated by dividing the rhizomes in spring or fall. Grow in rich, well-drained soil, high in organic matter, full sun to part shade. Zones 3–8.

Blue flag

Iris versicolor

Also called flag lily, water flag, iris, liver lily, snake lily, poison flag **Family** Iridaceae **Parts used** Rhizomes, roots

> *If something is blocked in the body, blue flag can probably clear the path.*

Organs or systems affected Intestines, liver, lungs, lymphatic system **Therapeutic actions** Alterative, cathartic, diuretic, stimulant, cholagogue **Nature** Pungent, bitter, sweet **Plant constituents** Alkaloid, salicylic acid, acids, volatile oil, polysaccharides, phytosterols, tannin, resin, gum **Flower essence** Encourages the flow of artistic creativity

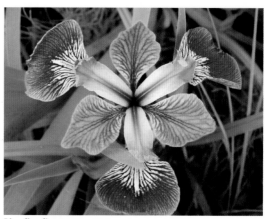
Blue flag flower

Medicinal uses

Opens secretory pathways Blue flag can help clear secretory pathways that are blocked or slow and underperforming—such as diminished intestinal secretions and gastrointestinal discomfort, or lymphatic stagnation causing hardened or swollen lymph glands.

Stimulates liver Blue flag stimulates a sluggish liver that struggles with detoxification and helps clear blocked bile ducts and regulate function. Other herbs perform this function as well, but blue flag works in a gentler way.

Helps clear skin eruptions When liver function improves, the skin usually benefits, and blue flag helps with both. Its ability to support the liver naturally aids in clearing the skin, but it also helps cleanse the blood, which directly reduces skin eruptions and blemishes.

Tones the endocrine system Blue flag can help reduce mood swings, thyroid excess, and hot flashes.

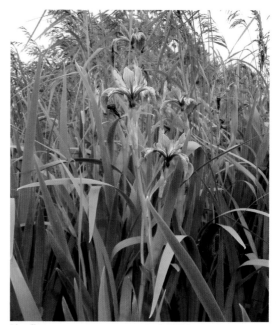
Blue flag

Contraindications Blue flag should not be used long-term.

MEDICINE CABINET

Decoction ½ to 1 teaspoon per cup, simmer 10 to 12 minutes covered, once per day as needed
Tincture 3 to 15 drops, 1 or 2 times per day as needed

Identification and cultivation

Stems are stout and straight, 2 to 3 feet, with narrow, sword-shaped leaves. Purple-blue flowers have three large and three smaller petals, united at the base, white or yellow at base of the sepals. Grows abundantly in swamps, low ground, and freshwater ponds. Harvest in the fall. Perennial. Best used in flower and water gardens, along edges of ponds, and in areas where it may naturalize. Grow in heavy, rich, moist soil, full sun. Zones 5–9.

Blue vervain

Verbena officinalis

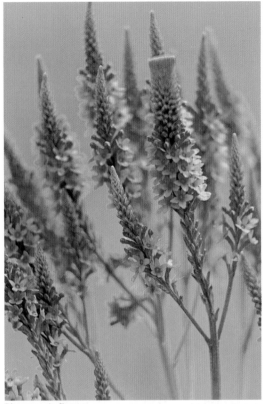
Blue vervain flowers

Also called vervain, verbena, herb of the cross, pigeon's grass, wild hyssop, herb of grace, simpler's joy **Family** Verbenaceae **Parts used** Aerial parts

> *Blue vervain helps release tension to improve the body's functions.*

Organs or systems affected Brain, skin, central nervous system **Therapeutic actions** Antispasmodic, diaphoretic **Nature** Bitter, slightly pungent, cool **Plant constituents** Bitters, volatile oil, alkaloids, mucilage, tannins **Flower essence** Good for those who are inflexible, overbearing, and extreme; helps create balance within the individual

Medicinal uses

Disperses tension Long regarded as a comprehensive herbal treatment, blue vervain's dispersing effect makes it excellent for any condition in which tension or constrained energy creates pathology. For a feverish ailment when sweating is unobtainable, blue vervain helps open restraints in the skin. It is an ideal treatment for those who live in their heads, who have high

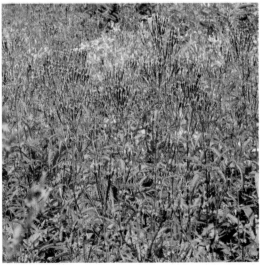
Blue vervain

expectations of themselves, striving for perfection and imposing those ideas onto others. Such behavior causes tension throughout the body that blue vervain can help to release. Tension can also affect the liver. In Chinese medicine, the liver is considered the house of the emotions. When emotions run high, a person feels constrained or internalized, which creates a physical burden on the liver. Blue vervain is also helpful for headaches and neck pain caused by extreme tension.

Eases hot flashes and PMS Blue vervain has been used for centuries as an excellent women's herb. Those suffering from hot flashes will benefit from its cooling astringent properties. It can help balance progesterone levels, which typically drive PMS-C (premenstrual syndrome cravings disorder).

Improves milk flow New mothers are often under significant stress, which can result in a lack of milk production. Blue vervain helps reduce tension and improve milk flow.

Contraindications Large quantities may induce nausea, but its extremely bitter quality makes this issue unlikely.

MEDICINE CABINET

Infusion 1 teaspoon per cup, steep 8 to 10 minutes, 2 or 3 cups per day or as needed for tension

Tincture 5 to 30 drops, 1 to 3 times per day

Identification and cultivation

Lobed and toothed leaves are arranged oppositely on angular stems. Small, pale lilac flowers are borne on spikes. Found in waste ground and along roadsides. Harvest before flowering and dry promptly. Perennial. Start seedlings inside in spring or fall. Grow in well-drained soil, full sun. Zones 4–8.

Bogbean

Menyanthes trifoliata

Also called buckbean, bog myrtle, marsh clover
Family Menyanthaceae **Parts used** Leaves

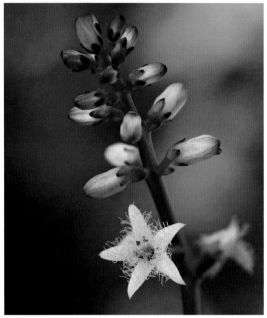

Bogbean flower

This aquatic plant targets the lymphatic tissues of the body, clearing obstruction and waste.

Organs or systems affected Gallbladder, kidneys, liver, lungs, stomach, lymphatic system **Therapeutic actions** Tonic, cathartic, deobstruent, febrifuge **Nature** Bitter, pungent, cold, dry **Plant constituents** Alkaloids, bitter glycoside menyanthin, rutin, hyperin, essential oil, alcohol, carotene, ascorbic and other acids, tannins, saponins, fatty oil, manganese, iodine **Flower essence** Helps one refrain from judgment and accept change, including changes in point of view

Medicinal uses

Supports lymphatic system Bogbean's strength is its ability to clean out the lymphatic system. The lymphatics are like garbage workers—they drive around the body and pick up all the trash. Sometimes the trash is overflowing and the lymphatics are congested, resulting in swollen lymph nodes and, more importantly, an excess of old acids and wastes in the body. When wastes accumulate, rheumatism, skin afflictions, kidney insufficiency, back pain, sciatica, and liver congestion all worsen. Bogbean can help the body purge waste for effective symptom relief.

Relieves shingles Mathew Wood (2008) reports this treatment for shingles: steep 1 ounce of bogbean in 1 pint of water, and take 4 tablespoons several times a day. The constituent menyanthin normalizes the central nervous system, which is perhaps why bogbean is helpful for treating shingles. I would consider prescribing bogbean for other viral conditions as well.

Cleanses and tones liver and gallbladder Bogbean is a supreme bitter. As with most, it is a reputable herb to cleanse and tone the liver and gallbladder.

Regulates female hormones In Germany, bogbean is referred to as moonflower, indicative of its use as a women's hormone regulator—probably because of its strong effects on the liver, which regulates hormones.

Alleviates lung problems Taken as syrup or smoked, it has been used to alleviate chronic lung conditions.

Contraindications Bogbean is known to thin the blood, and moderate doses can cause diarrhea.

MEDICINE CABINET

Fomentation 3 tablespoons per pint, steep at least 1 hour, strain, and apply saturated cloth to affected area.

Infusion 1 or 2 teaspoons per cup, steep 10 minutes, 1 to 3 cups per day

Syrup 1 teaspoon as needed for bronchial conditions

Tincture 10 to 30 drops, 1 to 3 times per day

Identification and cultivation

Stems are smooth, erect, to 12 inches. Leaves are alternate, trifoliate. Delicate white flowers are starlike and abundant. Semiaquatic plant grows at the shallow margins of lakes and along slow-flowing rivers, ponds, bogs, and dune slacks. In some areas, bogbean is a threatened or endangered plant, so check before you collect, or grow your own. Aquatic perennial. Best planted in a container, because it can become invasive. Plant directly in water, maximum 6 inches deep, in acidic, peaty soil, full sun; not tolerant of shade. Zones 3–10.

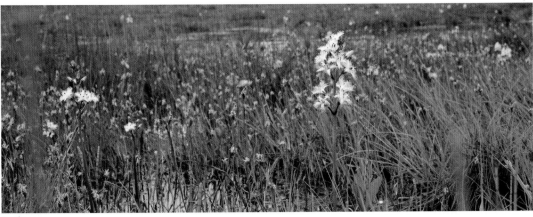

Bogbean

Boneset

Eupatorium perfoliatum

Also called thoroughwort, Indian sage, crosswort, feverwort **Family** Asteraceae
Parts used Leaves, stems

> *When you need to break a fever, bring in boneset.*

Organs or systems affected Respiratory system
Therapeutic actions Diaphoretic, tonic, febrifuge, expectorant, nervine **Nature** Bitter, cool **Plant constituents** Bitters, glycosides, flavonoids, inulin, volatile oil, acids, sterols, vitamin D1
Flower essence Assists those who are over-emotional, yet holding back their feelings

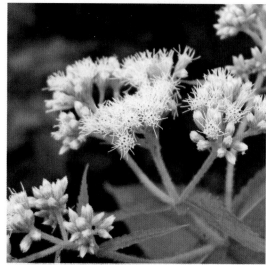

Boneset flowers

Medicinal uses

Breaks fevers A go-to for fever with chills and aches in the bones. Boneset will break a fever, aiding the body with a diaphoretic action to draw out what is ailing the person.
May help heal broken bones Despite its name, boneset has never been traditionally used to help heal broken bones, but some folks use it as a treatment for such and claim success.
Contraindications Generally regarded as safe.

MEDICINE CABINET

Infusion 1 or 2 teaspoons per cup, steep 10 minutes covered, 1 to 3 cups per day, or 4 ounces every hour for fever
Tincture 1 to 3 dropperfuls, 1 to 6 times per day

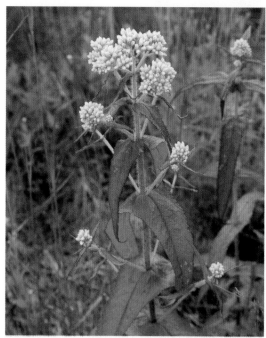

Boneset

Identification and cultivation

Stems, 1 to 6 feet, are round, pubescent, branching at the top. Thin leaves are perfoliate, arranged oppositely, 3 to 10 inches long. Small white flowers grow in dense clusters above the foliage. Grows in low ground, in open spaces, and next to rivers and swamps. Perennial. Divide the root ball or sow directly. Grow in any soil, full sun. Zones 3–9.

Borage

Borago officinalis

Also called burrage, bugloss **Family** Boraginaceae **Parts used** Flowers, leaves

> *Borage has a big effect on those who are stressed and exhausted.*

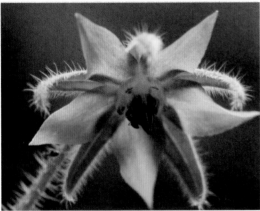

Borage flower

Organs or systems affected Brain, heart, respiratory system **Therapeutic action** Relaxant, demulcent, tonic, galactagogue, febrifuge **Nature** Sweet, salty, moist, cooling **Plant constituents** Mucilage, unsaturated pyrrolizadine alkaloids, gamma-linolenic acid, calcium, silicon, potassium **Flower essence** Helps those with heavy-heartedness or grief, who lack confidence in facing difficult circumstances and who are depressed

Medicinal uses

Nourishes endocrine and central nervous systems
In small doses, borage can restore deficiencies within the endocrine system and relax the nerves. The silicon content of borage nourishes the central nervous system, which influences the endocrine system higher up in the brain, enhancing communication between the central nervous system, the pituitary gland, and the hypothalamus gland. This results in nourishing the chronically deficient lower endocrine systems, particularly the thyroid and adrenals. Adrenal

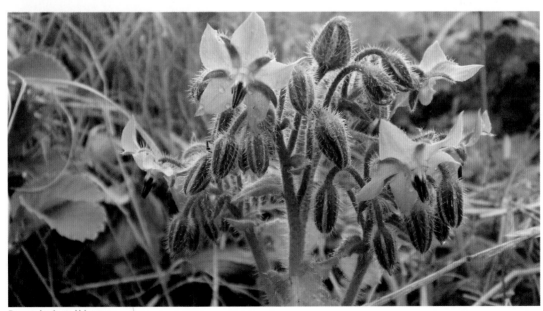

Borage buds and blooms

stress often presents as the overworked, completely exhausted person who has been on the go (physically or emotionally) for a long time. At times, a chronically fatigued person will present with melancholy and depression. Treating with borage in such cases can give them a bit of spark.

Soothes respiratory issues Borage contains mucilage, a wonderful ingredient to add to throat and cough syrups to soothe the respiratory tract. Overall, in small doses borage fortifies the entire respiratory system.

Contraindications Handling fresh leaves may provoke contact dermatitis. Constipation may occur after administration. Hepatotoxicity has been reported following chronic administration. Should not be taken during pregnancy.

MEDICINE CABINET

Infusion 1 teaspoon per cup, steep 8 to 10 minutes, 1 cup per day

Syrup 1 to 3 teaspoons per day with acute illness

Tincture 1 dropperful, 2 times per day, for short-term use only

---

Identification and cultivation

Round, hollow stems, 12 to 24 inches. Bristle-covered leaves alternate on branched stems, are deep green, broadly ovate, with pointed tips, 3 to 5 inches long. Bright blue, star-shaped flowers hang in downward-facing clusters, distinguished by black anthers that protrude from the center. Borage is commonly naturalized in woodlands and pastures. Perennial. Rapid grower and self-seeder. Sow seeds or propagate by division of rootstock in early spring. Grow in light soil, full sun to part shade. Zones 2–8.

Buckthorn

Frangula alnus (also *Rhamnus frangula*)

Also called alder buckthorn, highwaythorn, waythorn, hartsthorn, ramsthorn **Family** Rhamnaceae **Parts used** Bark

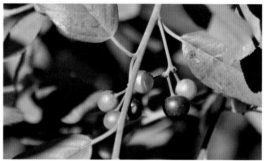

Buckthorn berries

> *Buckthorn's benefits are similar to those of cascara sagrada, but buckthorn motivates the bowels without irritation.*

Organs or systems affected Gastrointestinal system **Therapeutic actions** Alterative, laxative, antiparasitic, bitter, cathartic **Nature** Bitter **Plant constituents** Hydroxyanthraquinone glycosides, tannins, flavonoids

Medicinal uses

Facilitates elimination Buckthorn is a great place to begin when a laxative is needed. Although it may not be as strong as cascara sagrada, that's what makes it preferable in some cases. In appropriate doses, it is safe for children and won't lead to gripping pain with elimination. Average transit time after taking is 8 to 12 hours, so it decreases the need to worry about having a bathroom close by. Take buckthorn at bedtime to encourage morning elimination.

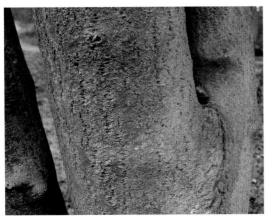
Buckthorn bark

using it medicinally. Consuming fresh bark can cause severe physical effects and is discouraged because of its emetic properties. Perennial shrub. Grow in neutral to acid soils, full sun to shade. Zone 3.

Bugleweed

Lycopus virginicus

Also called water bugle, sweet bugle, gypsyweed
Family Lamiaceae **Parts used** Flowers, leaves

> *A member of the mint family, bugleweed calms a rapid heart and is recommended for overactive thyroid.*

Organs or systems affected Heart, central nervous system, endocrine system **Therapeutic actions** Sedative, astringent **Nature** Bitter, cool, dry **Plant constituents** Flavonoids, bitters, tannins, volatile oils

Helps to stop bleeding and rid warts Apply a fomentation onto a wound to stop bleeding. Repeated applications are used to treat warts.
Soothes mouth and scalp irritations Buckthorn has been used both as a mouthwash for gum disease and as a hair rinse for scalp irritations.
Contraindications May cause loose stool. Consuming fresh bark can induce vomiting.

```
─── MEDICINE CABINET ───
Decoction 1 or 2 teaspoons per cup, simmer
10 to 12 minutes covered, take before bedtime
   Fomentation or hair rinse 3 tablespoons
per pint, steep at least 1 hour, strain, and apply
saturated cloth to affected area, or rinse entire
  infusion over hair and massage onto scalp
  Tincture 30 to 60 drops, taken as needed
```

Identification and cultivation
Tall, black-brown, smooth stems. Ovate leaves are arranged alternately. Small, green-yellow flowers are borne in dense clusters. Flowers are hermaphrodites (with both male and female organs) and are insect-pollinated. Pea-sized, black fruit is shiny when ripe. Collect and remove bark from fallen branches rather than removing from the trunk, which damages the tree. Cut bark into small pieces, dry and store it for a year before

Medicinal uses
Calms racing heart Bugleweed is used to relax a rapid heartbeat and slow down excited circulation, especially for the overextended and anxious person whose heart races, but with little force behind the beat—like the fluttering of a bird's heart when it is frightened. Bugleweed can also help a person return to sleep if the heart picks up in pace as a result of fright, stress, or worry. When an increased heart rate is experienced with a fever, bugleweed is a good choice.
Reduces thyroid hormone output In the early twentieth century, bugleweed was studied to determine its effects on hyperthyroidism, the overstimulation of the thyroid gland. When taken internally, bugleweed reduced thyroid hormone output. Many also use bugleweed oil topically to treat hyperthyroidism.

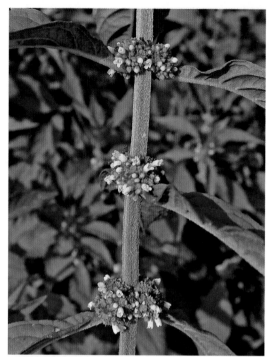
Bugleweed blooming

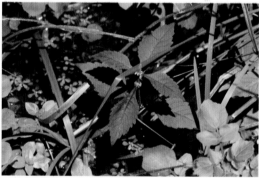
Bugleweed

Contraindications Those who have an underactive thyroid condition should not use this herb. It can also affect blood sugar levels.

MEDICINE CABINET

Infusion 1 or 2 teaspoons per cup, steep
15 minutes, 1 or 2 cups per day
Tincture 10 to 30 drops, 3 times per day

Identification and cultivation

Quadrangular and hairy stems, 6 to 24 inches. Lanceolate, toothed leaves are arranged oppositely. White flowers with purple flecks are borne in clusters along the spike. Found along streams and in low, damp, shady woodlands. Early to pop up in the spring and late to flower. Perennial. Divide in spring or fall. Grow in well-drained soil, full to part shade. Zones 3–9.

Burdock

Arctium lappa

Also called lappa, clotbur, thorny burr, cockle buttons, beggar's buttons **Family** Asteraceae **Parts used** Roots

> *Burdock is a tried-and-true liver and skin tonic.*

Organs or systems affected Kidneys, liver, skin **Therapeutic actions** Alterative, tonic, diuretic, diaphoretic, cholagogue **Nature** Bitter, sweet, cool **Plant constituents** Bitter glycosides, flavonoids, polysaccharides, antibiotic substances, vitamins A and C, minerals **Flower essence** Helps release intense anger and frustration

Medicinal uses

Supports and tones the liver Burdock has long been one of the most frequently used herbs for liver complaints. Its innate energy provides stability, while it gently cleanses the liver to support its natural function. As a tonic, it can be made to be liver-specific, but it is also used to increase overall well-being.

Cleanses the blood Burdock is good at cleansing the blood of toxic elements. Whenever you are working with tonifying the liver and blood,

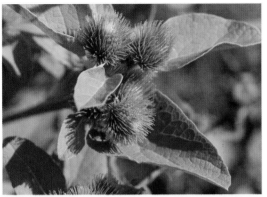
Spikey burdock bracts

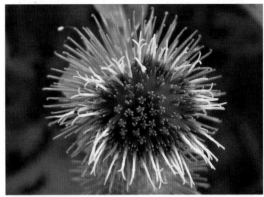
Burdock flower

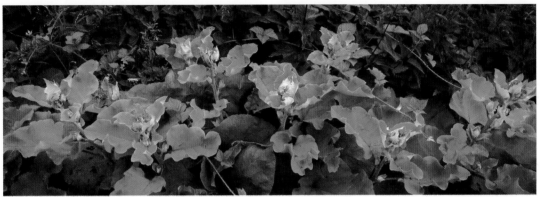
Burdock

skin outbreaks commonly arise, and this means the process is working. During this transition, burdock can help support the kidneys with elimination, and adding nettles or dandelion leaf can encourage this process.

Clears skin outbreaks Burdock is useful for treating hormone imbalance, the cause of many skin outbreaks.

Improves liver and gallbladder function Burdock breaks apart congestion in the body and is helpful with bile constraints. Drinking burdock tea or taking the tincture improves the function of the liver-gallbladder relationship, promoting better digestion and absorption throughout the digestive process.

Contraindications Generally regarded as safe.

MEDICINE CABINET

Decoction 1 or 2 teaspoons per cup, simmer 10 to 12 minutes covered, 1 to 3 cups per day
Tincture 10 to 30 drops, 1 to 3 times per day

Identification and cultivation

Short, stocky branches spread 2 to 6 feet. Large, coarse, heart-shaped leaves grow alternately. Round purple flowers are surrounded by spikey bracts. Grows in wastelands and woods. Often where you see nettle, burdock will be close by. Biennial. Listed as an invasive or noxious plant in some areas, so check before planting. Sow seeds in spring as soon as the ground can be worked. Grow in sandy, well-drained soil, full sun to part shade. Zones 2–10.

Calamus

Acorus calamus

Also called sweet flag, flag root, sweet sedge, sweet rush, sweet cane, gladdon, sweet myrtle, myrtle grass, cinnamon sedge, vacha **Family** Acoraceae **Parts used** Rootstock, rhizomes

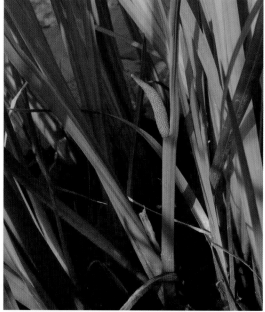
Calamus

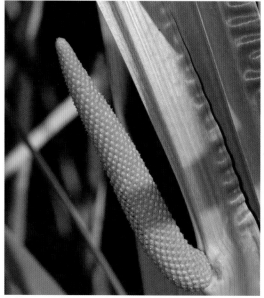
Calamus spadix

> *Calamus brings bright consciousness and the return of vacha, or voice.*

Organs or systems affected Brain, stomach, throat
Therapeutic actions Carminative, tonic, stimulant
Nature Bitter, pungent, acrid, warm, dry **Plant constituents** Volatile oil, terpenes, amines, tannins, resin, mucilage, gum, starch, acorin bitter glucoside, beta-asarone

Medicinal uses

Restores the throat and voice Based on the doctrine of signatures, the calamus rhizome

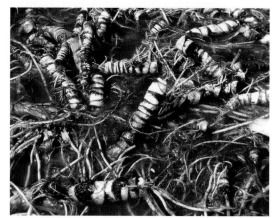
Calamus roots

resembles the trachea. It has been a traditional favorite herb of singers and performers.

Improves cognitive function In Chinese medicine, the closely related species *Acorus gramineus* is known to return clear thought and comprehensibility to cognitive function by removing stagnant phlegm type material. In clinical practice, calamus has been used with head trauma patients to reduce fogginess and help the patient concentrate. No studies have been performed with calamus and dementia, but it may be worth investigation.

Supports the gastrointestinal tract The high volatile oil content in calamus is helpful in treating flatulence and digestive complaints. It is used specifically for water brash, when acrid watery matter is regurgitated into the mouth. Chewing one small piece of root quickly cures such conditions.

Contraindications Extremely high doses have elicited hallucinogenic effects.

MEDICINE CABINET

Decoction 1 teaspoon per cup, simmer 10 to 12 minutes, 1 cup per day as needed
Fresh application On his website (herbcraft.org), herbalist Jim McDonald recommends chewing 1 or 2 tablespoons of the root per day as needed
Syrup 1 teaspoon, 3 or 4 times per day
Tincture 1 dropperful as needed

Identification and cultivation

Tufts of erect and sword-shaped basal leaves emerge directly from a spreading rootstock. Leaves resemble those of iris, but are greener, and are flattened on one side, with smooth margins and parallel veins. Some leaves develop a cylindrical semi-erect spike or spadix, 2 to 4 inches long, covered with tiny greenish yellow flowers in a diamond-shaped pattern. Each flower has six sepals and six stamens. A green spathe, or hood, wraps around the flower spike. Shallow branching rhizomes are stout and knobby, with a brown exterior and white interior. Grows on the banks of shallow, clay-bottomed lakes, rivers, and ponds. When it is not flowering, calamus looks a lot like yellow iris but is easy to identify by the pleasant lemony smell of its aromatic oil. Semi-aquatic perennial. Easy to establish from rhizome. Grow in wet, mucky, rich soil, full sun to part shade. Zones 2–10.

Cedar

Thuja occidentalis

Also called tree of life, arbor-vitae, American arbor-vitae, yellow cedar, false white cedar
Family Cupressaceae **Parts used** Leaves, young twigs

> *The cedar's use as a medicinal herb dates back to early American eclectic physicians who used it to treat tumors, cancer, and phlegm accumulation.*

Organs or systems affected Bladder, colon, lungs, skin, uterus **Therapeutic actions** Alterative, stimulant, anticatarrhal, astringent, antifungal, anti-inflammatory, astringent **Nature** Spicy, bitter, warm **Plant constituents** Flavonoid glycosides, mucilage, resin, tannins, volatile oil, vitamin C
Flower essence Helps to purify negativity, clearing energy for new beginnings and protecting energy from others when one is unable to set clear boundaries

Medicinal uses

Dissolves phlegm Cedar is a natural decongestant that helps alleviate built-up or stuck phlegm in the body, as occurs with sinus infections and head colds. It promotes the expectoration of phlegm. It is also used to treat cystitis, removing bacteria that is often accumulated in the bladder due to a warm, damp condition. Its antimicrobial and astringent actions often help expel the infection and work to increase overall tone in the bladder.

Stimulates uterus Cedar's stimulating action may cause the uterus to contract, or perhaps because it stimulates the gastrointestinal tract, the nearby uterus contracts as well. Either way, it can bring on menstruation and should not be taken during pregnancy.

Slows cancer growth Research is providing many uses for cedar in the treatment of cancer. In a lab, cedar seems to increase phagocytosis, a process in which bacterial cells are engulfed and digested by other cells. It also shows antiviral activity. The eclectic physicians of the late nineteenth and early twentieth centuries administered cedar internally and externally to patients, not only to slow down cancer growth but to eliminate it altogether. Some practitioners use it specifically for colon cancer and certain types of uterine cancers, injecting it directly into the affected areas.

Treats warts and fungal infections Cedar has long been used for the external treatment of warts and fungal infections such as ringworm. Grieve (1931) stated that an injection of cedar directly into venereal warts caused them to disappear.

Contraindications Should not be taken during pregnancy. Avoid in excessively large quantities because of the presence of thujone, which may be toxic. Persons with dry, irritating coughs should not take cedar. The herb can also cause tachycardia (faster than normal heart rate).

MEDICINE CABINET

Infusion 1 teaspoon per cup, steep 15 minutes covered, 1 or 2 cups per day
Tincture 1 to 4 dropperfuls per day, not to be consumed long-term. For warts, cover with tincture 2 times per day until gone.

Identification and cultivation

Fanlike branches with scaly, slender leaves. Bark is red-brown, furrowed, and peels in narrow strips. Cones are slender, yellow-green and ripen to brown; scales overlap. Leaves and twigs can be harvested year-round, but summer is best. Grows in swamps, along streams, in rocky soils. Evergreen conifer. Plant in spring. Grow in slightly acidic, moist soil, full sun. Zones 2–8.

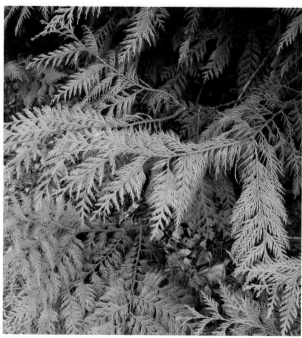

Cedar foliage

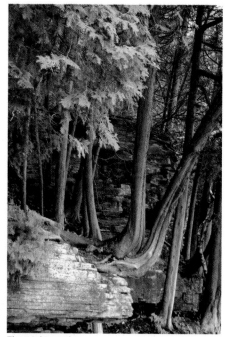

The mighty cedar

Centaury

Centaurium erythraea

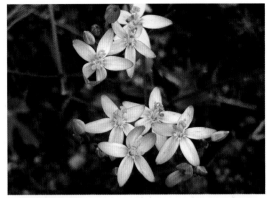

Also called European centaury, centaurium, century, feverwort, bitter herb, banwort, bloodwort, Christ's ladder **Family** Gentianaceae **Parts used** Flowers, leaves, stems

> *Centaury brings balance to the gastrointestinal system and vitality to the body.*

Organs or systems affected Gallbladder, heart, stomach **Therapeutic actions** Tonic, bitter, febrifuge **Nature** Bitter **Plant constituents** Bitter glycosides, alkaloids, volatile oil, acids, resin, flavonoids, magnesium **Flower essence** Indicated for those who need to act from strength of inner purpose and who need help saying "no" when appropriate

Medicinal uses

Aids the digestion Like gentian, centaury aids the digestion by helping the body secrete the appropriate balance of gastric juices and enzymes. It also works on the gallbladder in releasing bile and supports the liver's detoxification functions.
Tonifies the body At one time, centaury covered European hillsides and was used by farmers and households as a health tonic to increase vitality.
Contraindications Generally regarded as safe.

Centaury flowers

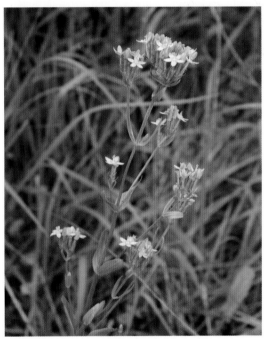

Centaury

┌─────────────── MEDICINE CABINET ───────────────┐

Infusion For digestion, 1 or 2 teaspoons per cup, steep 8 to 10 minutes, 1 to 3 cups per day
Tincture For digestion, 10 to 30 drops, 1 to 3 times per day

└───┘

Identification and cultivation

Erect stems are branched at the top. Ribbed leaves are triangular and arranged oppositely. Pink, petite flowers are starlike, with five petals and yellow anthers. Best collected in midsummer. Found in barren fields and wastelands. Annual. Sow seeds in fall. Grow in sandy, loamy, well-drained soil, full sun to part shade. Zones 4–9.

Chaga

Inonotus obliquus

Also called clinker polypore **Family** Hymenochae-taceae **Parts Used** Entire fungus

> *This mycelium has a strong ability to regulate immune function.*

Organs or systems affected Blood, liver, immune system **Therapeutic actions** Stimulant, adaptogen **Nature** Bitter, sweet **Plant constituents** Inotodiol, betulin, melanin, active polysaccharides **Flower essence** Indicated when rigid belief systems have diminished one's vitality and energy

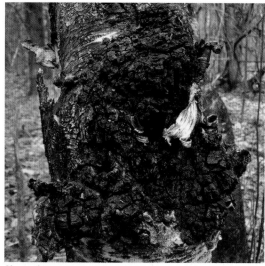
Chaga closeup

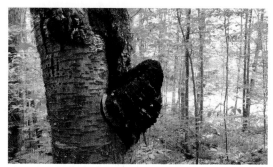
Chaga growing on bark

Medicinal uses

Lowers cholesterol, balances blood sugar Several constituents make researching chaga and its uses interesting: betulin and polysaccharides, for example, can lower cholesterol, balance blood sugar, and support regular metabolistic function.
Provides antioxidants Chaga constituent melanin, a natural antioxidant, is very important in reducing inflammation and maintaining proper cellular regeneration—and, of course, it is an essential part of the anti-aging regime.
Stimulates the immune system The polysaccharides and the adaptogen effects of chaga are considered valuable for stimulating the immune system to respond in a healthy way, especially when trying to rid the body of a cold or bacterial infection. Chaga also seems to help those with autoimmune dysfunction. New research indicates that it can regulate and reestablish an appropriate immune response when antibodies are functioning improperly.
Contraindications Diabetics using insulin should closely monitor blood sugar levels if taking chaga, because it can lower or raise these levels.

MEDICINE CABINET

Infusion 4 tablespoons per quart, steep overnight. Drink 3 cups per day. Do not infuse in water above 125°F (52°C), because this can damage its medicinal properties.
Tincture 1 dropperful, 1 to 3 times per day

Identification and cultivation

This parasitic fungal mycelium is typically found on yellow or white birch trees. Its outer surface resembles burnt charcoal, dark brown to black, with a deeply cracked texture. Slow growing and at risk of overharvesting, it can be cultivated using a mushroom-growing kit.

Chaparral

Larrea divaricata

Also called creosote bush, greasewood, black bush, gobernadora, *hediondilla* **Family** Zygophyllaceae **Parts used** Leaves, stems

> *The Spanish name for chaparral, hediondilla, means little stinker, and this strong-smelling desert herb helps remove trapped toxins from the body.*

Organs or systems affected Bladder, kidneys, liver, stomach **Therapeutic actions** Astringent, stimulant, alterative, diuretic, depurative **Nature** Bitter, pungent, salty, dry **Plant constituents** Essential oil, flavonoids, terpenes, acids, gum, resin, protein, sucrose **Flower essence** Helps clean out old, stored up emotions

Medicinal uses

Detoxifies the body Chaparral has been used for centuries to detoxify the liver and the body. The oils within the plant can decrease inflammation in both the gastrointestinal and respiratory tracts. Chaparral seems to travel throughout the body, clearing out thick, stuck residue. This in turn supports the lymphatic system by helping dissolve toxins.

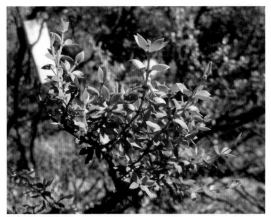
Chaparral leaves

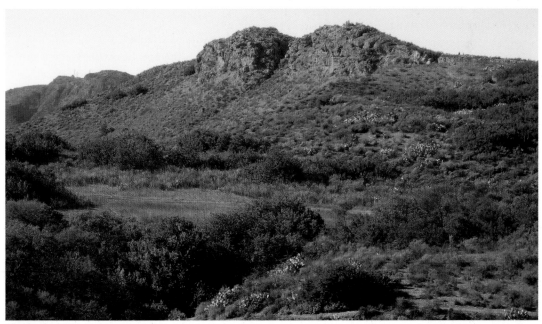
Chaparral

Rebuilds damaged tissue Chaparral works as an astringent and helps rebuild damaged tissue. Because of this and its anti-inflammatory characteristics, it is often recommended for arthritis when tissues have been damaged due to overuse, autoantibodies, or chronic inflammation.

Tones bladder and kidneys Whenever toxins are being released from the body, the bladder and kidneys work overtime. Chaparral's astringent nature tones up these systems during excessive burden.

Helps heal wounds In stronger external applications, chaparral works well for hemorrhoids, boils, bedsores, bruises, or wounds. Applying a fomentation 2 or 3 times per day can ease pain and expedite healing. Chaparral has also long been used to treat tumors and growths.

Contraindications Induces vomiting with large internal doses. Those with liver disease should not take chaparral.

MEDICINE CABINET

Douche 1 tablespoon of infusion per cup of water
Infusion ½ to 1 teaspoon per cup, steep 10 minutes, 1 or 2 cups per day
Sitz bath or fomentation 3 tablespoons per pint, steep 1 hour
Tincture 1 dropperful, 3 times per day

Identification and cultivation

Tangled, brittle stems, 2 to 9 feet. Leaves are olive green, small, resinous, divergent. Yellow flowers, ½-inch wide, bloom in spring. Harvest any time, but plants are best harvested when seeds are past maturity. Usually found at 5000 feet or lower elevations in desert regions. Evergreen shrub. Grow in loose, fine, sandy, well-drained soil, full sun. Zones 7–11.

Chickweed

Stellaria media

Also called starweed, stitchwort, scarwort
Family Caryophyllaceae **Parts used** Flowers, leaves, stems

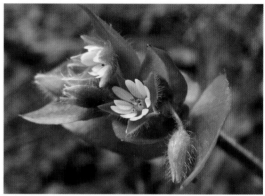
First spring bloom of chickweed

A sure sign of spring's arrival is the delicate chickweed, packed with trace minerals and nutrients.

Organs or systems affected Intestines, kidneys, lungs, stomach **Therapeutic actions** Demulcent, emollient, tonic, alterative **Nature** Sweet, salty, cool, moist **Plant constituents** Saponins, oils, flavonoids, rutin, coumarins, calcium, potassium, magnesium, iron, silicon, zinc, molybdenum, phosphorus, manganese, vitamins A, B, and C **Flower essence** Helps one embody tolerance, compassion, and divinity

Medicinal uses

Heals wounds As a cool and moist herb, chickweed is extremely healing to any wound, burn, or skin disease. A simple poultice, fomentation, or salve will work wonders.

Supports respiratory system A demulcent by design and moistening by nature, chickweed aids dry and constrained respiration problems, including dry coughs, asthma, and allergic irritations.

Reduces internal bleeding and inflammation A nutrient-rich herb, chickweed helps the body assimilate trace minerals and vitamins. This function creates overall vitality at the cellular level but can also aid in the cessation of bleeding from ulcers, intestines, or rectum. Its cooling nature also helps reduce inflammation.

Supports kidneys Chickweed balances water in the body, and this supports kidney function. Some have reported that it reduces water weight and water accumulations, and that it can reduce cysts in the body. When water is being properly regulated in the body, the metabolism usually functions normally.

Contraindications Generally regarded as safe.

MEDICINE CABINET

Infusion 1 to 3 teaspoons per cup, steep 10 to 12 minutes, 1 to 3 cups per day
Poultice, fomentation, or salve As needed
Tincture 1 to 3 dropperfuls, 1 to 3 times per day

Identification and cultivation

Clumps of flimsy stems, 4 to 6 inches, are covered in fine hairs on one side. Small ovate leaves are oppositely arranged. Tiny white flowers grow in terminal clusters. Grows nearly everywhere, at the bases of trees, in yards, woods, flower boxes, and gravel roads. In moist, temperate climates, harvest young shoots almost year-round. Annual. Collect seedpods when flowers fade and allow them to dry. Directly sow outdoors in fall or after last frost. Grow in any soil, part shade. Zones 3–8.

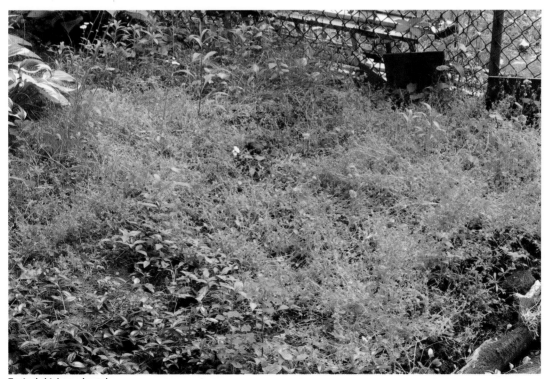

Typical chickweed patch

Chicory

Cichorium intybus

Also called succory, wild succory, hendibeh, *barbe de capucin* **Family** Asteraceae **Parts used** Roots

This gentle gastrointestinal healer has flowers of blue.

Organs or systems affected Gallbladder, gastrointestinal system **Therapeutic actions** Tonic, laxative, diuretic **Nature** Bitter, sweet, cooling, slightly moist **Plant constituents** Inulin, terpenes, flavonoids, beta carotene, vitamins C and K **Flower essence** Used when possessive or manipulative behaviors disguised as love are present, and for those who are demanding or emotionally needy, who seek attention through negative behavior, or who suffer from self-centeredness

Medicinal uses

Optimizes digestive process Chicory shines in its ability to optimize the digestive process, easing the breakdown of food to nutrient or waste. Once this is accomplished, it aids the blood in delivering nutrients to the body and in their absorption into the cells. As a result, the blood has less residual toxins, which reduces stress on the body's detoxification systems.

Supports bile production Chicory's bitter principle is helpful for stubborn or chronic gallbladder congestion. It helps open up the bile ducts, decreasing gallbladder colic.

Contraindications Generally regarded as safe.

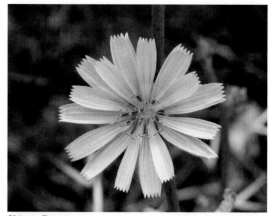
Chicory flower

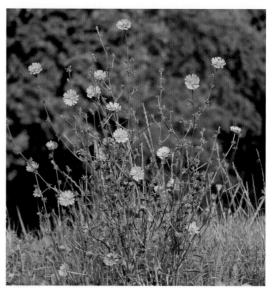
Chicory

Identification and cultivation

Stems are erect, 2 to 3 feet, multibranched. Similar to dandelion but smaller, lanceolate leaves are coarsely toothed and covered with hairs. Bright or light blue flowers grow in clusters of two or three, opening with the sunrise and closing by midday. Found in open or grassy areas, along roadsides and parking lots. Perennial. Keep well watered to prevent them from seeding too quickly. Grow in well-drained, fertilized soil, full sun. Zones 4–11.

MEDICINE CABINET

Infusion 1 or 2 teaspoons, steep 10 to 20 minutes depending on bitter preference, 1 to 3 cups per day

Tincture 1 to 3 dropperfuls per day, or 1 dropperful after meals

Cleavers

Galium aparine

Also called clivers, goosegrass, giraffe grass, burweed, bedstraw **Family** Rubiaceae **Parts used** Flowers, leaves, stems

> *A gentle lymphatic tonic, this plant grabs on and attaches to you as you walk through the woods.*

Organs or systems affected Bladder, kidneys, lymphatic system **Therapeutic actions** Diuretic, tonic, alterative **Nature** Sweet, salty, cool **Plant constituents** Acids, anthraquinones, saponins, coumarins, chlorophyll, tannins, trace minerals **Flower essence** Supports attachment and appropriate bonding, keeping relationships flowing and love strong

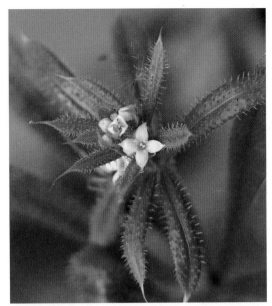

Cleavers flower

Medicinal uses

Tones and decongests lymph nodes Cleavers act very similarly to poke root, but they work in a milder and gentler way. They help relieve congestion in swollen lymph glands and nodules in the body. Their cleansing action supports the elimination of waste material and purifies the blood.

Supports kidneys and bladder Any time an herb has an affinity for the lymphatic system, it will probably complement the kidneys and bladder as well, because their tissues are similar and all serve the elimination process. Cleavers are useful for kidney or bladder stones, suppression of urine, obstructions, or irritations in these organs due to inflammation, infection, dysfunction, or other causes.

Contraindications Because of its diuretic principles, cleavers should not be taken by those with diabetes.

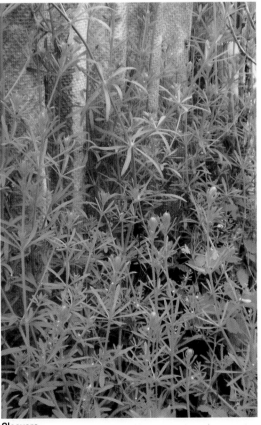

Cleavers

Identification and cultivation

Quadrangular-shaped stems, to 3 feet, are covered with tiny hooked hairs and sprawl along the ground and up other plants. Lanceolate leaves, also covered in hairs, in whorls of six to eight. The hairs on the plant stick to passersby. Tiny white flowers bloom in early spring to summer. Look for them in the woods, in moist thickets and wetlands, and along river banks. Harvest from spring through fall as new starts come on continuously. Annual. Considered a noxious weed in some areas, so check before planting. Directly sow outdoors in the fall or after last frost. Grow in moist, neutral soil, full to part shade. Zones 3–9.

Couch grass

Elymus repens

Also called dog grass, quack grass **Family** Poaceae **Parts used** Rhizomes

This common weed helps with kidney and bladder troubles.

Organs or systems affected Bladder, kidneys, skin, lymphatic system **Therapeutic actions** Diuretic, demulcent, astringent **Nature** Sweet, moist **Plant constituents** Carbohydrates, saponins, acids, glycosides, iron, silica, vitamins A and B **Flower essence** Assists those who are unable to let go of beliefs that are no longer serving them

Medicinal uses

Supports kidneys and bladder A definite go-to herb for any kidney or bladder complaint, couch grass helps to dissolve and relieve kidney stone discomfort. Because of its ability to relax and soothe the renal passageways, it can be helpful with most any kidney or bladder trouble. Couch grass has proven its worth in treating interstitial cystitis (IC), the irritation of the bladder wall that presents much like a bladder infection, but when tested shows no bacteria present. It

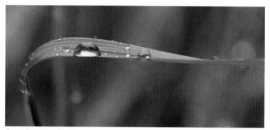
Couch grass leaf

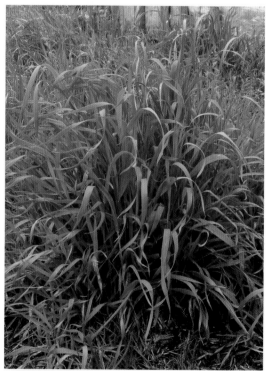
A clump of couch grass

is my opinion that IC is the result of long-term bladder irritation and inflammation, leading to tiny holes in the bladder lining. When irritants continue to pass through the bladder, these tiny holes become agitated, leading to bladder infection–type symptoms. Using couch grass, along with pipsissewa and goldenrod, can heal these punctures and soothe irritations.

Controls blood sugar Often when an herb works on the kidneys, the blood sugar may be balanced because of the herb's effect on the kidney and its release of erythropoietin, a hormone that helps modulate glucose metabolism.

Contraindications Use caution if taking it long-term because of its diuretic effects and the potential loss of potassium through increased urinary output.

MEDICINE CABINET

Decoction 3 teaspoons in 1 pint of water, simmer 15 minutes, 4 ounces every 30 minutes as needed

Infusion 1 or 2 teaspoons per cup, steep 3 to 4 hours, 1 to 3 cups per day

Tincture 1 or 2 dropperfuls, 1 to 6 times per day, or 1 dropperful every 30 minutes until acute symptoms subside

---

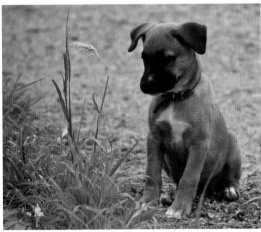

Dogs love to eat couch grass.

Identification and cultivation

Erect stems, 1½ to 3 feet, are branched at the base. Short-bladed leaves are smooth on top, hairy on the bottom. Dense flower spikes produce twenty-five seeds per stem. Follow your canine friend to find this grass, because dogs love to eat couch grass and it has naturalized almost everywhere. Collect the roots and rhizomes in spring. This plant is considered a noxious weed in many areas. Do not grow it in your garden. It can be extremely difficult to eradicate, spreads quickly, and absorbs more than its share of soil nutrients.

Cowslip

Primula veris

Also called fairy cups, key to heaven, herb peter, horse buckles, key flower **Family** Primulaceae **Parts used** Flowers, leaves, stems

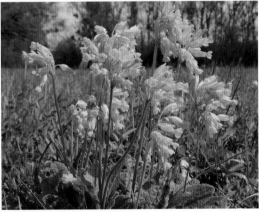

Cowslip

> *This gentle remedy creates a great calming effect.*

Organs or systems affected Heart, lungs, central nervous system, vascular system **Therapeutic actions** Sedative, antispasmodic **Nature** Bitter, sweet, pungent **Plant constituents** Glycoside, bitters, volatile oil **Flower essence** Nurtures the individual to feel safe and supported in life

Medicinal uses

Eases anxiety and tension held in the body As stress rises, so does tension in the body, causing restriction in breath, heart rate, blood flow, and even brain function. If you were to fall ill, this increased tension can have detrimental effects on the recovery process. One example could be increased tension in the chest cavity resulting from long-term stress while battling a chest cold, which can cause further complications in respiration. Cowslip helps relax the tensions held in the central nervous system, heart, vascular system, and lungs. It's a great choice for kids who need to relax a bit or who have undergone a stressful situation in their precious emotional development. Anywhere tension is exacerbating physical pain, cowslip is appropriate.

Relieves headaches Cowslip is often compared to wood betony for its ability to relieve head pain and complaints. I like to prescribe both to relieve headaches, migraines, mental agitation, and insomnia.

Improves the skin Cowslip gives the surface of the skin shine and gloss, can help reduce spots and wrinkles, and relieves sunburn discomfort.

Promotes calm A wine made from the flowers provides sedative qualities.

Contraindications Generally regarded as safe.

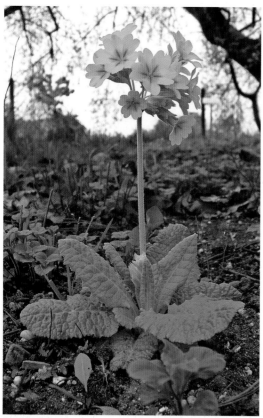

Cowslip flowers

MEDICINE CABINET

Infusion 1 or 2 teaspoons per cup, steep 8 to 10 minutes covered, 1 to 3 cups per day
Tincture 10 to 30 drops under the tongue, 1 to 3 times per day

---

Identification and cultivation

Downy, green, scalloped leaves form rosettes at the base of the plant. Clusters of ten to thirty yellow flowers per stem in the spring. Grows in old meadows, pastures, and grasslands. Best collected in early spring. In times past, a sign of a well-fertilized pasture was the presence of cowslip. Perennial. Sow seeds in late autumn, because they need a season of chill to break dormancy. Grow in slightly alkaline soil, full sun. Zones 3–9.

Cranesbill

Geranium maculatum

Also called crowfoot, wild geranium, wild alum root, spotted geranium **Family** Geraniaceae **Parts used** Roots

> *Cranesbill is a gentle astringent for drying out runny noses and other excessive discharges.*

Organs or systems affected Intestines, skin, stomach, respiratory system **Therapeutic actions** Astringent, tonic, styptic **Nature** Sweet, cool **Plant constituents** Tannins, acid, sulfates, calcium oxalate **Flower essence** Helps one feel safe and loved

Medicinal uses

Helps restrain excessive discharges Cranesbill is a premier astringent, restraining fluids that are flowing excessively, such as a constant runny nose with a cold, increased mucus production in the stomach, or excessive vaginal discharge. It acts to tone the tissue to restrain the fluid release.
Gently controls diarrhea A good choice for loose stools or diarrhea, this gentle astringent herb works well for children. It is not irritating or nausea producing as some astringents can be.
Reduces signs of aging in skin Traditional herbalists considered cranesbill a superior anti-aging herb. Using it in a cream or lotion helps reduce wrinkles, pores, and cystic acne.
Contraindications Generally regarded as safe.

MEDICINE CABINET

Decoction 1 or 2 teaspoons per cup, simmer 10 to 15 minutes covered, 1 to 3 cups per day
Tincture 1 to 30 drops, 1 to 3 times per day

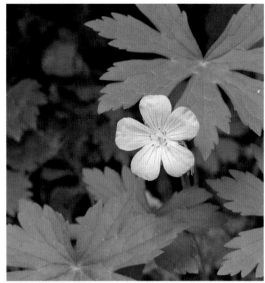
Cranesbill flower

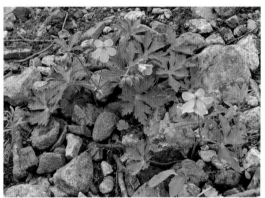
Cranesbill

Identification and cultivation

Round, greenish gray stems. Leaves palmately lobed with five or seven deeply cut and toothed lobes. Blooming in late spring and early summer in loose clusters, flowers are pinkish purple, 1 or 2 inches wide, with five petals. Grows in forests, open areas, or along roadsides. Harvest roots in the fall. Perennial. Best to purchase and grow established plant. Grow in acidic, rich, moist soil, full sun to part shade in cooler climates and full to part shade in warmer climates. Zones 3–8.

Culver's root

Veronicastrum virginicum

Also called black root, speedwell, tall veronica, bowman's root **Family** Plantaginaceae **Parts used** Roots

> *Culver's root can often relieve gallbladder pain and liver discomfort.*

Organs or systems affected Gallbladder, liver **Therapeutic actions** Cathartic, stimulant, hepatic, cholagogue **Nature** Bitter **Plant constituents** Bitters, glycosides, saponins, volatile oil, tannin, citric acid **Flower essence** Helps one release past failures, romantic attachments, and harsh self-judgments

Medicinal uses

Reduces congestion in liver and gallbladder Culver's root stimulates both the liver and gallbladder into action by gently forcing the organs to clear out stagnation of toxicity and bile. This in turn usually stimulates the bowels for proper elimination. This action is considered a tonic for the liver and is helpful for those whose eyes or skin appear discolored or jaundiced.
Contraindications Generally regarded as safe, but beware that it is purgative. Best taken in small, frequent doses.

MEDICINE CABINET

Decoction 1 or 2 teaspoons per cup, simmer 10 to 12 minutes covered, drink 4 ounces every 3 or 4 hours as needed
Tincture 1 to 3 dropperfuls every 3 hours until hepatic discomfort is resolved

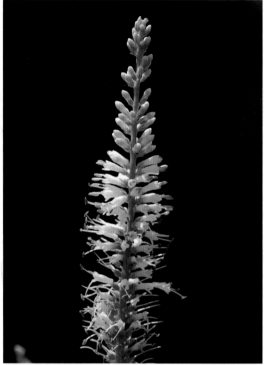
Culver's root flower

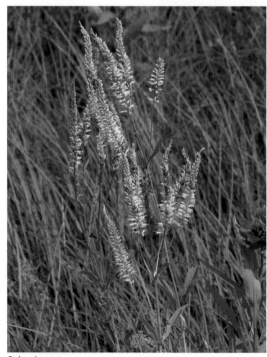
Culver's root

Identification and cultivation

Erect stems, 2 to 6 feet. Thin leaves are serrated and arranged in whorls of three to seven. Small, white to pale blue flowers grow in slender raceme spikes, midsummer to early fall. Widely naturalized, grows in low ground, thickets, and moist meadows, but is threatened or endangered in some areas. Drought-tolerant perennial. Propagate by dividing rhizomes or tubers in fall. Grow in mildly alkaline soil, full sun to part shade. Zones 3–8.

Echinacea

Echinacea purpurea

Also called black Samson, Sampson root, pale purple cornflower, comb flower, hedgehog **Family** Asteraceae **Parts used** Leaves, roots

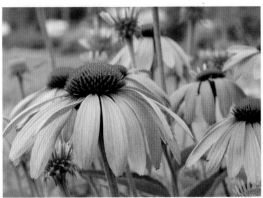

Echinacea flowers

> *Echinacea is a blood purifier and digestive stimulant for those regaining their health.*

Organs or systems affected Blood, immune system, lymphatic system **Therapeutic actions** Alterative, antiseptic, stimulant, tonic, diaphoretic **Nature** Sweet, salty, cool **Plant constituents** Glycosides, volatile oil, mucopolysaccharides, echinolone, betaine, tannins, resins, enzymes, fatty acids, phytosterols, vitamin C, trace minerals **Flower essence** Helps one maintain a strong sense of self, especially when challenged by stress or disease

Medicinal uses

Purifies blood As a strong alterative and antiseptic, echinacea root is traditionally used to clear the blood of toxic matter. It is often used for blood poisoning resulting from internal infection, an external wound, or a snake bite.

Reduces infection Applied externally as a poultice or fomentation, it is quite soothing and reduces infection and pus formation in wounds.

Stimulates digestion In folk medicine, echinacea was used to help those severely depleted from illness. It seemed to help return the appetite and improve digestion, which is important in attempting to return to good health.

Stimulates immune system Echinacea root seems to have an immune-stimulating action, although there is great debate over echinacea's true nature and how and when it should be used.

Increases white blood cells Research indicates that echinacea root helps increase white blood cell production. Therefore, I consider it a wise herb to use if you have been exposed to contagious illness or are feeling the very beginnings of illness. I advise using echinacea for a day or two. Many other herbs can be used to obtain the same results. For colds that last longer than two days, it is best to discontinue echinacea and begin a new formula that is in direct relation to your symptoms and constitutional type.

Contraindications Those suffering from leukemia should not take this herb.

Identification and cultivation

Stems are simple, erect, and covered with light hairs. Lanceolate leaves grow alternately and are also covered with hairs. Purple to pink, large, cone-shaped flowers bloom in summer. Grows in meadows or open pastures. Harvest the roots in the fall from mature plants that are a minimum of 2 years old. Perennial. Deer-resistant. Sow directly in spring, or self-sows freely. Grow in any soil, full sun to part shade. Zones 2–10.

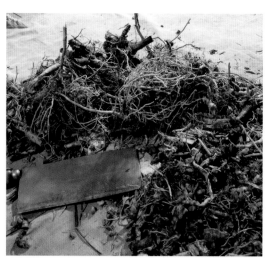

Harvested echinacea roots

Elder

Sambucus nigra

Also called black elder, European elder, boretree, pip tree, devil's wood **Family** Adoxaceae **Parts used** Berries, flowers, leaves

| *The medicine chest for the common people.*

Organs or systems affected Immune system, musculoskeletal system, respiratory system **Therapeutic actions** Berries: diaphoretic, diuretic, antiviral, laxative. Flowers: diaphoretic, anticatarrhal, pectoral. Leaves: emollient, vulnerary, purgative, expectorant, diuretic, diaphoretic **Nature** Pungent, sweet, cool, dry **Plant constituents** Flavonoids, sugar, acids, tannin, vitamins C and P, anthrocyanic pigments, volatile oil **Flower essence** For those who need to stimulate the powers of recovery and renewal of the vital life energies

Medicinal uses

A complete medicine chest Elder offers an abundance of medicine. The berries work to remove viruses from the body and remove deep congestion, whether it be in the lungs, kidneys, or joints. The flower promotes sweating, resolves phlegm in all areas of the body, and promotes the draining of it through the bladder. The leaf is excellent in cooling tissues inside and out and is used to make a soothing wound salve. The leaf is also good for eyewashes and compresses.

Supports immune system Recent research focusing on elder indicates that it has antiviral effects and can help knock out such viruses as H1N1 (swine flu). I prescribe elder as a tonic for the entire immune system, not just for the flu. Berries are packed with vitamin C and flavonoids, which support day-to-day cellular health and immune function. As a virus fighting, diaphoretic, and anticatarrhal herb, elder gives any mucus-invading virus a run for its money. Elder products have been extremely well marketed, so be sure to look at ingredients when purchasing products to ensure that added ingredients such as excess sugars and flavoring are not included.

Supports respiratory system Elder is supportive to the respiratory system, with its ability to open the body, induce mild sweating (flower and leaves), reduce fever, and dissolve phlegm. Phlegm tends to be a hot, sticky, stagnant situation, and when all parts of the elder are used together, they can be beneficial to resolve these issues.

Contraindications Generally regarded as safe.

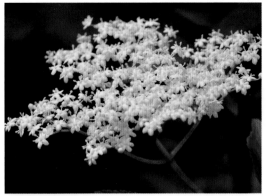
Elder flowers

MEDICINE CABINET

Decoction 2 teaspoons berries in 12 ounces water, simmer on low, covered, for 10 minutes, 1 to 3 cups per day
Infusion 1 or 2 teaspoons per cup, steep 3 or 4 hours or overnight, 1 to 3 cups per day
Tincture 1 or 2 dropperfuls, 1 to 3 times per day

Identification and cultivation

Large shrub or small tree, to 20 feet, with coarse, gray, furrowed bark. Pinnate, compound leaves arranged in opposite pairs. White, star-shaped flowers grow in clusters, 4 to 10 inches wide, in late spring to midsummer. Drooping berries produced in the fall. Grows in moist woodlands, thickets, and fencerows. Deciduous shrub. Elder is tolerant of pruning and can be cut to the ground in late winter to help keep the shrub healthy. Grow in well-drained, moist soil, full sun. Zones 4–7.

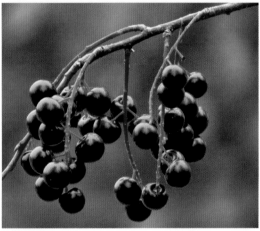
Elderberries

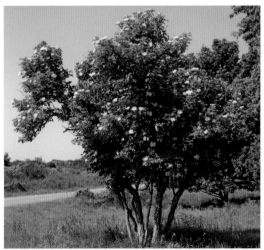
Elder shrub

Elecampane

Inula helenium

Also called scabwort, elf dock, yellow starwort, wild sunflower, horse heal, velvet dock **Family** Asteraceae **Parts used** Rhizomes, roots

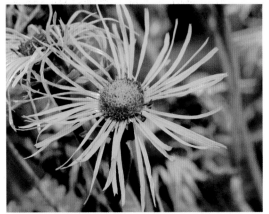

Elecampane flower

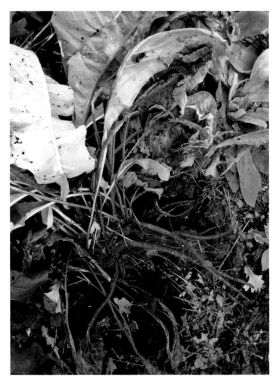

Elecampane roots

> *This disc of golden sun reaches into the depths of our lungs and being to rehabilitate and cleanse the tissues.*

Organs or systems affected Liver, lungs, spleen, stomach **Therapeutic actions** Tonic, expectorant, diaphoretic, carminative, diuretic, alterative, antiseptic, astringent **Nature** Sweet, bitter, dry, aromatic, pungent, warm **Plant constituents** Inulin, bitters, triterpenes, essential oil, alkaloid, mucilage, resin, sodium, calcium, magnesium **Flower essence** Helps one move through and move on, and overcome deeply ingrained fears or grief

Medicinal uses

Rehabilitates lungs Elecampane is my number one favorite herb for the lungs, especially to rehabilitate them after years of smoking, illness, or chronic pathology. It is very efficient at driving out old, deep, and stuck mucus from the pulmonary tract. At times, with initial use it can drive a cough deeper into the chest, resulting in an increase in mucous discharge—but this is a positive reaction, because it indicates that the herb has reached the depths of old hardened mucus to get it up and out of the body. My mentor, Linda Quintana, often recommended elecampane when she and I worked together in Bellingham, Washington, near a General Mills paper plant. Chlorine was used to bleach the toilet paper manufactured there, and many employees experienced pulmonary complaints as a result. Elecampane is my *crème de la crème* herb when it comes to healing the lungs. I often recommend it for children with asthma.

Cleans the liver and bowels The presence of sodium phosphate and potassium chloride in elecampane helps to clean the liver and bowels and dissolve hardened mucus. It creates a gentle

detoxification for the body, along with clearing skin conditions and balancing the hormones. **Supports the lymph system** This cleaning effect is also thought to support the lymph system and the gut, clearing toxins and unhealthy bacterial colonies that may be present. Sixty percent of your immune system resides in the lining of the gut, hence the need to support and nourish the lining. Matthew Wood (2008) states that elecampane has shown affinity for the lymphatics in reducing chronic swollen cervical glands.
Contraindications Should not be taken during pregnancy.

MEDICINE CABINET

Decoction 1 tablespoon per cup, simmer 10 to 15 minutes covered, 3 cups per day

Steam 1 ounce per quart of water in stockpot, simmer until hot, remove from stove. Cover pot with towel, and when ready, and water is not too hot, inhale slowly and deeply for 5 to 10 minutes.

Syrup 1 teaspoon, 1 to 3 times per day

Tincture 30 drops, 3 to 4 times per day

Identification and cultivation

Thick stems, 3 to 5 feet tall. Large ovate leaves, 10 to 18 inches long and wooly underneath, are arranged alternately. Large, solitary golden yellow flowers, 2 to 5 inches across, bloom in midsummer. Rhizomes are gray-brown on the outside, lighter brown internally. Grows in pastures, along roadsides. Perennial. Divide plants about every 3 years to maintain vitality. Grow in loamy, moist soil, full sun to shade. Zones 5–8.

False unicorn

Chamaelirium luteum

Also called helonias, starwort, drooping star wort, fairy wand **Family** Melanthiaceae **Parts used** Roots

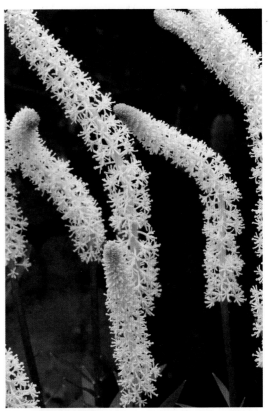

False unicorn flowers

False unicorn targets the uterus and ovaries to provide tone and regenerative function.

Organs or systems affected Ovaries, stomach, uterus **Therapeutic actions** Tonic, diuretic **Nature** Bitter, cool, dry **Plant constituents** Saponins, glycosides, resins

Medicinal uses

Tones female reproductive organs False unicorn was traditionally used by Native Americans to provide tone to an atrophied uterus. It is useful in prolapse and sterility, where the uterine ligaments have proven too weak to continue proper function.

Prevents miscarriage It is often administered in times of threatened miscarriage or to prevent habitual miscarriage. Tincture dosage for habitual miscarriage would be 2 to 3 dropperfuls, 3 times per day, starting 2 weeks before the typical miscarriage week. Dosage to prevent threatened miscarriage is 1 or 2 dropperfuls every hour until bleeding or cramping subsides and you can get to your care provider.

Stimulates digestion False unicorn is almost always tolerated by a stomach that is refusing everything, whether caused by illness or food poisoning. It helps to stimulate and restore the appetite and is soothing to the gut lining.

Contraindications Generally regarded as safe, though extremely large doses may cause nausea.

MEDICINE CABINET

Decoction 2 or 3 teaspoons per cup, simmer 10 minutes covered, 1 to 3 cups per day
Tincture 1 or 2 dropperfuls, 1 to 3 times per day

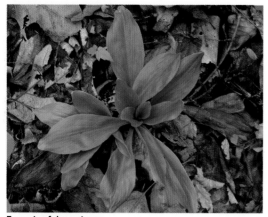

Emerging false unicorn

Identification and cultivation

Smooth stalks, 12 to 24 inches. Leaves, 4 to 9 inches long, grow in a basal rosette. Plumed flower stocks emerge in summer, bearing small white flowers on a raceme. Large, bulbous, grayish brown roots. Unfortunately, once harvested, the plant does not grow back, and because it has been overharvested in the wild, it is listed as an endangered or threatened plant in several areas. Try to grow it yourself. Herbaceous perennial. Rhizome can be divided, or sow seed. Grow in moist, acidic soil, full to part shade. Zones 4–8.

Fennel

Foeniculum vulgare

Also called sweet fennel, large fennel **Family** Apiaceae **Parts used** Seeds

> *Fennel's sweet taste quickly calms an upset stomach and reduces intestinal pain.*

Organs or systems affected Gastrointestinal system, respiratory system **Therapeutic actions** Carminative **Nature** Sweet, aromatic, warm **Plant constituents** Volatile oil, fixed oils, tocopherols, flavonoids, coumarin, silica **Flower essence** Provides support for clarity in leaving the past behind and moving on

Medicinal uses

Aids digestion Fennel's sweet and aromatic qualities make it one of the best herbs to use when digestion issues arise. Safe for children and adults, fennel seed tea is a quick tummy-ache reliever. Its carminative actions help relieve bloating, gas, and intestinal pain. Any time my little girl mentions her tummy hurts, I reach for

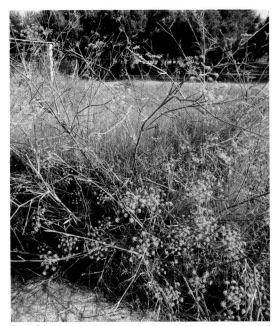

Fennel

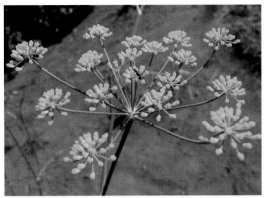

Fennel flowers

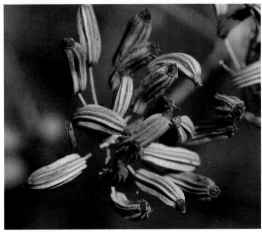

Fennel seeds

fennel essential oil. She loves the ritual of lying down and having me rub 1 drop of the oil over her belly in a circular motion. As young children are moving from their emotional world into more of the physical world, particularly around ages 4 and 5, they literally begin to feel things in their body. This often manifests as a tummy ache.

Calms coughs Fennel is as soothing to the respiratory tract as it is to the stomach. It helps with a dry cough or tickle in the throat that won't go away and works great as a syrup.

Contraindications Should not be taken during pregnancy, because it can stimulate the uterus.

Identification and cultivation

Branched stems are bright green, hollow, 4 to 6 feet. Leaves grow in feathery fronds. Tiny yellow flowers are borne in terminal umbels. Fennel grows freely in fields, meadows, and abandoned lots. Listed as an invasive or noxious plant in some areas, so check before growing. Collect seed heads as they form and are still green. Perennial. Sow seed directly in ground in spring. Grow in moist, well-drained soil, full sun. Zones 4–9.

MEDICINE CABINET

Essential oil 1 drop massaged over abdomen
Herbal oil (not essential oil) 1 or 2 teaspoons massaged over abdomen as needed
Infusion 1 teaspoon per cup, steep 10 to 12 minutes, 3 cups per day or as needed
Syrup 1 or 2 teaspoons as needed
Tincture 5 to 30 drops as needed

Gentian

Gentiana lutea

Also called yellow gentian, bitterwort, Sampson's snakeroot, felwort, balmoney **Family** Gentianaceae **Parts used** Roots

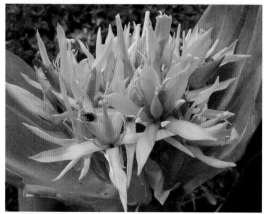

Gentian flowers

> *A simple bitter with powerful effects, gentian revitalizes the gastrointestinal tract, liver, and endocrine system.*

Organs or systems affected Gallbladder, liver, gastrointestinal system **Therapeutic actions** Tonic, stimulant, febrifuge, emmenagogue, antiparasitic, antiseptic, antispasmodic **Nature** Bitter, acrid, cold, dry **Plant constituents** Glycosides, flavonoids, alkaloids, xanthones, phenolic acids **Flower essence** Ideal for those who have trouble handling and moving through setbacks, who feel hopeless and believe things are not going to get better

Medicinal uses

Improves digestion Gentian is considered one the best herbs for creating general wellness, as demonstrated in research time and time again. Its primary action occurs in the stomach and gastrointestinal system. A principle bitter, its affinity is naturally to the entire gastrointestinal system, where it optimizes levels of hydrochloric acid and digestive enzymes, leading to improved digestion and food absorption. Gentian is excellent for those who are weak, either physically or functionally, and need strong support to gain nutrients from the food they are eating. Gentian stores high levels of oxygen in its roots, which creates feelings of revitalization. It also supports the blood vessels, big and small, particularly in the abdomen. As it improves digestion, it decreases the burden on the liver, causing a toning effect. But the interesting piece about its relationship to the liver is that it does not seem to stimulate the gallbladder and secretion of bile, which is helpful for those who need to tone the digestion and liver but experience gallbladder colic, which most bitters stimulate.

Stimulates endocrine system Some have experienced a stimulating effect on the endocrine system with the use of gentian. In my clinical practice I have often attributed hormone imbalances (thyroid, reproductive, or adrenal) with digestion insufficiency. When this is present, the body often pulls energy away from other bodily systems, including the endocrine system, to the digestive function to aid the insufficiency. Therefore, it makes sense that, with improved function of the gastrointestinal system and the increase of vital nutrients through proper absorption, the endocrine system is returned to balance.

Contraindications Avoid gentian if diarrhea is present due to gastrointestinal weakness. Avoid if on H2 receptor antagonists, such as Tagamet, Zantac, or other antacids. These drugs inhibit the release of stomach acid, and gentian stimulates and corrects digestive acid deficiency.

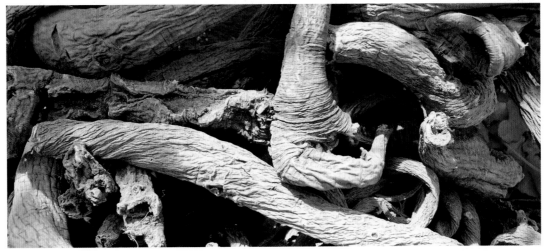
Gentian roots

Identification and cultivation

Hollow, erect stems, 2 to 4 feet. Yellow-green leaves are broadly lanceolate, almost embracing the stem at their bases. Clusters of yellow-orange flowers in midsummer. Collect the rhizomes and branching roots of plants at least 3 years old, preferably when the plants are in flower. Found mostly in alpine regions but can grow elsewhere. Perennial. Plant in fall (with cold frame) or spring. Grow in rich, well-drained soil with pH of 6.5 or higher, full sun to part shade. Zones 3–9.

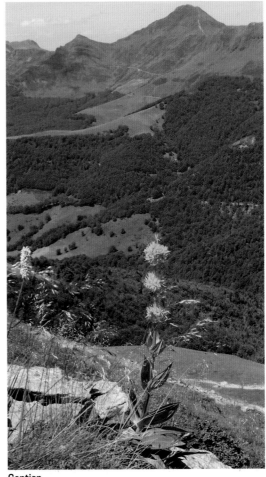
Gentian

Goat's rue

Galega officinalis

Also called professor's weed, French lilac **Family** Papilonaceae **Parts used** Aerial parts

> *Goat's rue helps new mothers relax and let it all flow.*

Organs or systems affected Blood, mammary glands, pancreas **Therapeutic actions** Galactagogue, diuretic, diaphoretic **Nature** Sweet **Plant constituents** Flavonoids, saponins, galegine

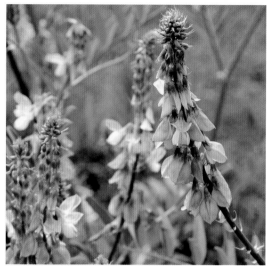
Goat's rue flowers

Medicinal uses

Stimulates breast milk flow As a galactagogue, or breast milk enhancer, goat's rue is effective in stimulating both the production and flow of milk. It has been shown to increase milk output by up to 50 percent.

Reduces blood sugar levels Since the Middle Ages, goat's rue has been used in the treatment of diabetes mellitus. Goat's rue contains an alkaloid, galegine, that was found in clinical trials to decrease blood sugar and insulin resistance. This led to the development of metformin, which is currently used in the treatment of diabetes.

Contraindications Contraindicated with diuretic prescriptions.

MEDICINE CABINET
Infusion 1 or 2 teaspoons per cup, steep 15 minutes covered, 1 to 4 cups per day
Tincture 1 or 2 dropperfuls, 3 times per day

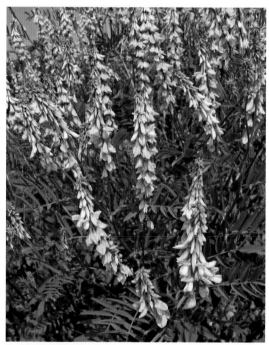
Goat's rue in bloom

Identification and cultivation

Hollow, smooth stems. Pinnate leaflets spaced alternately in six to ten pairs, with terminal leaflet. Purple to white flowers borne on stalks in summer. Grows in cropland, pastures, fence lines, and often wherever livestock is present. Perennial. Goat's rue is considered a noxious weed in most areas, so it should not be grown in the garden.

Goldenrod

Solidago canadensis

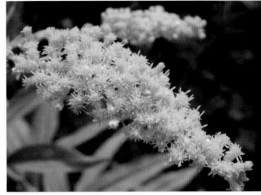

Goldenrod flower spike

Also called woundwort, blue mountain tea **Family** Asteraceae **Parts used** Leaves, stems

> *Goldenrod resonates with the lungs and bladder to support and tonify their function.*

Organs or systems affected Bladder, kidneys, respiratory system **Therapeutic actions** Astringent, antiseptic, anti-inflammatory, vulnerary **Nature** Bitter **Plant constituents** Volatile oil, tannins, saponins, flavonoids, glycosides, bitters **Flower essence** Helps to instill a strong and secure sense of individuality

Medicinal uses

Heals the bladder As a supporter of the mucous membranes, goldenrod works wonders on both the bladder and respiratory tract. It is a good choice particularly for bladder incontinence. Its antiseptic, anti-inflammatory nature helps to cool and clean the bladder, but it also has a strong healing quality on the bladder wall. With chronic bladder irritation, small holes can appear and are often irritated, causing incontinence. Goldenrod helps to heals the bladder wall, reducing the symptoms of urgency and discomfort.

Soothes allergies Goldenrod's affinity for the respiratory tract helps with old stuck conditions after colds and flus by moving things up and out. Goldenrod is also a good option to consider for allergies that are affecting the lungs. Some use an infusion of goldenrod as an eye wash for itchy, swollen, and painful eyes affected by seasonal particulates.

Contraindications Generally regarded as safe.

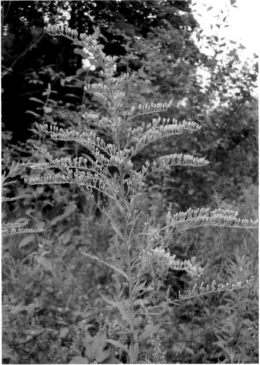

Goldenrod

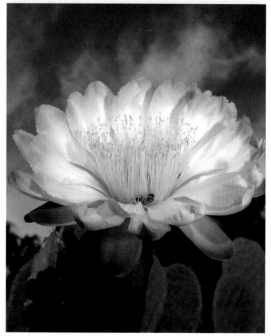

Grand cactus bloom

Identification and cultivation

Spiky stems, 2 to 3 feet. Tapered, pointed leaves are arranged alternately. Golden terminal flowers bloom in early fall, in panicles held above the foliage. Goldenrod grows in forests and fields and along roadsides. Perennial. Goldenrod is considered an invasive weed, so it should not be grown in the garden.

Grand cactus

Selenicereus grandiflorus

Also called night-blooming cactus, night-blooming cereus, vanilla cactus, sweet-scented cactus **Family** Cactaceae **Parts used** Green stems

This tonic heals the heart from the inside out by replenishing heart muscle.

Organs or systems affected Heart **Therapeutic actions** Tonic, relaxant **Nature** Sweet, bitter, cool, dry **Plant constituents** Resins, alkaloid, flavonoids, rutin **Flower essence** Helps one recognize inner wisdom and uncover long-stored abilities that were never allowed to surface

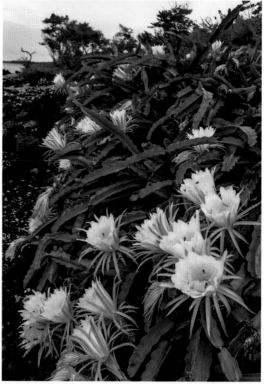

Grand cactus

Medicinal uses

Restores the heart Grand cactus is incredibly helpful any time there is an insufficiency of function or a weakness of the heart itself. If the heart has valve issues, grand cactus will not repair the actual valve, but its use can help ensure that the heart function does not diminish. It is said to strengthen the heart muscle itself, including contraction and electrical communications. It is recommended for those suffering with specific pathologies of the heart and emotional suppression of the heart, as well as the elderly who suffer from relative heart weakness.

Relieves chest restriction Grand cactus helps relieve chest and breath restriction.

Contraindications Should be avoided by those with mitral value disease or excessively high blood pressure.

```
─────── MEDICINE CABINET ───────
Tincture 10 to 60 drops, 1 to 3 times
       per day for tonic effects
```

Identification and cultivation

Five or six angled, branched arms are covered with clusters of tiny spines in a radiating arrangement. Large white flowers, with a fragrance that resembles vanilla, appear one night and close by sunrise but can bloom several times over the summer months. Grows in desert regions. Harvest midsummer and prepare tincture fresh. Cactus. Non-invasive and fast-growing. Grow in well-drained soil, full sun to part shade. Zones 12–15.

Gravel root

Eupatorium purpureum

Also called queen of the meadow, joe-pye weed, trumpet weed, kidney root, motherwort, feverweed **Family** Asteraceae **Parts used** Rhizomes

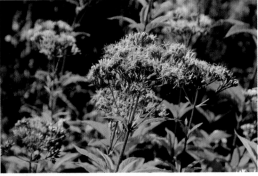
Gravel root

> *Gravel root is famous for helping to dissolve and dispel painful stones formed in the kidneys.*

Organs or systems affected Bladder, kidneys, uterus **Therapeutic actions** Diuretic, nervine, astringent, stimulant, tonic, antiseptic **Nature** Bitter, cool **Plant constituents** Resins, flavonoids, saponins, tannins, volatile oil, calcium oxalate **Flower essence** Helps those who are lonely or fear being alone, relieving anxiety over relationships and friendships

Medicinal uses

Relieves kidney and bladder stones Gravel root is extremely helpful in the relief of stones, or gravel, in the kidneys and bladder. It helps dissolve and break apart such accumulations and opens up the pathway of elimination to help reduce pain when stones are passed. As a result, the tissues are protected, reducing scarring and inflammation.

Dissolves toxic mineral buildup Gravel root's dissolving action works throughout the body in joints and small capsular spaces to remove toxic mineral buildup that may be causing joint pain or reduction in movement.

Helps prevent miscarriage Midwives have traditionally used gravel root to prevent miscarriage during the first trimester as well as to prepare the mother for labor.

Contraindications Generally regarded as safe.

MEDICINE CABINET

Decoction 1 or 2 teaspoons per cup, simmer 10 to 15 minutes covered, 1 to 3 cups per day
Tincture 1 to 3 dropperfuls, 1 to 3 times per day

Identification and cultivation

Graceful green or purple-tinted upright stems, 3 to 6 feet. Whorls of four oblong leaves, 8 to 12 inches long, grow at each node. Clusters of dull pink, lavender, or white florets bloom late summer to early fall. Found in low meadows, woods, gravelly lots, and near water. Harvest the rhizomes in the fall. Bag seed heads to capture ripening seeds and sow in the spring. Perennial. Grow in well-drained soil with a neutral pH, full sun to part shade. Zones 5–10.

Greater celandine

Chelidonium majus

Also called common celandine, garden celandine, tetterwort, swallowwort **Family** Papaveraceae **Parts used** Entire plant

> *An acute remedy, greater celandine is a strong supporter of gallbladder and liver function.*

Organs or systems affected Blood, gallbladder, liver **Therapeutic actions** Alterative, diuretic, purgative **Nature** Bitter, pungent, dry **Plant constituents** Alkaloids, bitters, essential oils, acids, enzymes, resin, histamine, vitamin C, calcium **Flower essence** Supports all types of information input and enables one to be more articulate and organized with thoughts

Medicinal uses

Detoxifies liver and gallbladder Greater celandine seems to have a direct affinity for the liver and gallbladder, aiding in the elimination of stagnant and congested materials, referred to as a damp heat condition in Chinese medicine. Greater celandine dredges the toxic buildup and drains the damp. Think of a cesspool of bile and gunk

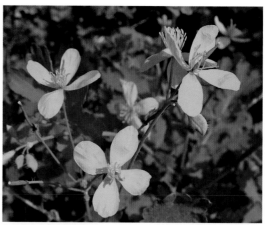
Greater celandine flowers

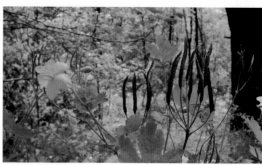
Greater celandine

stuck in the body, which causes symptoms such as jaundice, migraines, and chronic liver pathologies such as hepatitis. Greater celandine dredges out all of this, like a septic system flush. It is also historically known to help dissolve and eliminate gallstones and any other gallbladder inflammatory type complaints.

Eliminates skin problems Topically, the fresh juice can be used to eliminate warts, ringworm, tumors, and cysts. Cut a fresh picked stem to reveal the plant's bright orange juice. A fomentation is an excellent application with greater celandine that avoids the risk of skin irritation. Fomentations are also good for relieving other inflammation problems, such as hemorrhoids, ulcers, and sprains. In the past this juice was mixed with milk to make an eye cream for the white spots that can appear on the cornea. I like this correlation, because the eyes in Chinese medicine theory are correlated with the liver.

Contraindications Should not be taken during pregnancy. Those with glaucoma should avoid greater celandine. Topical application of juice may irritate skin.

MEDICINE CABINET

Fomentation 3 tablespoons per quart, steep at least 1 hour, strain, apply saturated cloth to affected area

Infusion 1 teaspoon per cup, 1 or 2 cups, as needed

Juice Topical application, as needed

Tincture 10 drops, as needed

Identification and cultivation

Slender, round, slightly hairy stems. Drooping, graceful, deeply lobed leaves, 6 to 12 inches long. Four flowers, each with four yellow petals, appear in loose umbels. Found commonly along walls, cultivated, or in natural hedges. Perennial. Seeds form on plants in about 3 weeks. Grow in any soil, part shade. Zones 5–8.

Hawthorn

Crataegus laevigata

Also called English hawthorn, haw, May blossom, Maybush, quick-set, whitethorn **Family** Rosaceae **Parts used** Berries, flowers, leaves

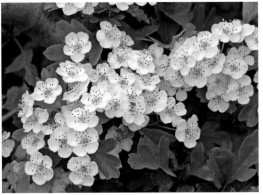

Hawthorn flowers

Just seeing the hawthorn tree with its full berry bounty is enough to calm the heart.

Organs or systems affected Blood, heart, central nervous system, cardiovascular system **Therapeutic actions** Cardiotonic, diuretic, astringent, tonic **Nature** Sweet, sour, dry **Plant constituents** Flavonoids, oxyacanthin, procyanidins, amines, tannins, pectin, calcium, vitamin C **Flower essence** Provides a strong and vital force that imparts power, courage, and bravery

Medicinal uses

Improves heart and cardiovascular system performance Hawthorn flowers, leaves, and berries are all potent at dilating the blood vessels around the heart and body, improving function and blood flow. It is often used to address high blood pressure issues, especially with hardened arteries. Hawthorn is also used for cases of angina

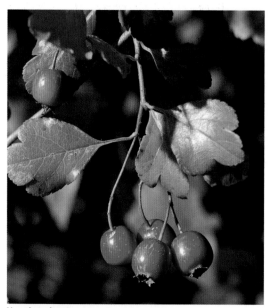
Hawthorn berries

MEDICINE CABINET

Decoction 1 or 2 teaspoons of berries per cup, simmer 10 to 15 minutes covered, 1 to 3 cups per day or as needed
Infusion Leaves and flowers: 1 or 2 teaspoons per cup, steep 12 to 15 minutes, 1 to 3 cups per day or as needed
Syrup 1 or 2 teaspoons as needed
Tincture 1 or 2 dropperfuls, 1 to 3 times per day

Identification and cultivation

Hawthorn trees can grow to 30 feet tall. Branches have sharp, straight thorns. Leaves are frequently lobed with serrated margins. Fragrant flowers are typically white but may be pink, forming in clusters. Found in woodlands, hedges, and urban areas. Flowers bloom and can be collected in spring, and the berries form in early autumn. Deciduous tree. Water new trees during dry spells and feed them annually for the first 3 years; then every other year. Grow in various soils, full sun. Zones 4–8.

and rapid heart rate. Poor circulation can lead to a host of issues, including varicose veins, cold hands and feet, and poor memory or decreased cognitive function. Hawthorn is indicated with any of these as a good choice to increase blood flow to areas that need it.

Treats diarrhea Hawthorn berries possess a strong astringent action that works on tough cases of diarrhea and loose stool.

Relieves anxiety Herbalists consider using hawthorn any time mental stress, anxiety, or fear upsets the heart. It calms the central nervous system, decreases agitation, and soothes heart palpitations. I have a beautiful hawthorn tree on my property. Whenever I feel particularly stressed out, I often find myself drawn to it, so much so that I've created a sitting garden around it. After sitting for a few minutes underneath this tree, I am often calm with a revived sense of balance. When you've worked with herbs for a while, you'll begin to notice that just being in their presence can have healing effects.

Contraindications Generally regarded as safe.

Hops

Humulus lupulus

Family Cannabaceae **Parts used** Strobiles

> *If you're looking for that relaxed feeling, it's time for some hops.*

Organs or systems affected Heart, intestines, stomach, central nervous system, respiratory system **Therapeutic actions** Nervine, sedative, tonic, analgesic, astringent **Nature** Bitter, dry, cool, pungent **Plant constituents** Bitters, volatile oil, alkaloids, flavonoids, vitamin C **Flower essence** Stimulates growth, both spiritually and physically

Medicinal uses

Calms and relaxes nerves and organs Hops are a strong sedative that can calm an overactive central nervous system, with symptoms of anxiety, insomnia, overthinking, and body twitches. Their relaxing effects can help relieve constricted lung issues, such as with asthma, and dry, spasmodic coughing.

Supports stomach Those who have not made healthy dietary choices often have stomach issues. The same goes for those who feel every emotion in their stomach. Hops are a good herbal remedy for both complaints, helping to relax tension and normalize the gastric juices for better gastrointestinal health.

Reduces pain Hops are helpful to reduce pain and inflammation with boils and toothache.

Supports healthy male reproductive issues Hops have been cited as helpful in male reproductive complaints such as painful and overactive urination and excessive nighttime seminal emissions.

Contraindications Contraindicated for those with depression or those who take pentobarbital.

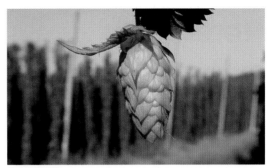

Hops strobile

MEDICINE CABINET

Infusion 1 or 2 strobiles per cup, steep 3 to 30 minutes covered, 1 to 3 cups per day

Pillow For insomnia, fill a small pillow with hops, use during sleep

Poultice or fomentation Apply over boils or painful swellings

Tincture For insomnia, 2 dropperfuls 30 minutes before bed, and 2 more at bedtime. For stomach, 10 drops, 1 to 3 times per day.

Identification and cultivation

Flexible stems of this climber twist around anything nearby. Heart-shaped leaves, arranged oppositely, are covered in rough hairs. Flowers are dioecious (female and male flowers grow on different plants). Female plants produce scaly strobiles, cone-shaped structures that hang from

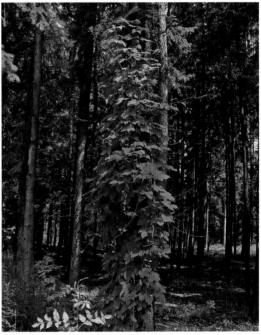

Hops

the plant, which can be harvested in late summer. Hops are cultivated for beer brewing. They also grow in hedges and open woods, climbing up trees, shrubs, or other vertical structures. Annual stems, perennial roots. Start seed indoors 6 weeks prior to the last frost date in soil temperature of about 70°F (20°C). If planting rhizomes, keep them cool and dry until ready to plant. Climbing plants need support. Grow in moist, well-drained soil with a pH of around 6.5, protected from wind, full sun. Zones 5–9.

Horehound

Marrubium vulgare

Also called hoarhound, white horehound
Family Lamiaceae **Parts used** Aerial parts

Horehound's army of herbal constituents fight for your respiratory health.

Organs or systems affected Heart, liver, lungs, kidneys, stomach **Therapeutic actions** Expectorant, tonic, stomachic, diaphoretic, bitter, pectoral, hepatic **Nature** Bitter, pungent, salty, warm **Plant constituents** Bitters, alcohols, flavonoids, alkanes, phytosterols, essential oil, mucilage, tannins, choline, pectin, resin, iron

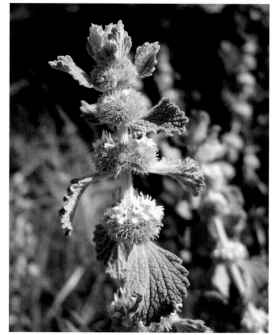
Horehound flowers

Medicinal uses

Soothes coughs and sore throats Singers and performers have long treasured horehound to soothe strained vocal cords and to help them carry on the show. Despite the US Food and Drug Administration (FDA) banning the use of horehound in commercially produced cough lozenges in 1986 (for lack of evidence that it was effective), it is the primary ingredient in many cough lozenges bought and sold in Europe. Luckily, we can still purchase European-made products in the United States, and some lozenges are available here as candy, so we can still find this wonderfully healing throat soother. We can also consume it as tea, tincture, or syrup, or make our own lozenges at home.

Helps expel phlegm Culpepper (1653) considered horehound one the best herbs for breaking apart and expelling stuck or hard phlegm from the chest. Horehound is a prime example of how an entire plant and its constituents work together to achieve health. With a lower respiratory infection that includes cough, congestion, and fever, horehound's constituents work on all three

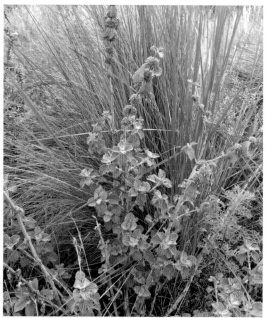
Horehound

complaints simultaneously. First the bitters stimulate secretions that thin and break apart thick phlegm to help rid it from the body. Within these secretions are new healthy immune fighter cells, which target the bacterial or viral invader. Horehound's diaphoretic action opens up the skin to allow perspiration to flow freely. And tannins ensure that the tissues involved are left astringed and toned to return to normal function.

Contributes to cancerous cell death A study performed in January 2006 took a look at horehound leaf and its effects on colorectal cancer cells. Aware of horehound's traditional use for anti-inflammatory conditions exhibiting symptoms such a cold, fever, and sore throat, scientists wanted to examine its potential on other cell lines. The study indicated that not only did horehound help inhibit human colorectal cancer cell growths, but it also seemed to increase apoptosis, or cellular suicide.

Contraindications Extended use of horehound may cause hypertension. Large doses can cause vomiting.

MEDICINE CABINET

Infusion 1 or 2 teaspoons per cup, steep 10 to 12 minutes, 1 to 3 cups per day

Lozenge As needed to soothe throat irritation

Syrup ½ to 1 teaspoon, 1 to 4 times per day

Tincture 10 to 30 drops, 1 to 3 times per day

Identification and cultivation

Square stems are covered with white, wooly hairs. Bluntly toothed leaves are nearly round, wrinkled, and somewhat hairy on the upper surface. Pungent white flowers are borne just above the leaves in dense clusters, from summer to fall. Look for horehound in dry and sandy fields. Harvest the entire plant in spring and summer. Perennial. Listed as an invasive or noxious plant in some areas, so check before growing. Direct sow, shallowly. Grow in any soil, full sun. Zones 3–10.

Horny goat weed

Epimedium grandiflorum

Also called fairy wings, bishop's hat, barrenwort
Family Berberidaceae **Parts used** Flowers, leaves, stems

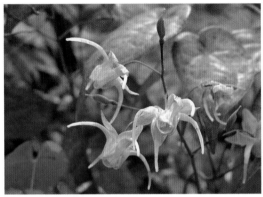

Horny goat weed flowers

> *Horny goat weed's name pretty much says it all.*

Organs or systems affected Kidneys, reproductive system **Therapeutic actions** Aphrodisiac, diuretic, tonic **Plant constituents** Fats, saponins, volatile oil, polysaccharides, flavonoids, sterols, alkaloids

Medicinal uses

Boosts libido Horny goat weed's actions were first observed, and probably used, to increase sexual libido in goats, hence its name. Research has found that this herb not only increases libido in humans, but it also helps with fertility issues and impotence. It tends to open the vessels to the brain and sexual organs, supporting and increasing blood supply. For men, in particular, studies indicate that it tones the liver and perhaps in turn balances out sexual hormone production. Erectile dysfunction studies have demonstrated positive outcomes in the use of this herb to increase blood supply to the penis, maintain erection, and aid in reaching climax.

Strengthens bladder and kidney function Studies in China indicate that horny goat weed strengthens and tones the bladder sphincter, leading to better urine retention. It can also improve kidney function, particularly regarding serum creatinine levels and blood urea nitrogen.

Contraindications Those who suffer from benign enlargement of the prostate should avoid this herb.

MEDICINE CABINET

Infusion 1 or 2 teaspoons per cup, steep 10 to 12 minutes, 1 or 2 cups per day

Tincture 5 to 30 drops, 1 to 3 times per day

Identification and cultivation

Bright red stems, to 12 inches tall. Undersides of heart-shaped leaves are slightly hairy. Pink, white, or purple long-spurred flowers. This plant may be cultivated in North America but is naturalized only in Asia. Deciduous perennial. Grow in acidic soil, full to part shade. Zones 4–8.

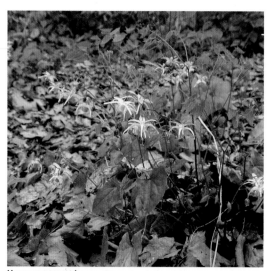

Horny goat weed

Horse chestnut

Aesculus hippocastanum

Also called buckeye **Family** Sapindaceae
Parts used Husks, seeds

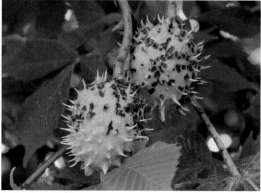

Horse chestnut fruits

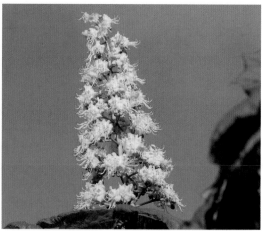

Horse chestnut flowers

> Horse chestnut is used to relieve swollen and congested venous pathways.

Organs or systems affected Cardiovascular system **Therapeutic actions** Astringent, tonic **Nature** Bitter **Plant constituents** Saponins, flavonoids, tannins, coumarin, fatty oil, protein, starch **Flower essence** Helps one cultivate life's wisdom and gain intelligence from personal experience

Medicinal uses

Improves vein health Horse chestnut works as an astringent with an affinity for the veins and cardiovascular system. It helps remove blockages, improve flow, and pull back laxity in tissues. Apply it topically to tortuous varicose veins to reduce pain and swelling.

Relieves hemorrhoids Horse chestnut is an excellent reliever of hemorrhoids and the accompanying symptoms. It can be infused into an oil or made into a suppository for direct application.

Mineralizes teeth Although I've no experience with such, some recommend chewing horse chestnut husks to mineralize the teeth.

Contraindications Should not be used by those on blood thinners. Use internally short term only.

MEDICINE CABINET

Lotion 1 teaspoon, applied externally 2 times per day for cardiovascular support

Tincture 3 to 10 drops in 1 ounce water, 3 times per day for 2 weeks

---

Identification and cultivation

A mature horse chestnut can reach 50 to 70 feet tall. Leaves are palmately compound with five to seven leaflets. White flowers grow in erect panicles. Several fruits develop on each panicle, and the seeds, or conkers, are glossy brown with a whitish scar at the base, sheathed in a spiky green capsule. Trees are widely cultivated in streets and parks throughout temperate regions. Harvest the seed and husks in the fall. Deciduous tree. Sow seed in the fall. Grow in moist, fertile, well-drained soil, full sun to part shade. Zones 3–8.

Hydrangea

Hydrangea arborescens

Also called sevenbark **Family** Saxifragaceae **Parts used** Roots

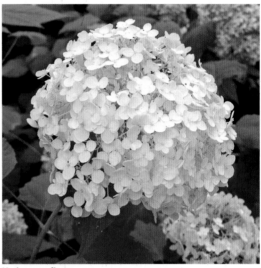

Hydrangea flowers

This showy flowered herb gets to the root of the problem of most bladder and kidney ailments.

Organs or systems affected Bladder, kidneys, prostate, skin **Therapeutic actions** Diuretic, cathartic, tonic **Nature** Pungent, sweet, cool, bitter **Plant constituents** Glycosides, alkaloid, saponins, resins, volatile oil, calcium, trace minerals **Flower essence** Provides loving and gentle support to help release repressed and internalized emotions

Medicinal uses

Supports bladder and kidney function Hydrangea works particularly on the bladder and kidneys, helping with complaints of stones, lower back pain, edema, and frequent urination. It does a superior job of cleansing the urinary tract, dissolving gravel and soothing inflamed mucous membranes.

Relieves prostate inflammation Reports have been documented of using hydrangea to relieve severe swelling of the prostate.

Helps heal eczema When an herb works to improve the elimination functions of the bladder and kidneys, it often helps relieve the body of excessive water or dampness. In many cases, eczema is caused by this over-accumulation of dampness, leading to congestion in the tissues. Hydrangea has been showed to be helpful when this is its cause.

Identification and cultivation

Heart-shaped, serrated, and deeply veined leaves hug the main stem. White flowers grow in rounded clusters in late spring to midsummer. Unlike other hydrangeas, this species' flower color is not affected by soil pH. Perennial shrub. Grow in moist soils, full to part shade. Zones 3–9.

Jamaican dogwood

Piscidia piscipula

Also called Florida fishpoison tree, fishfuddle
Family Papilionaceae **Parts used** Bark, root bark

> *A strong sedative that is extremely helpful with nerve pain.*

Organs or systems affected Lungs, central nervous system **Therapeutic actions** Sedative, astringent **Nature** Bitter, pungent, cool **Plant constituents** Isoflavones, organic acids, beta-sitosterol, tannins **Flower essence** Promotes a sense of freedom and opening within the body when one is feeling confined or constricted

Medicinal uses

Relieves tension With pain due to tension, Jamaican dogwood is an excellent choice. When a body is in an extreme state of discomfort, cortisol is released, which serves to alleviate pain but sometimes can make it nearly impossible for any

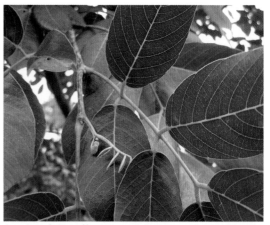
Jamaican dogwood leaves

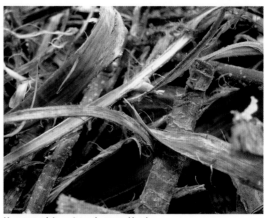
Harvested Jamaican dogwood bark

other type of treatment to be effective. This is the time for Jamaican dogwood, which can relax the tension and help with sleep if the discomfort is causing insomnia.

Supports the nervous system Jamaican dogwood seems to have an affinity for the central nervous system and all ailments that affect it, such as migraines, sciatica, mental stress, inflammatory conditions, and neuralgia.

Contraindications Because of its depressive action, it is not recommended for those suffering from depression or for elderly people who have limited physical movement. It is toxic in high doses, creating symptoms of nausea and headache. Do not use as a long-term remedy. Use sparingly in acute situations only. Best used in a formula.

MEDICINE CABINET

Decoction 1 teaspoon per cup, simmer 10 minutes covered, drink 6 ounces as needed, not to exceed 3 times per day
Tincture 1 dropperful as needed, not to exceed 4 times per day

---

Identification and cultivation

Trees reach 40 to 50 feet when mature. Pinnately compound leaves arranged alternately, with five to eleven leaflets per stalk, with the undersides of each leaflet covered in white hairs. White flowers often tinged in red or pink, blooming in midsummer. Brown seedpods have four projecting longitudinal wings. Grows in coastal areas. Collect bark and root bark from dead trees or downed branches year-round. Do not harvest from a live tree or you will damage or kill it. Deciduous tree. Moderately fast growing. Grow in moist, well-drained limestone or calcareous sandy soil, part shade. Zones 10–11.

Juniper

Juniperus communis

Also called juniper bush, ginepro, enebro **Family** Cupressaceae **Parts used** Bark, berries, leaves

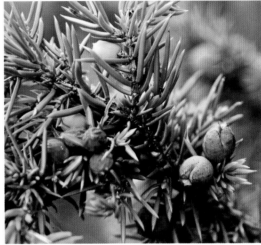
Juniper berries

> *This sweet and astringent berry targets the kidneys.*

Organs or systems affected Bladder, kidneys, stomach, uterus **Therapeutic actions** Diuretic, diaphoretic, stimulant, carminative, analgesic, emmenagogue **Nature** Pungent, aromatic, bitter, sweet **Plant constituents** Essential oil, flavonoids, resin, tannins, bitter, acids, calcium, magnesium, vitamin C **Flower essence** Helps to release ancestral patterns

Medicinal uses

Stimulates kidneys and bladder Most herbalists consider juniper a good choice whenever there is excess fluid in the body and the kidneys are sluggish (but not impaired) to expel it. Juniper stimulates both the kidneys and the bladder, and although slightly irritating, it dilates tissues to increase urine flow and reduce excess mucus production. With heart disease, diabetes, and other pathologies, fluid accumulation can place a true burden on the body. Juniper can be helpful in such cases. And although stimulating, it also seems to have a tonifying effect to the entire genitourinary (genital and urinary) system, making it helpful with incontinence and stones.

Stimulates mucous membranes Juniper supports the gastrointestinal system, uterus, and lungs. Whenever congested damp mucus conditions are present in smooth muscle, juniper is a good consideration.

Strengthens brain Herbalist John Christopher (1976) used juniper to strengthen the brain, memory, and optic nerve. This makes sense considering its mucus-clearing effects. In Chinese medicine, phlegm is said to be the predominating cause of brain fog and mental disruptions.

Fights tumors Juniper leaves contain the antibiotic podophyllotoxin, which has been found to be effective against tumors.

Contraindications Should not be used long-term, so discontinue use after 6 weeks. Those suffering from kidney disease should not take juniper because it may be too stimulating.

MEDICINE CABINET

Fresh application 3 to 5 berries, eat to reduce stomach upset
Infusion ½ to 1 teaspoon crushed berries in 8 ounces water, steep 1 to 3 hours, 1 or 2 cups per day
Tincture 1 or 2 dropperfuls, 3 times per day

Identification and cultivation

Evergreen shrub or tree grows to 40 feet. Awl-shaped, scaly leaves in whorls of three, ⅓ to ½ inch long. Small cones. Found on dry slopes, open aspen woods, and clearings. Think twice about planting junipers if you or your neighbors grow pears, because pear rust is a common fungus that affects pears and junipers in alternating years. Grow in well-drained soil, full sun. Zones 2–9.

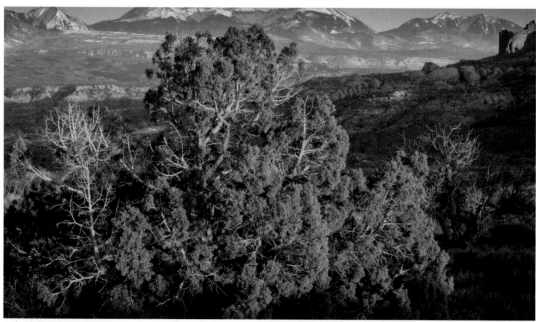

A magnificent juniper tree

Lady's slipper

Cypripedium pubescens (also *Cypripedium parviflorum*)

Also called nerve root, American valerian, moccasin plant, Noah's ark **Family** Orchidaceae **Parts used** Rhizomes

> *A hidden gem that provides pain relief and support for menstruation.*

Organs or systems affected Central nervous system, reproductive system **Therapeutic actions** Nervine, antispasmodic, tonic, relaxant, diuretic **Nature** Sweet, bitter, pungent, cool **Plant constituents** Volatile oil, glycoside, resins, tannins, acids, gums, starch, potassium, magnesium **Flower essence** Helps to promote higher purpose in alignment with work

Medicinal uses

Supports women's reproductive health Lady's slipper has historically been used for women suffering from pelvic congestion leading to irregular menstruation, bleeding, and menstrual pain.

Supports nervous system A wonderful relaxant to the nervous system, lady's slipper is also called American valerian because of the properties it shares with *Valerian officinalis*, but lady's slipper is much milder and more specific to overstimulated nerves than muscles. It can be helpful in times of insomnia resulting from stress and anxiety.

Relieves pain It possesses natural pain relieving properties, particularly when tension is causing obstruction through vessels and tissues. It helps to relax the area and promote positive blood and oxygen flow to relieve discomfort.

Contraindications Generally regarded as safe.

MEDICINE CABINET

Decoction 1 tablespoon per cup, simmer 10 minutes covered, 1 to 4 cups per day **Infusion** Cold infusion, 1 to 3 teaspoons per cup, steep for 12 hours, 1 or 2 cups per day **Tincture** 10 to 60 drops, 1 to 3 times per day

---

Identification and cultivation

Round, leafy, hairy stems, 12 to 24 inches. Broad leaves are oval, many veined, clasping at the base, 3 to 6 inches long. Yellow orchid flowers resemble

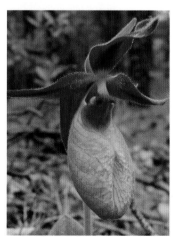

Lady's slipper orchid

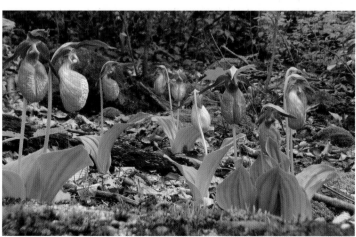

Lady's slippers

a slipper or moccasin. Rhizomes are orange-brown and fleshy. Lady's slipper is an endangered plant; do not collect lady's slippers in the wild. Use a homeopathic preparation unless you grow them yourself. If you are lucky enough to find it growing in moist woods or meadows, stand in its glory, because it truly is a prize to see. Offer gratitude and blessings for a revival, and allow it to stay where it grows. Perennial orchid. Grow in evenly moist, humus-rich soil that is slightly acid, full to part shade. Zones 3–8.

Larch

Larix occidentalis

Also called western larch, hackmatack, western tamarack **Family** Pinaceae **Parts used** Inner bark, gum

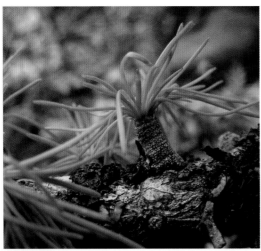

Larch needles

The bark of this statuesque tree produces prebiotics that strengthen the immune system and improve digestion.

Organs or systems affected Gastrointestinal system, immune system, upper respiratory system **Therapeutic actions** Stimulant **Nature** Sweet **Plant constituents** Arabinogalactans, flavonoids, resins, volatile oil, lignans **Flower essence** Relates to self-confidence for a negative state, which usually stems from infancy, for a child who grows up believing in the certainty of failure

Medicinal uses

Improves digestion and strengthens immune system Lately, arabinogalactan is earning a solid reputation for stimulating the immune system as well as healing the gastrointestinal tract. The powdered extract from the bark of the larch tree is made up of 98 percent arabinogalactan, which is a prebiotic, a nondigestible food that stimulates the production of positive bacteria in the gut. About 60 percent of your immune system is in your intestines, so the big payoff of using larch arabinogalactan is digestion improvement with increased immune strength. Arabinogalactan has been showed to inhibit ammonia generation in the intestines, therefore reducing the harmful effects of ammonia on the colon cells. Typically, the liver aids in elimination of generated ammonia, but when liver disease is present or overburdened, larch can be beneficial.

Helps reduce tumor cells One area of research that holds larch in particular interest is oncology and the immune system. Larch arabinogalactans have been used in studies and show consistent results of reducing tumor cell colonization, increasing macrophages and natural killer cells through stimulation of interferon gamma, which helps make cells resistant to viral infections.

Helps heal ear infections Larch arabinogalactan can be used to help treat and heal middle ear infections in children.

Contraindications Generally regarded as safe.

Identification and cultivation

Mature larch trees can reach more than 100 feet tall. Mature tree bark is thick and deeply furrowed. Leaves grow in clusters of fifteen to thirty slender, soft, spirally arranged needles, 1 to 2 inches long. Leaves turn bright yellow in the fall and drop off the tree, with new leaves forming the following spring. Cones are ¾ to 2 inches long and slender, often remaining on the tree for many years. Find larch in mountain valleys and lower slopes of cool, moist areas of western North America. Deciduous conifer. Sow seed in late winter in pots in a cold frame. Grow in well-drained, mineral rich soil, in light shade first year, and then full to part shade. Zones 3–7.

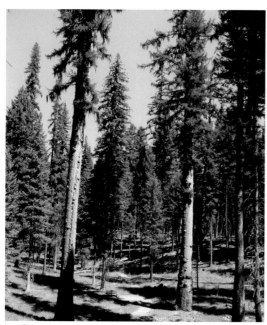

Larch

Lemon balm

Melissa officinalis

Also called bee balm, balm, sweet balm **Family** Lamiaceae **Parts used** Aerial parts

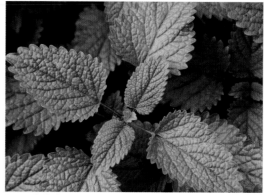

Lemon balm leaves

For the head and nerves, this fragrant nervine has been revered in works by Shakespeare and Homer as well as the Bible.

Organs or systems affected Skin, central nervous system **Therapeutic actions** Carminative, febrifuge, nervine **Nature** Sour, cool **Plant constituents** Volatile oils, labiate tannin, phenolic acids, triterpenes, monoterpene, glycosides, flavonoids **Flower essence** Eases the velocity of the mind, helps one wind down, eases fears and anxieties, and serves as a restorer after stress from modern civilization and being around too many people has stretched a person too thin

Medicinal uses

Calms the nerves Lemon balm has a longstanding reputation for calming the nerves, or spirit. It was a common herb in the eighteenth century, as Spirit of Melissa, a tonic made from lemon balm, was often kept in the house. As a member of the mint family with a sour quality, lemon balm works wonders on the overstimulated mind and body. For those who are always on the go, lemon balm is the perfect calming herb. It also works on other overactive conditions such as hyperthyroidism and hyperadrenalism. Any time the system is in overdrive, including the physical manifestations of heart palpitations, high blood pressure, manic thinking, and shortness of breath, lemon balm is advised.

Helps reduce fevers Because of its light diaphoretic tendency, lemon balm is wonderful for fever brought on by stress and for fever in children. It will gently open the skin to allow perspiration and help relax the sufferer.

Antiviral Lemon balm can reduce the infectivity of a variety of viruses, including herpes simplex virus (HSV) and HIV-1, the AIDS virus. The activity has been attributed to caffeic acid and its dimeric and trimeric derivatives, as well as to tannins.

Contraindications Some research cautions the use of lemon balm for patients with a propensity toward hypothyroidism, because the herb affects thyroid stimulation hormone (TSH) levels. And yet, James Duke (1997) states that lemon balm (and similar effective herbs) seems to normalize high or low thyroid hormone levels.

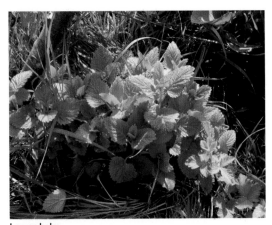

Lemon balm

MEDICINE CABINET

Herbal oil 1 teaspoon applied 1 or 2 times per day
Infusion (Fresh is best) 1 teaspoon per cup, steep 6 to 8 minutes, 1 to 3 cups per day or as needed
Tincture 1 to 10 drops or 1 dropperful, 1 to 3 times per day

Identification and cultivation

Square stems, 12 to 24 inches. Lemon-scented leaves are broadly ovate or heart-shaped. White or yellow-tinted flowers form small bunches in leaf axils in summer through early fall. Lemon balm is grown in many gardens. Harvest younger leaves year-round. Perennial. Sow seeds in early spring or fall. Grows freely in any soil, full sun to shade. Zones 4–11.

Licorice

Glycyrrhiza glabra

Also called liquorice, sweetwood, lick weed, lycorys **Family** Papilionaceae **Parts used** Dried rhizomes, roots

> *Licorice is fifty times sweeter than sugar cane.*

Organs or systems affected Endocrine system, gastrointestinal system, respiratory system **Therapeutic actions** Demulcent, expectorant, emollient, pectoral, stimulant **Nature** Sweet, neutral moist **Plant constituents** Flavonoids, isoflavonoids, chalcones, saponins

Medicinal uses

Soothes mucous membranes Licorice is one of the best known plants to soothe the nasal

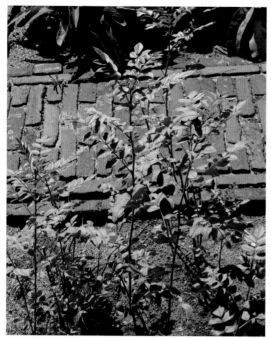
Licorice

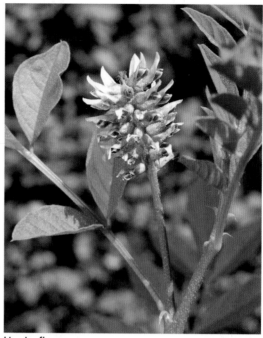
Licorice flowers

passageways, throat, lungs, stomach, and gastro-intestinal tract. It can soothe, soften, lubricate, and nourish the entire intestinal tract. It is an excellent choice for relaxing the spasms of irritating coughs or gut.

Stimulates the adrenal glands More and more research shows licorice's positive effects on the adrenal glands. One function of the adrenal glands is to secrete the hormone cortisol. Licorice can enhance adrenal function and cortisol production in the body, to balance blood sugar and decrease stress and inflammation. But keep this in mind: if you suffer from overworked adrenals, a syndrome known as adrenal fatigue, licorice is not the best choice. It will try to stimulate an exhausted gland and make you feel quite jumpy, like you've had more than enough coffee. It's like trying to jump-start an empty car battery: your engine might turn over, but you are running on false fumes.

Contraindications Should not be taken by those with high blood pressure.

MEDICINE CABINET

Infusion 1 teaspoon per cup, steep 10 to 15 minutes, 1 to 3 cups per day

Decoction 1 teaspoon per cup, simmer 8 minutes covered, 1 to 3 cups per day

Syrup 1 teaspoon, 3 to 5 times per day

Tincture 1 dropperful, 1 to 3 times per day

Identification and cultivation

Graceful branching stems, 2 to 5 feet. Smooth, pinnate leaflets arranged in pairs. Spikes of small pale blue, violet, or yellow-tinted flowers form in the leaf axils is spring, forming fruiting pods. Look for wild licorice in areas with rich soil, in native prairie near wetlands or coulee bottoms. Perennial. Sow seeds in spring or early summer, or grow from plant cutting. Grow in rich, moist, and sandy soil, full sun to part shade. Zones 6–10.

Linden

Tilia americana

Also called basswood, lime tree **Family** Malvaceae
Parts used Flowers

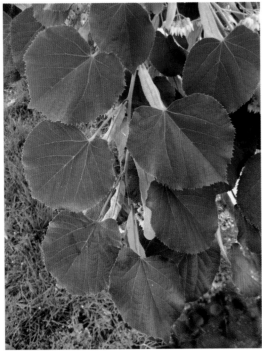

Linden leaves

| *This big, beautiful tree is regarded as safe for all in calming the heart and soul.*

Organs or systems affected Heart, central nervous
system **Therapeutic actions** Nervine, astringent,
diaphoretic **Nature** Sweet, cool **Plant constituents**
Volatile oil, saponins, flavonoids, acids, mucilage,
tannin, sugar, gum, chlorophyll, vitamin C **Flower
essence** Indicated when there is a need to calm
emotion turmoil

Medicinal uses

Calms central nervous system Linden is a universally safe nervine relaxant for people of all ages.
Children who tend to be hyperactive physically
or emotionally, from overstimulation, fear, or
fatigue, will benefit from the use of linden, as
will adults who are overworked or under high
amounts of stress. Linden helps them regain
emotional control and breath. If tension or pain
is involved, linden opens up and relaxes tension
pathways.

On a trip to Slovenia, I saw my first linden
tree. It was the European variety, but they are very
similar in appearance and function to the North
American lindens. Slovenians regard nature as a
religion, and this linden tree was most definitely
respected as a goddess. She was more than 100
years old, a beautiful presence in the middle of a
field. My dear friend Sasha told me that people
from all around knew of this particular tree and
often came to pay their respects. Whenever I've
had a particularly stressful day, I fill up my bath-
tub, pour in linden flowers, and imagine I'm in
the middle of that field under that tree.

Reduces heart tension Heart tension, which
presents as hypertension, angina, and a red
complexion can benefit from linden. Research
indicates that linden can relax tension around the
heart and help dissolve negative deposits that are
contributing to the tension.

Cools physically or emotionally Because of its
cooling nature, linden can help whenever there is
a need to cool down, whether that is physically or
emotionally.

Contraindications Generally regarded as safe.

MEDICINE CABINET

Infusion 2 teaspoons per cup, steep
10 to 12 minutes, 1 to 3 cups per day
Tincture 1 to 3 dropperfuls, 1 to 3 times per day

Identification and cultivation

Trees grow to 130 feet. Leaves are alternately arranged, ovate to cordate, 2 to 4 inches long, sharply serrated. Yellow-white fragrant flower droop in flattened clusters in summer. Typically found in pastures and urban landscapes in areas with cold winters and hot, humid summers. Deciduous tree. Grow in rich, moist, alkaline soil, full sun. Zones 3–8.

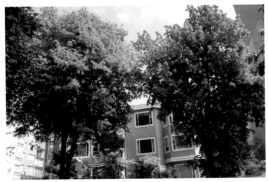

Linden trees

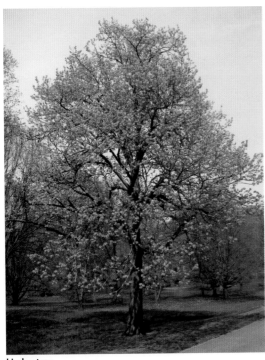

Linden tree

Lobelia

Lobelia inflata

Also called Indian tobacco, puke weed, asthma weed, gag root, eyebright, wild tobacco, bladder-pod **Family** Campanulaceae **Parts used** Aerial parts

> *If used wisely, lobelia clears obstruction to allow flow in breath and blood.*

Organs or systems affected Central nervous system, gastrointestinal system, respiratory system **Therapeutic actions** Emetic, expectorant, diaphoretic, anti-asthmatic, counterirritant **Nature** Acrid **Plant constituents** Alkaloids, gum, resin, volatile oil, fixed oil **Flower essence** Strengthens the throat chakra, allowing the truth to be spoken; helps those who may feel too timid to express their opinions

Medicinal uses

Relaxes the body Lobelia is known for its ability to relax the entire body. Taken in small doses, it can relax constricted areas that prevent blood flow and completely suspend the sympathetic nervous system, allowing the parasympathetic nervous system to take over so that the body relaxes and vessels dilate, literally forcing you to relax. Lobelia is a great choice to relax stomach spasms, bronchial irritations, gallbladder spasms, strangulated hernia, and bodily tension created by stress.

Increases blood circulation Lobelia's ability to relax blood vessels also increases circulation. A good use of lobelia is for persistent cold hands and feet. It can bring the warmth of blood flow. A fomentation can quickly draw out pain and is also valuable for fever reduction. Just a few drops of tincture in the ear can resolve stubborn pain and congestion.

Relieves constricted lungs Lobelia can greatly affect the respiratory system, with an affinity to help the constricted bronchioles of asthma. American herbalist John Christopher (1976) recounts the case of a man who had suffered from severe asthma for more than 20 years. It was so severe he wasn't able to lie down at night and needed to sleep propped up, sleeping only a few hours at a time. Christopher first administered a cup of peppermint tea to create a stimulating effect in the patient's body; 15 minutes later the patient was given 1 teaspoon of lobelia tincture, and in another 10 minutes, a second teaspoon. This led to the emetic principle being initiated, and the patient was able to bring up copious amounts of phlegm and other liquids from his lungs. The next evening, the man slept soundly for the first time in a decade. After reading this, I was intrigued and decided to try a similar approach on a young patient who suffered severely from asthma. With constant monitoring and communication with the child's mother, we administered a lobelia, fennel, catnip glycerite tincture for two days. She had one episode of nausea and a few days later one episode of vomiting. Recently, she went through her first winter without the need for her regular albuterol inhaler.

Purifies the stomach We can give credit to American herbalist Samuel Thomson (1769–1843) for our understanding of the value and principles of lobelia for stomach purification. Successive small doses (not enough to cause vomiting) were sufficient to relax the gastrointestinal organs to remove obstructions and eliminate congestion. When a patient was given an amount that produced vomiting, his appetite increased and he reported feeling lighter, stronger, and healthier all around.

Contraindications Should not be taken by those with hypertension. Should not be taken during pregnancy.

Identification and cultivation

Stems are covered in tiny hairs and reach 4 to 28 inches. Pale green, ovate leaves are arranged alternately and finely serrated. Flowers, pale violet-blue with yellow inside, bloom from midsummer to early fall. An annual plant in warm latitudes and a biennial in moderate and colder latitudes. Found in meadows, pastures, woods, and grassy places. To protect this sensitive wild species, direct sow in spring or autumn. Grow in slightly acidic soil, preferably clay, full to part shade. Zones 4–9.

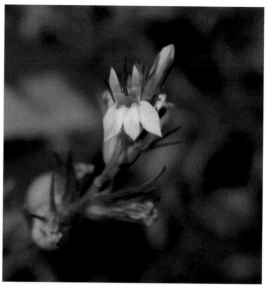

Lobelia flowers

Lovage

Levisticum officinale

Also called Old English lovage, Italian lovage
Family Apiaceae **Parts used** Leaves, roots

> *This plant acts as a stimulant
> for the entire body, to increase
> healthy organ functions.*

Organs or systems affected Kidneys, stomach, cardiovascular system, lymphatic system, reproductive system **Therapeutic actions** Stimulant **Nature** Bitter, sweet, salty, warm **Plant constituents** Salt, volatile oils, terpenes, coumarin, sterols, resin, gum, minerals **Flower essence** Helps promote confidence in taking action

Medicinal uses

Stimulates bodily functions Lovage is rarely used much these days, but it was once used often for stimulating various bodily functions. For example, it stimulates the lymphatic system when it is congested or not able to clear buildup. It also warms the stomach and digestive process, helping to increase the secretions and process food along the gastrointestinal tract. Lovage's high salt content drains edematous conditions and draws away excessive fluids that can intensify gout, arthritis, and bladder and kidney stones.

Warms the body In cold conditions such as irregular menses or with Raynaud's disease (a condition in which blood vessel spasms block blood flow to extremities), lovage can help warm the body and promote movement into blocked areas.

Contraindications Bladder irritation may result. Repeated use of lovage root has caused photosensitivity. Should not be taken during pregnancy because of its stimulating nature.

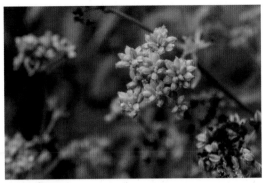

Lovage flowers

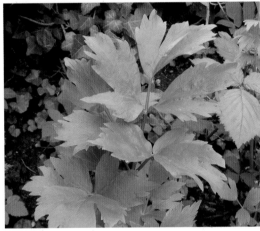

Lovage

MEDICINE CABINET

Decoction 1 or 2 tablespoons roots in 1 cup water, simmer 5 minutes covered, 1 to 3 cups per day
Infusion 4 tablespoons leaves in 1 quart cold water, steep overnight, 1 to 3 cups per day
Tincture 1 to 3 dropperfuls, 1 to 3 times per day

Identification and cultivation

Tall, erect stems to 8 feet. Shiny green, triangular shaped, divided leaves smell like celery or lime when crushed. Yellow flower heads borne atop stems in umbels in late spring. Perennial. Divide the rootball for planting tips or sow seed in the fall. Grow in well-drained soil, full sun to part shade. Zones 3–7.

Lungwort

Lobaria pulmonaria

Also called tree lungwort, lung moss, oak lung **Family** Lobariaceae **Parts used** Thallus (leaflike tissues)

| *The name says it all.*

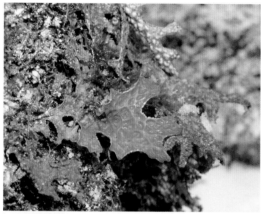

Lungwort thallus

Organs or systems affected Respiratory system
Therapeutic actions Antioxidant, secretolytic
Nature Bitter, sweet, cool **Plant constituents**
Vitamin C, mucilage, tannins, saponin, flavonoids, allantoin, menthol

Medicinal uses

Reduces irritation Studies show the positive effects of a lungwort infusion in reducing tissue inflammation in both the respiratory and gastrointestinal tracts. This may contribute to lungwort's ability to maintain healthy cells and improve white blood cell deficiency.

Supports lungs and improves sinusitis According to a Global Healing Center report, "The Lung Cleansing Benefits of Lungwort" (globalhealingcenter.com/natural-health/lung-cleansing-benefits-of-lungwort/), an 82 percent success rate was reported in resolving a sinusitis infection with the use of an herbal formula combining lungwort, cucumber sponge, and an oxidizing agent. The symptoms improved within four days and complete resolution was reported at two weeks.

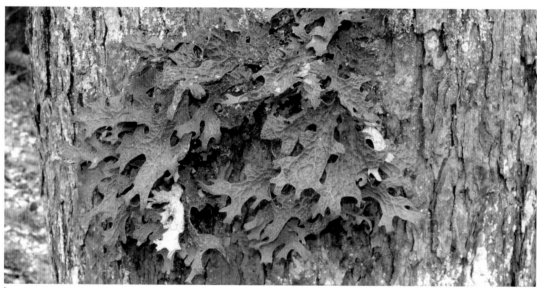

Lungwort

Supplies antioxidants The Global Healing Center report also cited a Russian study that used microbial test systems to evaluate the antioxidant properties of twenty different herbal extracts, which found that lungwort tested among the highest in the body and in the test tube. This is great news for all of those looking to retain the glow of youth.

Contraindications Generally regarded as safe.

MEDICINE CABINET

Decoction or infusion 1 tablespoon per cup, lightly simmer 5 minutes, steep 10 minutes, 1 to 3 cups per day

Tincture 1 or 2 dropperfuls, 1 to 3 times per day

Identification and cultivation

This large, leaflike lichen has a distinctive lobed growth form, bright green on the upper side when wet, but more olive-brown in dry conditions, with a creamy white underside. The thallus (vegetative tissue similar to a leaf) surface is covered in ridges and hollows, giving rise to the common name of lungwort in accordance with the doctrine of signatures: as formulated by herbalists in the Renaissance era, the use of plants was thought to be indicated by their physical form, and this lichen was used for treating respiratory problems because of its resemblance to the structure of a lung. It usually grows on the bark of broad-leaved trees such as oak, beech, and maple but will also grow on rocks. Lungwort takes 5 to 30 years to grow and is found in healthy ecosystems such as old-growth forests. It can be quite abundant in certain places. It grows well in mountainous areas or woods where water is close by. Harvest the thallus in the spring. Lungwort lichen is not available at nurseries, but a stroll in a damp wood may lead you to find this beauty.

Maitake

Grifola frondosa

Also called hen of the woods, ramshead, sheepshead **Family** Meripilaceae **Parts used** Entire fungus

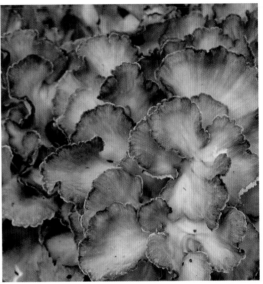

Maitake fungus

| *Nature's natural cancer-fighting agent.*

Organs or systems affected Central nervous system, immune system **Therapeutic actions** Adaptogen **Nature** Bitter **Plant constituents** Beta glucan, calcium, potassium, magnesium, amino acids, fiber, vitamins B1, B2, and D2

Medicinal uses

Activates cells that attack cancer Research indicates that maitake can increase macrophages, natural killer cells, and T-cells, the cell types that surround and attack cancer cells. It also walls off cancer cells until macrophages clear them from the body. Some research shows that it can inhibit or prevent the spread of tumors.

Boosts immune function As an adaptogen, maitake shines in reducing stress and raising overall immune function to protect the body from cold and flus. It seems to work on capillaries in helping them readily absorb trace minerals such as zinc via copper, which is often reduced in pathologies such as chronic fatigue syndrome.
Contraindications Generally regarded as safe.

MEDICINE CABINET

Decoction 1 teaspoon powder per cup, simmer 5 minutes covered, 1 to 3 cups per day
Tincture 1 dropperful, 1 to 3 times per day

Identification and cultivation

Maitake mushrooms grow in clusters around the bases of dead or dying oak or maple trees. They are variable in color, from pure white, to tan, brown, or gray, with curled, spoon-shaped caps. This fungus fruits in the fall. Some clusters can reach up to 50 pounds. Can also be cultivated using a mushroom growing kit.

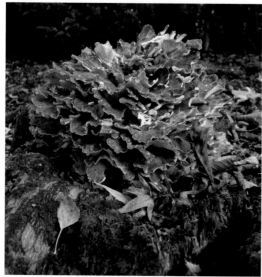
Maitake

Mistletoe

Viscum album

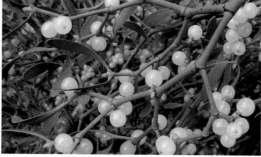
Mistletoe berries

Also called European mistletoe, birdle mistletoe, all heal, golden bough, devil's fuge **Family** Santalaceae **Parts used** Leaves, twigs

> *Even if you take it internally, mistletoe makes you feel like you've just been kissed.*

Organs or systems affected Brain, heart, reproductive organs, nervous system **Therapeutic actions** Nervine, antispasmodic, tonic, sedative **Nature** Bitter, sweet, cold, moist **Plant constituents** Mucilage, flavonoids, sugar, fixed oils, resin, tannins, various salts **Flower essence** Helps create positive love from the heart, especially in times of sudden loss or grief

Medicinal uses

Reduces convulsions, improves circulation Mistletoe is considered a gentle and safe nervine with powerful effects when used wisely. Having an affinity for the brain, it can reduce epilepsy, convulsions, and delirium. It appears to do so by opening up bodily blockages to improve circulation and reduce fluid accumulation. It is this action specifically that has made it common in the use for high blood pressure and edema.

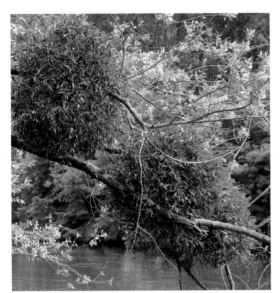
Mistletoe clusters

MEDICINE CABINET

Infusion 2 teaspoons per cup, steep
10 minutes, 1 to 3 cups per day
Tincture Must be made from green plant
material, 30 to 90 drops, 1 to 3 times per day;
for acute issues, take 5 to 10 drops
every 15 minutes

Identification and cultivation

This parasitic shrub grows on the stems of other trees. Leathery leaves are oblong-lanceolate but rounded at the apex, 1 or 2 inches long, arranged in opposite pairs. Tiny yellow flowers. Yellow or white berries form in late fall or spring. Mistletoe grows in the crowns of broad-leaved trees, particularly deciduous trees with soft bark, such as apple, linden, hawthorn, and poplar. Process plant parts into tincture right away, or dry them quickly and store in an airtight container. Parasitic evergreen. Harvest seed from ripe (white) berries in the spring. Smudge the berries against an apple, hawthorn, or poplar branch of at least 8 inches in diameter. Choose a branch that gets plenty of sunlight. Seeds germinate in 10 to 12 weeks and plants grow slowly.

Regulates heartbeat Mistletoe has been used by those who suffer from heart insufficiency that causes irregular heartbeat and cardiac obstructive diseases. Mistletoe drops administered under the tongue is said to return both heart and breath to regularity to allow the sufferer the ability to lie down and rest. Mistletoe also opens up obstructions resulting from disease or tension.

Relaxes pelvic muscle spasms Pelvic congestion, whether it be uterine or ovarian in women or prostate in men, may benefit from mistletoe. When disease or tension has caused the inability of fluids and blood to flow naturally to an area, pain often results. Mistletoe relaxes smooth muscle around such organs, creating greater function and reducing cramping and spasm pain. It can be taken in early labor to help support contractions without fear of creating spasms and is also helpful immediately post-labor to contract the uterus and support its return to normal size.

Contraindications Should not be taken during pregnancy because it can cause uterine contractions, unless induction is desired at appropriate time. Generally regarded as safe in appropriate dosages.

Motherwort

Leonurus cardiaca

Also called lion's tail, Roman motherwort, lion's ear, throwwort **Family** Lamiaceae **Parts used** Leaves, stems

Motherwort nurtures the uterus and calms the heart.

Organs or systems affected Heart, kidneys, uterus
Therapeutic actions Diaphoretic, antispasmodic, tonic, nervine, emmenagogue **Nature** Bitter,

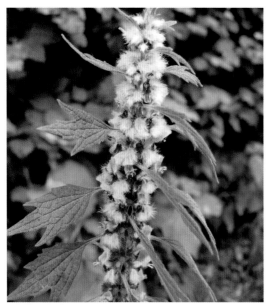

Motherwort flower spike

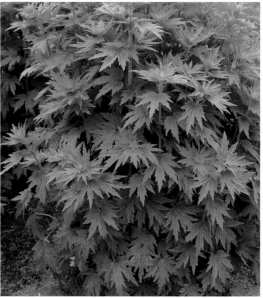

Motherwort

cooling **Plant constituents** Alkaloids, iridoid glycoside, diterpenoids, flavonoids (including rutin, quercitin), volatile oil, tannins, vitamin A **Flower essence** Promotes the development of healthy boundaries; facilitates the development of inner strength while allowing a soft, nurturing presentation

Medicinal uses

Calms the sympathetic nervous system Motherwort's ability to calm the sympathetic nervous system is probably due to its intense acrid bitters, which promote the transition from the sympathetic state to the parasympathetic state of relaxation. According to herbalist Matthew Becker (Wood, 2008), motherwort is excellent for those who move too quickly in thoughts, emotions, or actions that are not well thought out. Also good for anxiety and stress held in the gastrointestinal tract.

Calms the heart Traditionally used as a tonic to calm the heart and nerves surrounding it, motherwort can reduce palpitations caused by stress and anxiety. Herbalist Susun Weed says

that taking motherwort each day helps new blood vessels grow to the heart. She calls it "a bypass in a bottle." A dose of 10 to 20 drops of tincture, taken several times a day, can lower blood pressure, improve heart action, and strengthen electrical activity in the heart.

Stimulates uterus A well-documented herb used in women's health, motherwort is a uterine stimulant that aids the flow of menses and tonifies the uterine membranes. It is indicated for a cold uterus, a condition characterized in Chinese medicine as when the uterine lining doesn't respond appropriately to the warming hormone (progesterone). The vessels that supply blood to the uterus are constricted as a result of this cold response.

Reduces fever This highly underutilized herb is good for obstinate fevers and fevers that have left one drained. Drink 3 cups of infusion each day to reduce fever and return strength to the body.

Suppresses placenta According to Finley Ellingwood, a gynecologist and obstetric author of the late eclectic tradition, "Motherwort is superior to all other remedies in suppression of the lochia (afterbirth). By giving it internally and applying a fomentation of the herb over the lower abdominal region the author has used it with excellent results" (Wood, 2008).

Contraindications Motherwort is contraindicated for those taking pharmaceutical sedative prescriptions or heart medications. As with many herbs, it should not be taken during pregnancy and while a mother is breastfeeding. Motherwort's use during pregnancy is specific; because it is an emmenagogue, it can put the pregnancy in danger of termination, but only if it is taken in tincture form. The alkaloids in motherwort stimulate uterine contraction, but the alkaloids are alcohol-soluble, not water-soluble. Therefore, although the tincture of motherwort, both alcohol and glycerin, should be avoided during pregnancy, pregnant women can safely use the tea to treat anxiety.

MEDICINE CABINET

Fomentation 4 tablespoons per pint, steep at least 4 hours, soak cotton cloth in infusion and apply as needed
Infusion 1 or 2 teaspoons per cup, steep 8 to 10 minutes, 1 to 3 cups per day
Tincture 1 to 3 dropperfuls, 1 to 3 times per day

Identification and cultivation

Stems are square and slightly hairy. Palmately lobed leaves are wedge shaped with three points on basal leaves and five on upper leaves, dark green on top and pale underneath, opposite in orientation, rough, and downy. Pale pink, purple-pink, or white flowers grow in summer in whorls of six to twelve, in an alternating arrangement up the stem. Found in meadows, fields, yards, neglected gardens, open woods, floodplains, riverbanks, waste places, and along roadsides. Perennial. Seeds germinate easily whether sown inside or directly in the ground in fall or early spring. Typically flowers in the first year. Grow in moist, gravelly, or calcareous soil, full sun to part shade. Zones 4–8.

Mullein

Verbascum thapsus

Also called blanket herb, velvet dock, shepard's club, old lady's flannel, bullock's lungwort
Family Scrophulariaceae **Parts used** Flowers, leaves

> *A healer of the lungs for stubborn congestion and coughs.*

Organs or systems affected Respiratory system
Therapeutic actions Leaves: analgesic, antibacterial, antispasmodic, astringent, demulcent, diuretic, expectorant, sedative, vulnerary. Flowers: antispasmodic, demulcent, emollient, nervine, sedative **Nature** Bitter, salty **Plant consituents** Resin, saponins, glycoside (aucubin), flavonoids (hesperidin, verbascoside), choline, magnesium, mucilage, tannins, carotene, iron, magnesium, potassium, sulfur, calcium phosphate **Flower essence** Helps when one is unable to hear the truth, particularly around morals and values, when deceiving oneself

Medicinal uses

Brings moisture to respiratory tract Mullein is appropriate for a wide range of complaints of the upper and lower respiratory tract. Because it brings water into hardened, closed places, it is a good choice for dry and irritated tissues, or when water is trapped in the lungs. It can soothe a tickly cough and can help lung cilia function properly if a cough is chronic. Mullein is also indicated for constriction or tightness in the lungs or throat, making it useful for treating asthma.

Relieves earache An old favorite for earaches is mullein flower oil combined with garlic, for soothing pain and fighting infection. Drop 1 to 3 drops into each ear as needed and gently massage over and around the ear and neck.

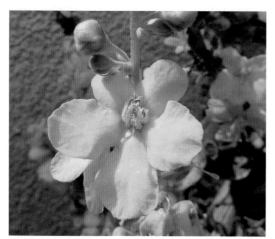
Mullein flower spike

Helps lubricate connective tissues Matthew Wood (2008) writes of mullein's ability to help with the lubrication of connective tissue in joints, which in turn supports healthy cartilage. It can be helpful in dealing with complex fractures and is used to support the spine.

Contraindications Generally regarded as safe.

MEDICINE CABINET

Ear drops 1 to 3 drops in each ear, 2 times per day
Infusion 1 or 2 teaspoons per cup, steep 10 minutes covered, 1 to 3 cups per day
Syrup 2 to 4 teaspoons per day
Tincture 1 or 2 dropperfuls, 3 to 6 times per day

Identification and cultivation

Erect, unbranched stems to 6 feet tall. Rosette of leaves emerge soft, fuzzy, and pale green. As it grows, the upper leaves are alternate and strongly clasp the stem, 5 to 8 inches long and 2 to 2½ inches broad. A corolla of flowers bloom in mid-summer, golden yellow and round, densely packed on a thick, wooly spike. Grows on stream banks, by roadsides or waste ground, in gravelly, sandy, or chalky soil. Biennial. Plant seedlings indoors in early spring. If you sow directly into the soil, they will be consumed by birds before they have the chance to germinate. Grow in slightly alkaline and dry soil, full sun to part shade. Zones 3–9.

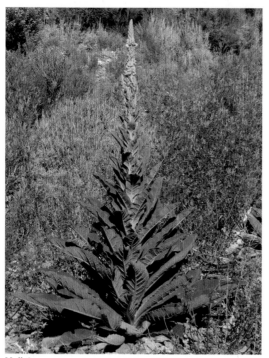
Mullein

Calms irritated nerves Author and herbalist Louise Tenney claimed that mullein is an excellent pain reliever, relaxing the mind and central nervous system to calm inflamed and irritated nerves, and it can be particularly helpful for those who are having difficulty sleeping (Wood, 2008).

Nettle

Urtica dioica

Also called stinging nettle **Family** Urticaceae
Parts used Leaves, roots, seeds

Despite nettle's sting, most herbalists will search high and low for a yearly supply of this valuable herbal tonic.

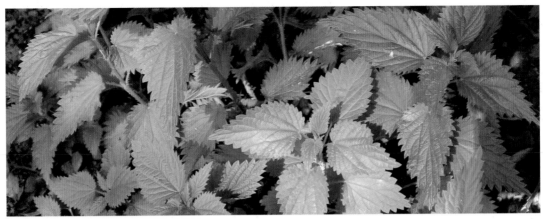
Nettle

Organs or systems affected Blood, kidneys, liver, lungs, bodily fluids **Therapeutic actions** Alterative, antiseptic, astringent, diuretic, expectorant, galactagogue, hemostatic, nutritive **Nature** Neutral, cool, dry, salty, slightly sweet **Plant constituents** Tannins, indoles, chlorophyll, flavonoids, protein, fiber, acetylcholine, mucilage, glycoside, vitamins C and B, beta-carotene **Flower essence** Often recommended for those who are irritated due to their inability to make life decisions

Medicinal uses

Supplies multitude of nutrients and proteins High in protein, nettle is also packed to the rim with nutrients for all aspects of physical form and function. Nettle is excellent at helping process protein within the body as well as removing toxic protein wastes. It seems to take from waste all that is still valuable and turn it into healing gold.

Tonifies the body Nettle is the perfect example of a nutritive tonic herb that is helpful in almost every situation. Considered safe for use with all ages, it has little record of negative side effects (except for those who pick it without gloves). It is a wonderful blood builder and nourisher. Those who suffer from anemia (even children) or have the Chinese medicine diagnosis of blood deficiency will often be recommended nettle. A woman who has scanty or absent menses will likely benefit from the use of nettle, which increases physical nutrients into the body. Nettle has been shown to improve bodily function, whether it be sluggish thyroid, kidney, nerves, muscles, or gastrointestinal. I typically always include nettle in my breastfeeding formulas to give the new mother all the nutrient support possible.

Relieves allergy symptoms Its anti-inflammatory effects also work on allergies. When particulates are inhaled, the body reacts to allergen proteins. Nettle is excellent at inhibiting this reaction and diminishing resulting symptoms such as excess mucus or an irritating itch. Most practitioners recommend freeze-dried nettle or fresh tincture for this purpose, but a nettle infusion works well, too.

Relieves inflammatory pain Studies indicate that nettle is valuable for pain relief, particularly from an inflammatory cause such as arthritis. Some tests used oral administration of nettle tea, capsules, or tincture, and others used the traditional application of topical nettle sting. Interestingly, most patients who endured the repeated topical stinging approach reported minimal discomfort with treatment and significant improvement afterward. This application causes minor irritation, thereby stimulating the area and increasing blood flow to reduce inflammation.

Supports and heals the nerves and surrounding tissues Although few studies have considered nettle's effects on nerve pain, it does seem to have an affinity for the nerves and has been documented to help relieve sharp, shooting pains often attributed to nerve pain such as sciatica. This effect could be due to the simple fact that bioavailable nutrients within the plant work to support and heal the nerves and surrounding tissues.

Stimulates and supports thyroid, kidneys, prostate, scalp Nettle seed is specifically indicated as a thyroid stimulant in subclinical hypothyroid function. Nettle root also helps with kidney dysfunction, prostate hyperplasia, and any condition with dampness being the primary cause of pathology. Roots and seed can also help stimulate hair growth.

Contraindications Some consider nettle to be too drying, leading to symptoms such as headaches or constipation. If this seems true for you, blend it with something moistening such as violet, which will lessen the drying effects and still provide the bountiful benefits of nettle.

MEDICINE CABINET

Fomentation 3 tablespoons per pint, steep 4 hours, soak cotton cloth and apply to affected area 2 or 3 times per day
Fresh application Place leaves directly on any paralyzed or nonresponsive area
Infusion 1 or 2 teaspoons per cup, steep 8 to 12 minutes, 3 cups per day
Tincture 30 to 60 drops, 1 to 3 times per day

Identification and cultivation

Hollow ribbed stems to 7 feet tall. Soft leaves are finely toothed, tapered, and covered with stinging hairs. Thin catkins of small white flowers are borne on the leaf axils. Nettles generally appear in the same location each year—in woodlands, thickets, disturbed areas, and along rivers and trails.

Harvest in early spring, before the flowering top develops. Sharp stinging, tiny hairs encompass the entire plant, but plants should be harvested fresh, so be sure to wear gloves. After nettle leaves are steamed or boiled, they can be eaten without fear (soaking nettles in water or cooking removes the stinging chemicals from the plant) and taste similar to spinach. If you want to impress someone, learn to pick a young leaf by folding it inward, and eat it right off the stem, avoiding the sting. Delicious! Perennial. Transplant young plants. Cut off flowering heads to reduce seed production. Grow in rich, moist soil, full sun to part shade. Zones 4–8.

Oatstraw

Avena sativa

Also called oatgrass **Family** Poaceae
Parts used Aerial parts

A delicate grass packed with nutrients.

Organs or systems affected Skin, central nervous system, musculoskeletal system **Therapeutic actions** Nervine, stimulant, antispasmodic, demulcent, nutritive **Nature** Sweet, oily, warm, moist **Plant constituents** Minerals, carotene, folliculin-like hormone, flavones, glycosides, polysaccharides, alkaloids, proteins, flavonoids, saponins, fixed oil, starch, vitamins B, D, E, and P **Flower essence** Ideal for anyone who is unable to make a choice; recommended during pivotal points in life when decisions need to be made to move in a positive direction

Medicinal uses

Strengthens tissues and nerves With its high silicon content, oatstraw is an excellent herb for strengthening the connective tissue, skin,

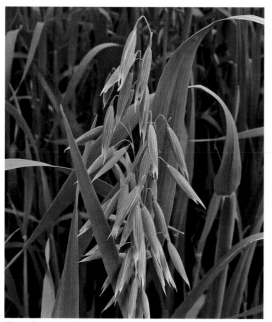
The milky tops of oats

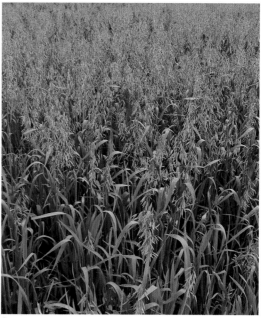
Oatstraw

mucous membranes, and nerve fibers. But silicon isn't the only supportive nutrient in oatstraw. This delicate herb is packed with trace minerals and vitamins to help build up the entire physical body, particularly for those suffering illness or overexertion.

Calm and relaxes the system Classified as a nervine, oatstraw helps relax and tone the central nervous system. It is a good choice for children to promote a sense of calmness.

Reduces skin irritation and inflammation A study was performed in 2012 regarding oatstraw and its use in dermatological conditions. As always, it's great to see what herbalists have known for centuries be legitimized by today's social standards of acceptance. Oatstraw can reduce arachidonic acid and stop the pro-inflammatory cascade in the body—in other words, oatstraw is great for reducing irritation and inflammation on the skin. It relieves itch and is specific for relieving the temporary symptoms of atopic dermatitis, psoriasis, and fungal and viral rashes. Oatstraw baths are a great choice for moisturizing the skin.

Contraindications Those with gluten sensitivity should avoid oatstraw.

MEDICINE CABINET

Bath Make an infusion with 4 tablespoons per quart, steep 2 hours, strain and then soak affected area

Fomentation 3 tablespoons per quart, steep 1 hour, strain, apply soaked cloth to area as needed

Infusion 1 or 2 teaspoons per cup, steep 10 minutes, 1 to 4 cups per day

Tincture 1 or 2 dropperfuls, 1 to 3 times per day

Identification and cultivation

Stems are smooth and erect. Sheathed leaves arise from the upper part of the stem. Oak grains are borne on a drooping panicle. Harvest the green grain in the early fruiting stage. The milky oat tops while still green are the best, but you can also use the entire plant as long as it is still in its early or immature phase and still greenish in color. Annual. Harvestable fifty days after sowing. Grow in most soils, full sun. Zones 5–10.

Oregon grape

Mahonia aquifolium

Also called mountain grape, Rocky Mountain grape, California barberry, berberis, holly-leaf marberry, trailing mahonia **Family** Berberidaceae **Parts used** Rhizomes, roots

> *A versatile shrub that supports the liver and gastrointestinal system and relieves the symptoms of constipation and diarrhea.*

Organs or systems affected Liver, spleen, gastrointestinal system **Therapeutic actions** Alterative, depurative, tonic, stimulant, hepatic **Nature** Bitter **Plant constituents** Alkaloids (berberine, berbamine, oxyacanthine, herbamine) **Flower essence** Assists those with paranoid or defensive behavior, expectation of hostility from others, and antagonistic projection

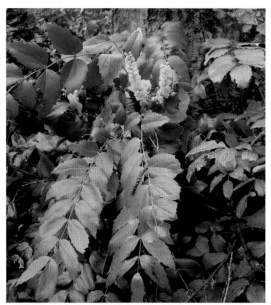
Oregon grape leaves and flowers

Medicinal uses

Improves digestion Oregon grape has an affinity for the digestion process, increasing appetite and improving digestion, assimilation, and metabolism. It stimulates hydrochloric acid (HCl) production, initiating proper digestion from the start, and increases the secretions of the liver and gallbladder.

Purifies blood Known in the Spanish-American tradition as the herb of the blood, Oregon grape is a superior blood purifier. Many believe that if the blood is clean, the patient is well. Oregon grape supports and liberates iron from the liver to enter the bloodstream to boost hemoglobin levels.

Fortifies skin tissue Oregon grape has a longstanding reputation for having a direct effect on the skin, in part due to its effects on the digestion process and liver function, but it also brings other

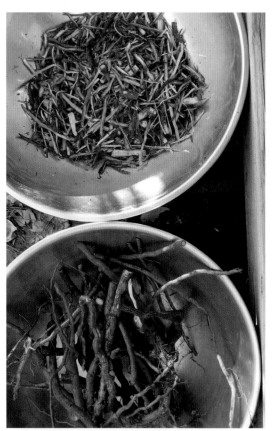
Harvested Oregon grape roots and rhizomes

aspects into balance. Each of us has within us the ability to build and break down cells, tissues, and hormones as needed. Oregon grape fortifies this process, building up what is needed to support the skin and breaking down the obstacles that are causing skin issues.

Helps with elimination issues Oregon grape is a go-to herb for sudden onset diarrhea because of its antibacterial action. It is also a great choice combined with cascara sagrada for chronic constipation resulting from slow liver function and atonic, dry bowels. A perfect example of an alterative, in the sense that it brings up what is down and brings down what is up.

Contraindications Caution is advised if taking liver-related medications.

MEDICINE CABINET

Decoction 1 or 2 teaspoons per cup, simmer 12 minutes covered, 3 cups per day or as needed
Tincture 1 dropperful, 1 to 3 times per day

Identification and cultivation

Evergreen shrub, grows to 3 feet. Leaves are variable, pinnately compound, with five to seven spiny, leathery leaflets that resemble holly. Flowers are borne in spring to early summer in dense clusters at the sides or tips of branches, developing spherical to elliptical-shaped, small, purple-black berries in grapelike clusters. Roots and rhizomes are yellow, branching, and knotty. Grows on dry slopes and in the understory of coniferous forests and oak woodlands. Evergreen shrub. Plant in spring from woody stem cuttings, soft stem cuttings, or simple layering. Grows in neutral soil, part shade. Zones 5–9.

Pennyroyal

Mentha pulegium

Also called pudding grass, hillwort, brotherwort, run-by-the-ground, pulegium, lurk-in-the-ditch, piliolerial **Family** Lamiaceae **Parts used** Aerial parts

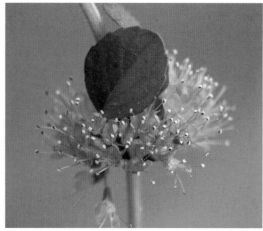
Pennyroyal flower

Another member of the mint family, this herb will bring on delayed menses.

Organs or systems affected Intestines, lungs, uterus **Therapeutic actions** Stimulant, astringent, emmenagogue, diaphoretic **Nature** Pungent, bitter, cool, dry **Plant constituents** Essential oil, tannins, flavonoids **Flower essence** Assists those who get lost in themselves, work, others, and life

Medicinal uses

Initiates menses Pennyroyal is one of the North American native plants that is rich in Native American history. Pennyroyal has been used safely for initiating menses when it is delayed due to stress, illness, or simple suppression. Some women have a shorter progesterone phase, which is the second half of a menstrual cycle. This can lead to pain with menstruation and drastic uterine spasms, lower pelvic and back pain, and clotting. Pennyroyal helps to assist the uterus by creating a smooth flow and thinning the uterine lining.

Soothes stomach Native Americans used pennyroyal to soothe an upset stomach and aid digestion.

Reduces fevers For people with sudden and extreme feverish conditions, pennyroyal can help bring on perspiration to reduce fever.

Contraindications Should not be taken during pregnancy. Many mistakenly believe that pennyroyal can induce abortion, but this is not the function of pennyroyal. Never ingest pennyroyal essential oil or use it topically, because it is toxic and can be lethal.

MEDICINE CABINET

Infusion 1 or 2 teaspoons per cup, steep 10 to 12 minutes, 1 to 4 cups for 1 or 2 days only
Tincture 15 drops, 1 to 3 times per day

Identification and cultivation

Square stems, 3 to 12 inches long. Gray-green leaves are oval, arranged oppositely on the stem, and slightly hairy. Violet-lavender flowers grow in whorled clusters. Perennial. Sow directly in ground after last frost. Grow in acidic to neutral soil, full sun. Zones 6–9.

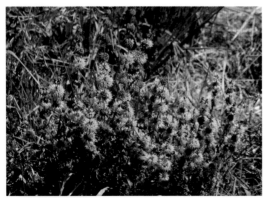

Pennyroyal in bloom

Plantain

Plantago major

Also called snakeweed, broad-leafed plantain, ribble grass, waybread, cuckoo's bread, Englishman's foot, white man's foot **Family** Plantaginaceae **Parts used** Aerial parts, roots, seeds

> *Watch where you step! This little weed is often underfoot and highly underutilized as a healer for all.*

Organs or systems affected Bladder, intestines, kidneys, lungs, skin **Therapeutic actions** Deobstruent, cooling alterative, emollient, astringent, diuretic **Nature** Bitter, cooling, moist **Plant constituents** Polysaccharides, lipids, caffeic acid derivatives, flavonoids, iridoid glycosides and terpenoids, alkaloids, vitamins C and K, beta-carotene, calcium **Flower essence** Transmutes emotionally sensitive situations and allays fears

Medicinal uses

Draws out toxins Plantain is often underutlized for all the power it posseses. It is one of the finest herbs for all poisonous afflictions of the body, inside and out. There are many accounts of using a poultice application of plantain in drawing out toxins of venomous snake and spider bites. I have seen it heal deep wounds by purifying the skin and injured tissue and pulling it together to heal. Matthew Wood (2008) recalls a 2-year-old whose neck swelled to an enormous size after being stung by a bee. He placed four bruised plantain leaves onto the area, and within an hour the swelling completely subsided.

Soothes respiratory tract Plantain is an excellent choice for irritation of the respiratory tract. It soothes and slightly moistens the mucous membranes and lifts up water and mucus from the lungs. It is also indicated for the irritating cough

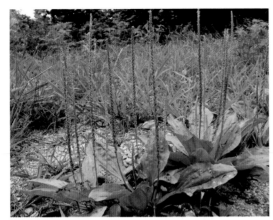
Plantain blooms

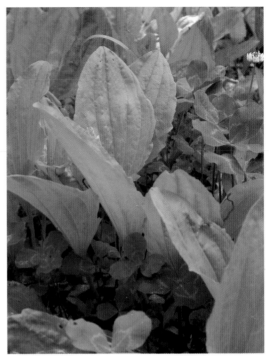
Broad plantain leaves

that at times arises from respiratory irritation.

Helps heal infections Both the roots and leaves create a slightly stimulating effect on the cardio-vascular system, which in turn benefits the glandular and lymph system to help with infection of the body. Plantain is also recommended for issues of the mouth, including thrush and painful or infected gums.

Contraindications If taking prescribed blood thinner medication, avoid taking large doses of plantain.

MEDICINE CABINET

Decoction For thrush, boil 1 ounce of seeds in 3 cups water, reducing to 2 cups, let sit for 1 hour and strain, add honey to taste. Use 1 tablespoon, 4 times per day.

Infusion 1 teaspoon per cup, steep 10 minutes, 1 to 3 cups per day.

Mouthwash For infected gums or absessed tooth, 3 tablespoons root powder per pint, steep 2 hours, swish 2 times per day

Powder For infected gums or absessed tooth, apply fine root powder to the area for 20 minutes, 2 times per day

Tincture 1 dropperful, 3 times per day

Topical Apply chewed or bruised leaves directly to affected area until symptoms resolve

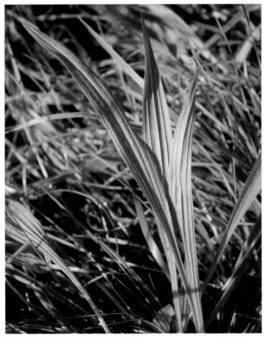
Lance-shaped plantain leaves

Identification and cultivation

Two common plantain species are used interchangeably in western herbal medicine: *Plantago majus* is the broad-leaved plantain, described here, and *Plantago lanceolata* is the narrow leafed species.

In the broad-leaved plantain, dense rosettes of heavily ribbed, ovate leaves are 4 to 10 inches long and 2 to 5 inches broad, growing from a short rhizome with long, straight, yellowish roots. Small, greenish-brown flowers with purple stamens are produced in a dense spike, up to 6 inches tall. As a common lawn weed, plantain can be found almost anywhere—unfortunately, you may see a neighbor spraying them like mad with a toxic weed killer. Perennial. Grows in any soil, shade or part shade. Zones 2–15.

Poplar

Populus tremuloides

Also called American aspen, white poplar, quaking aspen, trembling poplar **Family** Salicaceae **Parts used** Bark

> *This ancient medicine is beneficial for the sensitive bladder.*

Organs or systems affected Intestines, stomach, genitourinary (genital and urinary) system **Therapeutic actions** Astringent, febrifuge, tonic, anti-inflammatory, analgesic **Nature** Bitter, cool, dry **Plant constituents** Populin, essential oils, glycosides, acids, mannitol, oils **Flower essence** Helps relieve all states of fear, and helps those who tend to take on the negativity of others

Medicinal uses

Supports the bladder Poplar bark has a unique ability when working on the bladder, because it seems to target both the function and structure of the organ itself. In cases such as incontinence, when many variables come into play—overactivity, bladder wall punctuation, sensitivity, sphincter tone—poplar is an excellent choice for healing the entire bladder. Many practitioners use it for a bladder or kidney that is easily stimulated by emotions such as fear, nervousness, or anxiety.

Relaxes the body Poplar has a calming effect when the sympathetic nervous system is on overdrive, resulting in changes in physical function. For example, poplar's astringent, relaxing, and tonifying actions typically calm the intestinal tract to cease watery diarrhea due to long-term stress or anxiety. If the gastrointestinal tract is affected by perpetual tension and stress held in the abdomen, poplar can correct the resulting malabsorption and overall weakness.

Heals wounds, reduces fever, and eases headaches Poplar has long been used to heal wounds, reduce intermittent fevers, and ease typical headaches. Capitalizing on its salicylates, from which aspirin is derived, it is also helpful for minor aches and pains.

Contraindications Generally regarded as safe. Poplar should be taken for 12 to 20 weeks to create a sustained physical change within.

MEDICINE CABINET

Decoction 1 teaspoon per cup, simmer 12 to 15 minutes covered, 1 to 3 cups per day
Tincture 1 dropperful, 1 to 3 times per day

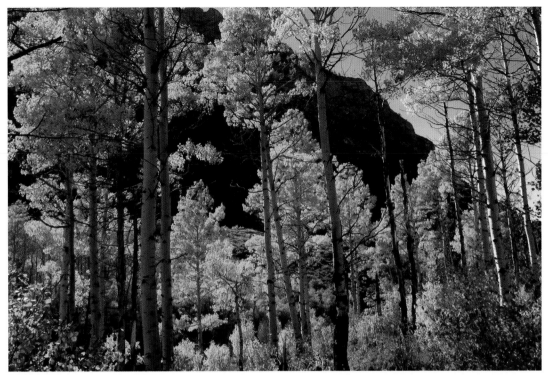

Poplar trees

Identification and cultivation

Mature trees reach 30 to 40 feet. Red-brown stems are slender, often with a waxy coating. Heart-shaped leaves are arranged alternately, simple, 1 to 3 inches long with fine-toothed margins. Light green catkins are covered with soft hairs. Fruit grows on catkins, with light green capsules containing small, hairy seeds. Bark is smooth initially, furrowing with maturity and dark at the base. Large poplar groves will have hundreds of trees, all originating from a single extensive underground root system. Grow in rocky, clay, or sandy soil, full sun. Zones 1–6.

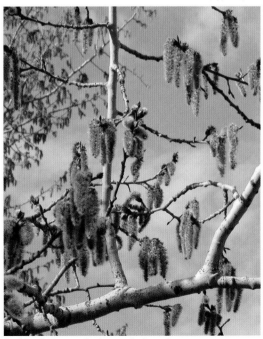

Catkins drying on a broken poplar branch

Purple loosestrife

Lythrum salicaria

Also called spiked loosestrife, flowering Sally, sage willow, rainbow weed, purple grass **Family** Lythraceae **Parts used** Flowers, leaves, stems

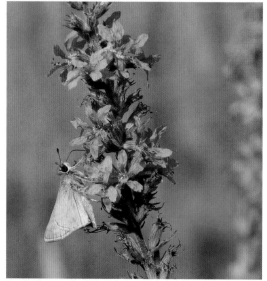

Purple loosestrife flowers

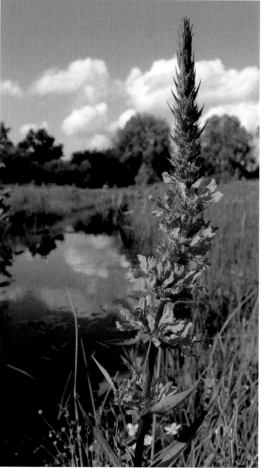

Purple loosestrife

> *One of the only herbs to possess both astringent and demulcent actions.*

Organs or systems affected Bladder, kidneys, liver, biliary system **Therapeutic actions** Alterative, antibiotic, antispasmodic, diuretic, diaphoretic, tonic, demulcent **Nature** Sweet, moist **Plant constituents** Glycosides, mucilage, salicarin, tannins, volatile oil, plant sterols **Flower essence** Helps promote a feeling that as old ways and forms pass away, new opportunities will appear; also helps one replace fear with trust

Medicinal uses

Helps clear dysentery and diarrhea With its natural antibiotic and astringent attributes, purple loosestrife helps clear infectious bowel issues such as dysentery or bacteria-caused diarrhea. Many herbalists also consider it a safe plant, in teaspoon doses, for infants struggling with diarrhea. The breastfeeding mother can also take 3 cups per day.

Reduces and heals inflammatory bowel disorders Purple loosestrife has potent astringent actions but does not dry out tissues. Instead, it creates a smooth mucus layer to reduce inflammation and heal tissues. It is helpful for Crohn's disease, inflammatory bowel disease, and other bowel inflammatory disorders.

Improves kidney and bladder function Because of its affinity for mucous membranes, it seems to work particularly well on the kidneys and bladder, offering its tonic actions to improve overall function.

Improves vision Many texts report the use of purple loosestrife for any type of vision issues, including cloudiness, reduced vision capability, or injured eyes.

Contraindications Generally regarded as safe.

MEDICINE CABINET

Decoction 3 teaspoons per 12 ounces water, simmer for 8 to 10 minutes covered, 1 to 3 cups per day
Eye wash 3 teaspoons per pint water, steep 1 to 4 hours and strain, rinse eyes with 1 ounce several times per day
Tincture 1 or 2 dropperfuls, 1 to 3 times per day

Identification and cultivation

Paired leaves are cordate, 2 to 4 inches long, on quadrangular stems, 2 to 4 feet tall. Purple terminal flower spikes bloom in early summer. Collect flowers, seeds, and stems from spring to late summer. Purple loosestrife is a highly invasive plant that threatens significant portions of natural wetland habitats across North America and should not be planted in gardens.

Queen of the meadow

Filipendula ulmaria

Also called bridewort, sweet hay **Family** Rosaceae
Parts used Flowers, leaves, stems

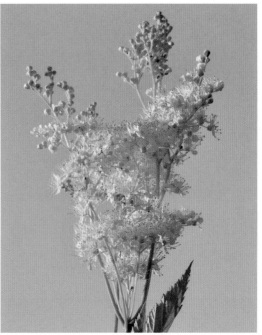

Queen of the meadow flowers

> *When ligaments and tendons are inflamed and weak, queen of the meadow can help.*

Organs or systems affected Bladder, connective tissue, intestines **Therapeutic actions** Astringent, diuretic, decongestant **Nature** Sweet, bitter, salty, cool **Plant constituents** Glycosides, salicylic acids, flavonoids, volatile oils, iron, sulfur, calcium, silica, vitamin C **Flower essence** Enhances energy flow throughout the body; helps to enhance intuition and ability to change direction

Medicinal uses

Relieves pain, fever, and inflammation The salicylic acid in queen of the meadow is a great pain reliever and fever reducer. This aspect works well in reducing overall inflammation. In conjunction with trace minerals such as silica, queen of the meadow is used to bolster the body's connective tissues, including ligament weaknesses from overuse, poor diet, or previous injury.

Helps release toxins, relieves gout Whenever a plant focuses on smaller spaces in the body and the connective tissues found there, it often has the ability to sweep those spaces clean of toxic build-up. The plant knows that there must be an out-with-the-old and in-with-the-new to correct imbalances of form and function. One example is the toxic accumulation of uric acid in small joints, which causes gout. Queen of the meadow works on multiple levels to accomplish many things, including inflammation reduction, pain support, and the draining of toxicity through natural pathways such as urination. It is also helpful for arthritis, rashes, rheumatism, and overall fatigue.

Eases diarrhea The astringent action of queen of the meadow is helpful with diarrhea and loose stool, helping to pull back water released in intestinal tissues.

Contraindications Extremely high doses may cause nausea. Some medications interact with salicylic acid and can cause skin irritations and other problems.

MEDICINE CABINET

Infusion 1 or 2 teaspoons per cup, steep 8 to 10 minutes, 1 to 3 cups per day
Tincture 1 to 3 dropperfuls per day

Identification and cultivation

Erect stems are 2 to 4 feet tall. Fernlike leaves are downy underneath and dark green on top, 1 to 4 inches long. White flower tufts borne atop erect stems. Collect the flowers in midsummer; the white tufts are hard to miss. Found in woodland gardens with dappled shade, bog gardens, moist banks, and meadows across North America. Perennial. Propagate by dividing the root ball. Grow in consistently moist soil, dappled shade. Zones 3–9.

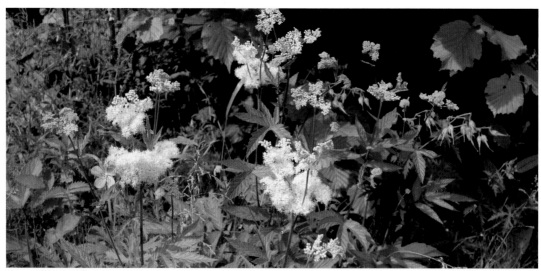

Queen of the meadow

Raspberry

Rubus idaeus

Also called American raspberry, wild red raspberry, hindberry **Family** Rosaceae **Parts used** Leaves

> *One of the oldest and wisest herbs for women's health.*

Organs or systems affected Lungs, uterus, gastrointestinal system **Therapeutic actions** Astringent, stimulant, tonic, alterative **Nature** Sweet, sour, cool **Plant constituents** Tannins, acids, vitamins C and A, calcium, phosphorus, iron, trace minerals **Flower essence** Assists those whose feelings are easily hurt or who have a touchy nature

Medicinal uses

Tones the uterus For centuries, herbalists and women have used red raspberry as a healing herb for the uterus. It not only nourishes the blood with its minerals and vitamins, but it specifically

tones the uterine tissues and helps to regulate the flow of menses. During pregnancy, if taken regularly, red raspberry will help prepare the uterus for labor. Similar to how you might prepare to run a marathon, taking red raspberry during pregnancy is like running several short distances in preparation for the long haul. It can also prepare for breastfeeding by enriching the breast milk and helping the uterus return to its normal size after birth.

Tones stomach and intestinal lining Having an affinity for smooth muscle and mucous membranes, red raspberry soothes and heals the tissues of the stomach and intestinal lining. It's

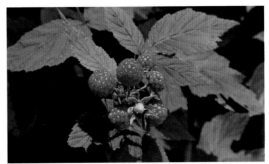
Raspberries

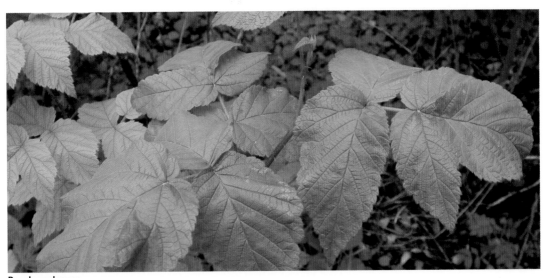
Raspberry leaves

a good choice if ulcers or inflammatory pockets are present. Typically such conditions are paired with a reduction in tone of the intestinal wall, allowing for increased flare-ups of Crohn's disease, inflammatory bowel disease, constipation, or diverticulitis. Red raspberry can help improve overall tone and pull tissues back together.

Eases constipation This herb is used for stubborn constipation, which can often be attributed to improper peristalsis, or the contracting motion of the intestines. Why the movement becomes impaired may not be known, but the result is slow transit time and difficulty passing stools.

Supports mucous membranes Mucous membranes of the mouth and lungs are also supported by red raspberry, because of its affinity for such tissues and the valuable nutrients it contains.

Contraindications Generally regarded as safe.

MEDICINE CABINET

Infusion 2 teaspoons per cup, steep 10 to 12 minutes, 1 to 3 cups per day

Tincture 1 to 3 dropperfuls, 1 to 3 times per day

Identification and cultivation

Stems are 3 to 6 feet long with fine prickles. Pale green, pinnate leaflets are rounded at the base, with serrated edges. Small, white, cup-shaped flowers grow in clusters of five. Grows in hedges, fields, abandoned lots, and thickets. Common throughout most of North America. To help differentiate plants from blackberries if berries are not present, raspberry brambles are much smaller than blackberry, averaging only 5 feet. Raspberries tend to have more prickles than blackberries, but blackberry prickles are more substantial. Perennial. Plant in the early spring (or late winter for warm zones) and prepare soil with compost or aged manure a couple weeks before planting. Grow in slightly acidic and moist soil, full sun. Zones 2–7.

Rauwolfia

Rauvolfia serpentina

Also called snake root **Family** Apocynaceae
Parts used Roots

> *Just two drops can usually lower blood pressure quickly in acute situations.*

Organs or systems affected Heart, cardiovascular system **Therapeutic actions** Hypotensive, relaxant **Nature** Bitter, cooling **Plant constituents** Alkaloids, phenols, saponins, tannins, flavonoids, calcium, phosphorus, sodium, potassium, magnesium

Medicinal uses

Lowers blood pressure High blood pressure most commonly occurs due to hardened residue in the vessels, reduced kidney function, and poor lifestyle choices. Although not a curative, rauwolfia does work to lower blood pressure in acute situations. Reserpine, the chief alkaloid in rauwolfia root, is the component responsible for this, as it relaxes the blood vessels around the heart so it doesn't need to work so hard. In small doses, rauwolfia works extremely well and very quickly. It was used with frequency in the United States in the 1950s as the main medication for lowering blood pressure but was discontinued because of misuse that had led to overdosing.

Relaxes the body for sleep As you might imagine, something that can lower blood pressure through the action of relaxation must also relax other nerves and tissues in the body. Rauwolfia is considered a mild relaxant. Mahatma Gandhi was reported to use rauwolfia often before bed to promote a peaceful night's sleep.

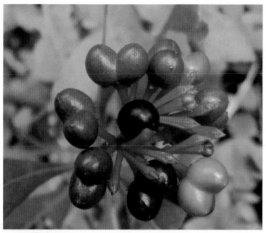
Rauwolfia berries

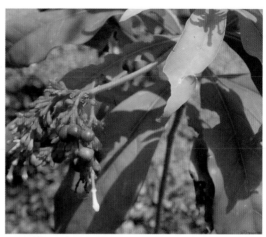
Rauwolfia

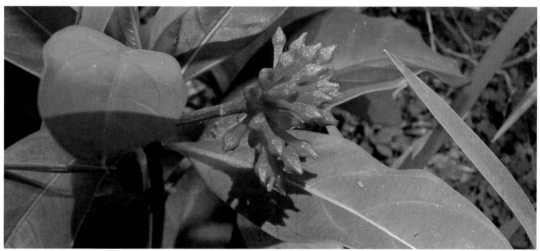
Rauwolfia flower buds

Calms agitation Many cultures, including Indian, African, and Chinese, often use this herb to help calm irrational mental states such as insanity and hysteria. They mix it with goat's milk and sugar.
Contraindications Excessive dosages can induce trembling and convulsions. Should not be taken during pregnancy or while breastfeeding.

> ——— MEDICINE CABINET ———
> **Tincture** 2 to 5 drops (not dropperfuls) as needed

Identification and cultivation
Lanceolate leaves grow in whorls of three, are bright green above and pale underneath. Flowers are white-tinged with violet on irregular cymes. Tuberous roots are pale brown. This valuable herb is not found in North America, but should you find yourself in India, be sure to seek it out. Subtropical evergreen perennial shrub. Can be propagated by seed, stem cuttings, and root cuttings. Harvest at approximately the eighteenth month. Grow in slightly acidic to well-drained soil. Zone 11, or in a greenhouse.

Red clover

Trifolium pratense

Also called wild clover, trefoil, purple clover, meadow clover **Family** Papilionaceae **Parts used** Flowers, leaves, stems

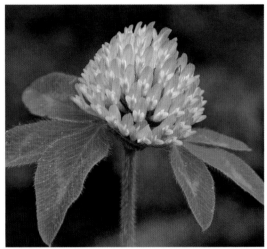
Red clover flower

| *Red clover stimulates a sense of calm and well-being, and improves cognitive function.*

Organs or systems affected Blood, brain, skin, central nervous system **Therapeutic actions** Alterative, sedative, tonic **Nature** Sweet, neutral temperature, moistening **Plant constituents** Volatile oils, acids, glycosides, coumarins, flavonoids, tannins, iron, chromium, molybdenum, vitamin C, tocopherol **Flower essence** Indicated for those who are easily influenced by group energy and get carried along with the crowd, instead of making their own decisions

Medicinal uses

Purifies blood Red clover has long been regarded as a blood purifier that helps to rid the body of toxic buildup and excessive waste. This action can been considered nutritive in action as it gently restores the cardiovascular system.

Purges lymphatic congestion Red clover seems to have an affinity for the lymphatic system, where it helps to purge the lymph nodes of congested materials to reduce hard, swollen, and painful nodules.

Improves cognitive function As a cardiovascular agent, red clover can not only clean the blood, but also help it move more effectively. It is reported to improve cognitive function, where memory had declined because of overwork. This may imply that red clover is working on the microcirculations of the body, or perhaps its purifying ability reaches the smallest capillaries in the body to improve overall function.

Contraindications Generally regarded as safe.

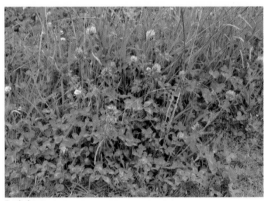
Red clover

MEDICINE CABINET

Infusion 1 or 2 teaspoons per cup, steep 8 to 10 minutes, 1 to 3 cups per day
Tincture 1 to 3 dropperfuls, 1 to 3 times per day

Identification and cultivation

Erect stems, 6 to 20 inches, are slightly hairy and branching. Three leaflets grow on alternate sides of stem. Round flowers are pinkish purple, spring to early fall. Found in fields, meadows, abandoned lots, and roadsides. Perennial root, annual stem. A great cover crop, red clover helps to build soil and replenish the nutrients in your garden. Grow in well-drained soil, full sun. Zones 4–8.

Red root

Amaranthus retroflexus

Also called amaranth, New Jersey tea, wild snowball, mountain lilac, snowbrush, deerbrush, walpole, buckbrush **Family** Amaranthaceae **Parts used** Roots, bark

A classic herb for spleen swelling and pathologies of a hot and congested nature.

Organs or systems affected Liver, lungs, spleen, uterus **Therapeutic actions** Astringent, antispasmodic, expectorant, sedative **Nature** Cold, dry, bitter **Plant constituents** Alkaloids, acids, quercitrin, oil, resin, tannin **Flower essence** Assists those who feel guilty when others suffer

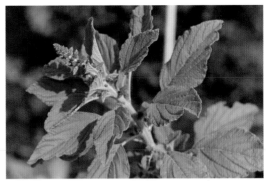
Red root

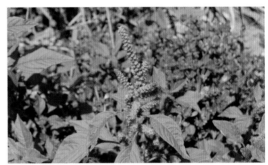
Red root in bloom

Medicinal uses

Supports spleen Red root has traditionally been used in the treatment of swollen spleen, often associated with malaria. In developed countries, red root is a signature treatment for mononucleosis and its history of leaving the patient with a swollen spleen after recovery. I thoroughly enjoy R. Swinburne Clymer's interpretation of red root's use in his 1963 book, *Nature's Healing Agents: The Medicines of Nature*, where he mentions that any time there is despondency and melancholy during illness, with soreness to the touch over the spleen area, red root is indicated. He also says that red root is for those who fall prey to the "artistic funk," or melancholy. And, by the way, if you aren't familiar with Clymer's work, you should be.

Cools and constricts blood vessels Red root is indicated for any hot and congested fluids and blood. It works to cool and constrict vessels, making it valuable in hemorrhage, uterine, and liver blood congestion; excessive cellular secretions; and lymph and liver stagnation.

Contraindications Rarely known to cause allergic reactions, but if so, swelling of the tongue is most common.

MEDICINE CABINET

Infusion and cold infusion 1 or 2 teaspoons per cup, steep 10 to 12 minutes, 1 to 2 cups per day
Tincture 3 to 90 drops, 1 to 3 times per day

Identification and cultivation

Stems are branching, woody, and erect. Dark green leaves are irregularly toothed, 2 or 3 inches long. A large inflorescence of white flowers grows in terminal clusters. Found in open, deciduous woods, woodland edges, oak savannahs, and dry prairies. Deciduous shrub. Collect seeds in late summer and early fall, or root greenwood cuttings in midsummer or late summer. Drought tolerant. Grow in any soil, full to part shade. Zones 4–9.

Reishi

Ganoderma applanatum (also *G. lucidum*, *G. oregonense*, *G. tsugae*)

Also called artist's conk **Family** Ganodermataceae **Parts used** Entire fungus

> *Are you catching every cold that comes by? Time for reishi.*

Organs or systems affected Central nervous system **Therapeutic actions** Adaptogen, stimulant, tonic, astringent **Nature** Salty, sweet **Plant constituents** Polysaccharides, phytosterols, terpenes, triterpenes, protein

Medicinal uses

Strengthens the immune response Reishi strengthens both the parasympathetic nervous system and the adrenal cortex in creating a better balance, physically, between reaction and relaxation. Reach for reishi when you seem to catch every cold that walks by your door. It can help when the immune system has been under fire and cannot respond appropriately.

Strengthens adrenal system Usually when stress goes up, immunity goes down. After a time of over-reactive adrenal responses, the immune system falters and can begin to deregulate, which can lead to autoimmune issues, where deficiency is the root cause. Reishi has been shown to work on the fire-building, or mineralocorticoid side, of immune and inflammatory response to stoke the fires of proper antibody reaction.
Contraindications Generally regarded as safe.

MEDICINE CABINET

Decoction Simmer a small piece about the size of your thumb for 15 minutes, covered, drink 1 to 3 cups per day
Tincture 1 to 3 dropperfuls, 1 to 3 times per day

Identification and cultivation

This mushroom grows on hardwood stumps and logs, including oak, elm, beech, maple, and more. *Ganoderma tsugae* seems to prefer conifers—mainly hemlocks. Fruiting bodies are kidney- or fan-shaped and reddish in color, with a wet, lacquered appearance when young. From summer to fall, look for them in damp, dark forests or on rotting logs. Can also be cultivated using a mushroom growing kit.

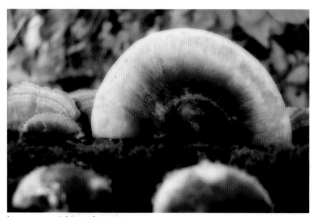
Immature reishi mushroom

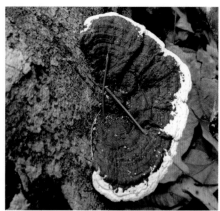
Mature reishi

Rosemary

Rosmarinus officinalis

Also called compass-weed, poplar plant, old man
Family Lamiaceae **Parts used** Leaves

> *Rosemary thrives in damp, cooler climates and treats the illnesses associated with such environments.*

Organs or systems affected Brain, heart, intestines, lungs **Therapeutic actions** Anti-inflammatory, antiseptic, astringent, carminative, diaphoretic, stimulant **Nature** Pungent, sweet, warm, dry **Plant constituents** Essential oils, saponins, flavonoids, acids, rosmaricine, tannins, resin, bitter, calcium, potassium, phosphorus, magnesium, iron, zinc, beta-carotene **Flower essence** Used to help find peace within, for those who struggle within themselves or with others

Medicinal uses

Supports heart and cardiovascular system Rosemary has been cited endlessly for its positive benefits on the heart and cardiovascular system. It is considered the ideal heart herb because it is toning and cleansing. It is also a good nerve tonic. Many clinicians have used it specifically for cardiac edema, noting its ability to move out stuck fluid. This removal of stagnated buildup extends to the extremities, stimulating the nerves and vessels along the way, opening up positive blood flow, and decreasing cold sensations, muscle stiffness, and inflammation due to oxygen deprivation.

Balances blood sugar Rosemary helps balance blood sugars in the body. It increases the breakdown of sugars and carbohydrates, improving metabolism and reducing the highs and lows of

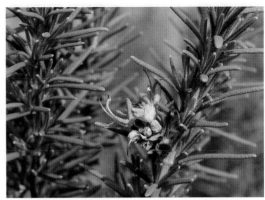

Rosemary leaves and flowers

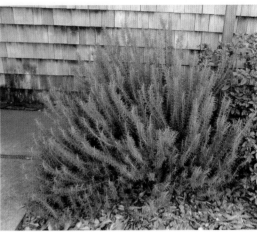

Rosemary

fluctuating blood sugar levels. This is helpful for dysglycemia and the symptoms that accompany it, including irritability, dizziness, and fatigue.

Helps warm the body Rosemary stimulates, motivates, and warms bodily systems, making it helpful for those who feel cold all the time or who have cold hands and feet. Weakness, or lacking the heat-driving forces necessary for the body, can occur when vessels are constricted and are unable to drive blood to warm an area. The result is slower reactions and poor physical function. Using rosemary in such situations is effective at warming up and stimulating the overall metabolic state.

Stimulates hair follicles Rosemary oil can be used on the scalp to stimulate hair follicles for potential growth. This is an old remedy but not outdated. Massage it into the scalp for 2 to 5 minutes, once per day.

Contraindications Those with hypertension should avoid rosemary.

Identification and cultivation

Woody stems are covered with needlelike, pungent leaves. Small purple-white flowers have protruding stamens. Rosemary is cultivated in gardens and available at most nurseries. Perennial. Grow from established plant or cuttings; difficult to start from seed. Grow in well-drained soil, full sun to part shade. Zones 6–9.

Sage

Salvia officinalis

Also called garden sage, meadow sage, sage **Family** Lamiaceae **Parts used** Leaves

> *Many herbalists have exhausted themselves listing all the uses for sage.*

Organs or systems affected Lungs, skin, uterus, gastrointestinal system **Therapeutic actions** Stimulant, tonic, carminative, diaphoretic, bitter, astringent **Nature** Pungent, dry **Plant constituents** Essential oils, saponins, tannins, flavonoids, bitters, triterpenoids, phenolic acid, resin, estrogenic sterols, calcium, iron, phosphorus, magnesium, zinc, vitamins A and C, riboflavin, niacin

Flower essence Helps those who are unable to move forward with life because they think they do not deserve good things, and those who have difficulty finding power and purpose in life

Medicinal uses

Balances bodily fluids Sage has a unique ability to balance fluids with the body, almost working in the way an alterative works—what is high it lowers and what is low it raises. Sage leaf's astringent action constricts fluids if someone is excessively perspiring, such as from menopausal night sweats or hot flashes. It can be taken hot to open up the pores and allow constrained fluids to flow from the body, such as with fever or for those who have difficulty mounting a sweat. In traditional Chinese medicine, blood is related to tendon health, and western herbalists often use sage for the person whose tendons seem sinewy and dried up. In the stomach and intestines, sage works as an astringent to lessen damp accumulations that present as gas, bloating, loose stools, and decreased appetite.

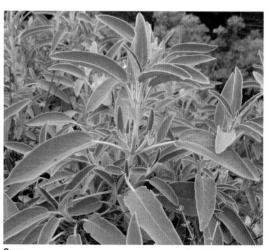

Sage

Supports gums, mouth, and throat When taken internally or as a gargle, sage is a go-to herb for mouth sores (cankers), gum disease, and sore throats.

Dissolves blood clots Matthew Wood (2008) has used sage in his clinical practice to treat blood clots. His experience is that sage dissolves clots safely without dislodging them, which would be the biggest concern with such treatment. Sage has a strong cardiovascular effect and has also been used to reduce painful varicose veins. Although I have no clinical experience with this, I would find it interesting to see its results on pathologies such as hemorrhagic cysts or endometriosis. It is also considered a heart tonic.

Calms anxiety Sage has traditionally been used to calm overly excited states such as nervousness, anxiety, and tremors. It promotes a calming sensation to the brain, which is particularly helpful for overthinkers.

Contraindications Sage is for short-term use only, unless combined in a formula. It should not be used for those suffering from epilepsy and should not be taken during pregnancy or if breastfeeding.

MEDICINE CABINET

Essential oil 1 to 3 drops, diluted with 1 ounce of a carrier oil, apply to abdomen, chest, or affected area as needed

Infusion 1 teaspoon per cup, steep 8 to 10 minutes covered, 3 cups per day

Tincture 1 dropperful, 1 to 3 times per day

Identification and cultivation

Quadrangular-shaped stems are covered with short hairs, as are the gray-green leaves, which are intensely aromatic, oval, to 3 inches long. Flowers are blue, lilac, or white, borne in racemes. Sage is typically cultivated in the garden. Perennial. Propagate stem cuttings in early spring. Grow in well-drained, sandy or loamy soil, full sun to part shade. Zones 5–8.

Schizandra

Schisandra chinensis

Also called Chinese magnolia vine **Family** Shisandraceae **Parts used** Berries

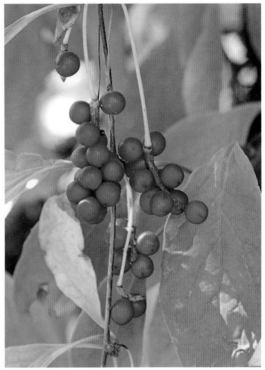

Schizandra berries

This adaptogen herb supports, nourishes, and balances adrenal function.

Organs or systems affected Adrenal glands, brain, heart, stomach, central nervous system
Therapeutic actions Tonic, astringent, stimulant
Nature Sour, pungent, bitter, salty, warm, dry
Plant constituents Essential oil, lignans, triterpenoids, acids, saccharides, sitosterol, tannins, resin, minerals, vitamins C and E

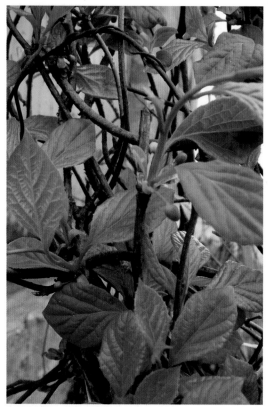

Schizandra woody stems

Medicinal uses

Supports adrenal glands Schizandra is indicated for the adrenal glands and hypofunction, often resulting in fatigue not relieved by sleep; body aches; light-headedness; loss of body hair; and digestive symptoms. The adrenals can be nourished with regular consumption of schizandra. In Chinese medicine, schizandra is called the five-flavored seed because it tastes sour, bitter, sweet, acrid, and salty. In the late 1950s, Russian holistic doctor I. I. Brekhman and his colleague I. V. Dardymov coined the term "adaptogenic" to refer to any herb that has a normalizing action regardless of the direction of the pathological state—in other words, what is high is lowered and what is low is raised within the body.

Helps promote sleep Schizandra has been used for centuries to help promote sleep and as a sedative. One study revealed a direct neurotransmitter effect on the brain, promoting sedation. GABA (gamma-aminobutyric acid, a neurotransmitter), dopamine, and serotonin were all affected, contributing to a sense of well-being. In Chinese medicine, schizandra is also known to calm the Shen, or the spirit of the person acting through the heart, leading to a peaceful body, mind, and heart. I believe its actions on the adrenals help decrease adrenal fatigue symptoms, one being insomnia.

Protects the liver Schizandra can be protective of the liver. It seems to function similarly to milk thistle and licorice root in providing direct support and nutrients to the liver cells themselves.

Contraindications Considered safe when ingested orally.

MEDICINE CABINET

Decoction 2 teaspoons per cup, simmer 10 to 15 minutes covered, 1 to 3 cups per day
Tincture 30 drops, 1 to 3 times per day

Identification and cultivation

Woody vines climb to 30 feet. Deep green, ovate leaves are arranged alternately. Sweetly scented flowers are small and white, produced in spring. Red berries form clusters in late summer to early fall. Schizandra does not grow wild in North America, but it can be easily obtained and is cultivated widely. Deciduous vine. Grow in slightly acidic, moist soil, deep shade. Zones 4–10.

Self heal

Prunella vulgaris

Also called heal-all, all-heal, wound wort, carpenter's herb **Family** Lamiaceae **Parts used** Flowers, leaves, stems

| *This plant helps us heal ourselves.*

Organs or systems affected Blood, mouth, skin **Therapeutic actions** Astringent, styptic, tonic, demulcent **Nature** Bitter, sweet **Plant constituents** Volatile oils, bitters, tannins, vitamins A and K, trace minerals **Flower essence** Helps one to make lifestyle choices that lead to wellness and wholeness

Medicinal uses

Reduces mouth and throat problems As a gargle or taken internally, self heal is regarded as a good choice to reduce dental decay, mouth ulcers, and tonsillitis.

Soothes wounds Self heal can soothe and heal wounds.

Treats animal bites Considered a necessity herb for all types of animal bites, self heal is often combined with other herbs to draw out bacteria or toxins as well as heal the tissue. Also recommended when an animal bites you in your dreams, to heal the dream wound.

Cleanses the blood In recent times, self heal has been used to draw out heavy metals from the body, perhaps indicating its relationship to cleansing the blood and supporting kidney and liver function.

Contraindications Generally regarded as safe.

MEDICINE CABINET

Infusion 1 or 2 teaspoons per cup, steep 8 to 10 minutes, 1 to 3 cups per day

Tincture 1 to 3 dropperfuls, 1 to 3 times per day. Gargle: 2 dropperfuls in 2 ounces of water as needed

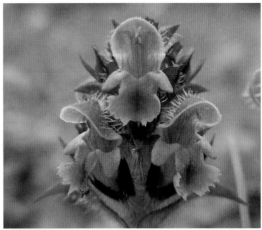
Self heal flowers

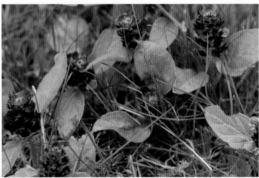
Self heal

Identification and cultivation

Creeping plants grow low to the ground on solitary or clustered stems. Lance-shaped leaves are serrated with reddish tips, growing in opposite pairs on short petioles. Purple, tubular, two-lipped flowers grow in clusters in summer. Abundant in pastures, farmland, waste ground, and lawns. Harvest in summer and fall. Listed as an invasive or noxious plant in some areas, so check before growing. Perennial. Grow in moist, rich soil, full sun to part shade. Zones 3–7.

Shiitake

Lentinula edodes

Also called Japanese mushroom, black forest mushroom, golden oak mushroom, oakwood mushroom **Family** Marasmiaceae **Parts Used** Enitire fungus

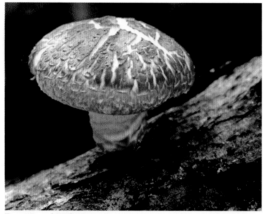
Emerging shiitake

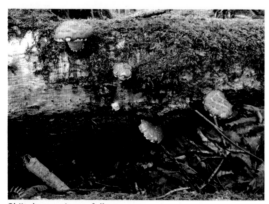
Shiitake growing on fallen trees

Another leader in the mushroom family that reduces cholesterol and has been reported to slow tumor growth.

Organs or systems affected Blood, liver, immune system **Therapeutic actions** Adaptogen, tonic, stimulant **Nature** Bitter **Plant constituents** Beta glucans, amino acids, volatile oil, protein, potassium, iron, vitamins A, B, and C **Flower essence** Assists those who feel stuck, stagnant, or uninspired in life

Medicinal uses

General cure-all In traditional Asian culture, herbalists have used shiitake to treat almost anything, for both people and their animals. Whether it was colds, flu, headaches, intestinal infestations, irregularity, cardiovascular insufficiency, or fatigue, shiitake was taken.

Lowers cholesterol Two of shiitake's principle constituents, eritadenine and beta glucan, have been heavily researched. Eritadenine in shiitake has been shown to reduce cholesterol levels by blocking the way cholesterol is absorbed into the bloodstream.

Slows or stops tumor growth Beta glucan helps fight off foreign cells and bacteria, and cancer researchers are noticing its immune-boosting effects as well. It has been reported to reduce tumor activity and lessen the side effects of cancer treatment. Another compound found in shiitake, lentinan, is believed to stop or slow tumor growth.

Contraindications Generally regarded as safe.

MEDICINE CABINET

Decoction 1 teaspoon powder per cup, simmer 5 minutes covered, 1 to 3 cups per day
Tincture 1 dropperful, 1 to 3 times per day

Identification and cultivation

The shiitake mushroom grows wild in Asia but is cultivated in North America. It is a medium-sized, umbrella-shaped mushroom, with a tan to brown cap, with edges rolled inward; the underside and stem are white.

Skunk cabbage

Lysichiton americanus

Also called western skunk cabbage, skunk weed, swamp cabbage, meadow cabbage **Family** Araceae **Parts used** Roots

> *This Native American plant is useful for respiratory illness and acute discomforts.*

Organs or systems affected Bladder, kidneys, central nervous system, respiratory system **Therapeutic actions** Nervine, stimulant, antispasmodic, diaphoretic, expectorant **Nature** Pungent, cool **Plant constituents** Volatile oil, lipids, resin, gum

Medicinal uses

Reduces lung congestion and coughs Although not used widely, this herb has earned its place as a useful respiratory agent, opening up the lungs, relieving congestion, and reducing bronchial spasms. Skunk cabbage has often been used in the acute stage of asthma to reduce symptoms. It is used similarly to treat spasmodic cough.

Heals ringworm Made into a salve, skunk cabbage is a traditional remedy for ringworm.

Reduces pain Although there is no scientific support for this use, Native Americans used skunk cabbage for the reduction of aches and pains, particularly musculoskeletal pain.

Contraindications Not indicated for long-term use.

MEDICINE CABINET

Decoction 1 teaspoon in 1 cup water, simmer 8 to 10 minutes covered, 1 or 2 cups per day
Poultice Apply to area as needed
Salve Apply to area as needed
Tincture 5 to 30 drops, 1 to 3 times per day

Identification and cultivation

Leaves are smooth, 15 to 20 inches long. Yellow flower spathes, to 15 inches tall, are among the first flowers to appear in spring. It gets its name from the bloom's distinctive skunky odor, which permeates the area where the plant grows. Found in moist woodlands and marshland areas and by streams and ponds. Biennial. Skunk cabbage grows from rhizomes. Propagate by division or separation. Divide offshoots and plant in the spring. Grow in moist, boggy soil, full sun to part shade. Zones 4–7.

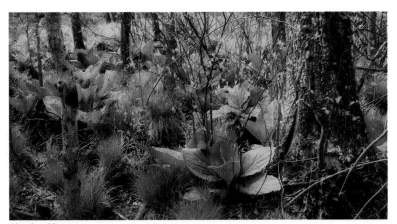
Skunk cabbage

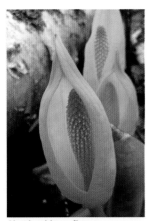
Skunk cabbage flower

Solomon's seal

Polygonatum biflorum

Also called true Solomon's seal, lady's seal
Family Asparagaceae **Parts used** Rhizomes

> *Solomon's seal provides appropriate*
> *tension and moisture to the body with*
> *an affinity for tendons and ligaments.*

Organs or systems affected Bladder, heart,
ligaments, tendons, uterus **Therapeutic actions**
Tonic, astringent, relaxant **Nature** Sweet, cool
Plant constituents Saponins, glycosides, mucilage,
tannins, trace minerals **Flower essence** Helps one
adapt to changes that have already occurred,
perhaps when one is struggling to adjust

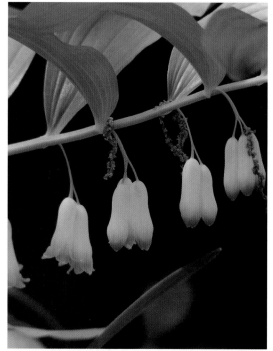

Solomon's seal flowers

Medicinal uses

Supports tendons and ligaments Solomon's seal
is a great example of the doctrine of signatures.
Much like the way tendons and muscles attach
around a bone, leaves and flowers of Solomon's
seal are attached around the stem. Solomon's seal
is known as a restorative and tonic for joints and,
in particular, tendons and ligaments. As we age,
tendons and ligaments often stretch and start
to deteriorate, leading to reduced joint lubrication and mobility issues. Solomon's seal can
strengthen tendons and ligaments and provide
lubrication to restore appropriate function and
support for joints, bones, and organs.
Helps heal uterine and bladder prolapse When
tendons and ligaments deteriorate, the uterus
and bladder can sag and prolapse. Solomon's seal
can help pull these organs back into their proper
place as it strengthens tendons and ligaments.
Balances heart rhythm Solomon's seal contains
some cardiac glycoside. Although it is not considered a heart tonic, it seems to promote calmness
to the cardiac rhythm.

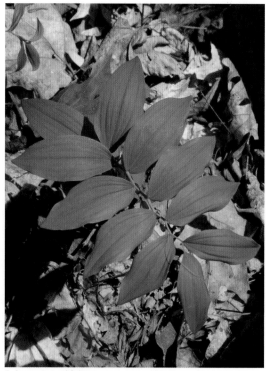

Solomon's seal foliage

Moistens dry conditions In Chinese herbal medicine, Solomon's seal is recommended for any type of dry condition in the body, such as dry tendons and ligaments, dry stool, dryness in the respiratory tract, or dry skin issues.

Contraindications Berries should not be eaten and can cause vomiting and diarrhea.

MEDICINE CABINET

Decoction 1 to 3 teaspoons per cup, simmer 10 minutes covered, 1 to 3 cups per day

Fomentation Steep 4 tablespoons per pint for 4 hours, or simmer 4 tablespoons in 3 cups for 10 minutes, covered, strain and soak cloth in infusion, apply as needed

Tincture 1 to 3 dropperfuls per day

Identification and cultivation

Slender, arching stems, 12 to 24 inches. Leaves arranged alternately on unbranched stalks. Small white flowers bloom in spring. Found in deciduous woodlands. Collect rhizomes in late summer or fall. Perennial. Propagate by dividing rhizomes. Grow in acidic soil, shade to part shade. Zones 3–9.

Sorrel

Rumex acetosella

Also called field sorrel, red sorrel, sheep sorrel **Family** Polygonaceae **Parts used** Flowers, leaves, stems

> *Sorrel has a long history of healing cysts and skin conditions.*

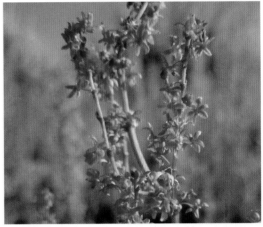
Sorrel flowers

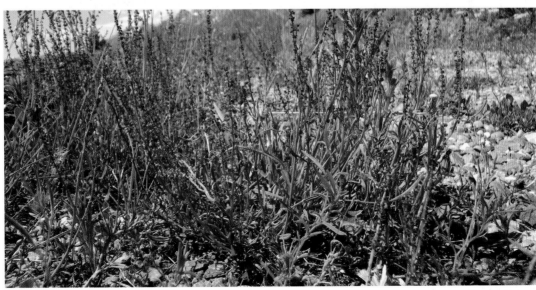
Sorrel

Organs or systems affected Skin, metabolic system **Therapeutic actions** Diaphoretic, diuretic, febrifuge, styptic **Nature** Cooling, bitter **Plant constituents** Glycosides, anthraquinones, oxalates, tannins, vitamins A, B complex, C, D, E, and K **Flower essence** Relieves the bitterness that arises when life seems desperately unfair

Medicinal uses

Treats cancer Sorrel's most common recognition has been for use in treating cancers. Originally cited for topical use with skin cancers, it can also be taken internally and is one of the original ingredients in essiac tea, used to treat certain types of cancer since the 1920s.

Relieves hot conditions Sorrel relieves hot conditions, reducing symptoms of excessive thirst, fever, or inflammatory conditions due to pathology.

Relieves skin afflictions Many skin conditions are hot in nature, such as boils and carbuncles. An external application of tincture or plant poultice is often helpful to pull out the driving cause of such complaints. When combined with vinegar, sorrel makes a wonderful treatment for ringworm.

Treats jaundice Taken internally, it has been helpful for treating transient jaundice.

Contraindications The presence of oxalic acid in the plant may pose risks for people with rheumatic-type complaints or kidney or bladder stones.

MEDICINE CABINET

Infusion 2 or 3 teaspoons per cup, steep 5 to 8 minutes, 1 to 3 cups per day
Poultice Apply as needed
Tincture 5 to 60 drops, 1 to 3 times per day, or externally as needed

---

Identification and cultivation

Long and slender, reddish stems grow 18 inches tall. Velvety leaves are arrow shaped. Male (yellow-green) and female (reddish) flowers develop on separate plants. Found in meadows, waysides, yards, woods, and pastures. When the plant is past its prime, the dried flowers and stems turn a deep red. Biennial. Listed as an invasive or noxious plant in some areas, so check before growing. Tolerates a range of pH levels. Grow in dry to medium soil, full sun to part shade. Zones 1–9.

Squaw vine

Mitchella repens

Also called partridge berry, checkerberry, winter clover, deerberry, hive vine, one berry **Family** Rubiaceae **Parts used** Aerial parts

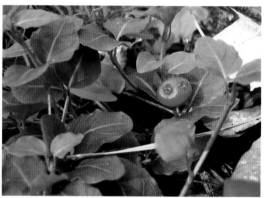

Squaw vine

> *Trailing along the forest floor, this little herb ensures a safe passage for both mother and child during labor.*

Organs or systems affected Bladder, uterus, gastrointestinal system **Therapeutic actions** Parturient, diuretic, tonic, astringent **Nature** Bitter, cool, dry **Plant constituents** Resin, wax, mucilage, dextrin, saponin **Flower essence** Provides support for initiating new beginnings

Medicinal uses

Supports uterus and pregnancy Squaw vine's most notable attribute is its ability to support and tone female reproductive organs, particularly throughout pregnancy.

Improves conception success Squaw vine helps to relieve congestion in the uterus and ovaries. Therefore, it can be helpful when conception is taking longer than desired by relieving constrained blood hormones or underfunctioning reproductive organs. This action has shown to alleviate pain associated with menses and may balance progesterone levels in the latter half of the menstrual cycle. Proper progesterone levels result in higher percentages of successful conception and maintaining conception.

Eases labor When taken in the weeks preceding labor, squaw vine helps create a smooth passage for both mother and baby during the labor process. During active labor, it stimulates and regulates contractions.

Tones bladder Squaw vine is used as a tonic for the bladder to help release urine retention and to tone the bladder muscle.

Resolves diarrhea Squaw vine's astringent action works well to help resolve diarrhea. I often blend it with Oregon grape for the sudden onset type of diarrhea with an unknown cause.

Soothes eyes Used as an herbal eyewash for tired, strained eyes. A good choice of herb to blend with chickweed after working too long on a computer.

Contraindications Do not take during the first and second trimester of pregnancy without a doctor's supervision.

MEDICINE CABINET

Infusion 1 or 2 teaspoons per cup, steep 10 to 15 minutes, 1 to 3 cups per day

Tincture 1 dropperful, 1 to 3 times per day, or 5 drops every 20 minutes until symptoms subside

---

Identification and cultivation

Slender, trailing vine, 12 to 24 inches. Dark green, shiny leaves arranged oppositely, oval shaped, evergreen. Trumpet-shaped, creamy white flowers with four petals bloom spring to fall. Red, edible fruit is dry and tasteless. Typically found in dry woods near hemlock. Harvest plants when in flower. This species is threatened and protected in some states, so check before harvesting in the wild. Perennial. Plant from seed or softwood cuttings. Grow in moist, acidic soil, shade to part shade. Zones 4–9.

St. John's wort

Hypericum perforatum

Also called goatweed, Klamath weed **Family** Hypericaceae **Parts used** Flowers

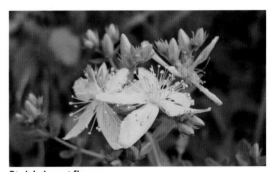

St. John's wort flower

A healer of troublesome wounds and nerve pain.

Organs or systems affected Bladder, heart, kidneys, liver, lungs, central nervous system **Therapeutic actions** Alterative, astringent, diuretic, nervine, vulnerary **Nature** Sweet, oily, warm, dry **Plant constituents** Phenolic compounds, terpenoids, hyperforin, hypericin

Flower essence A premier remedy that offers protection during the night and is indicated for a wide variety of sleep disturbances such as insomnia, nightmares, night sweats, and night-time incontinence

Medicinal uses

Soothes nerves Traditionally used for any ailment involving nerves and nerve pain, such as sciatica, radiating spinal pain, neuralgia, and rheumatic pains. In recent studies, St. John's wort has been helpful with neuralgia resulting from chemo-therapy. Everywhere nerves travel, including in the stomach and gastrointestinal tract, St. John's wort can be helpful. This also includes all the nerve bundles in the eyes, toes, teeth, and spine. It can be administered to support proper nerve firing and strengthen weak areas.

Detoxifies and strengthens organs St. John's wort has been used to strengthen the elimina-tive organs of the body. By focusing on the liver, it helps to clear morbid and toxic matter by encouraging it to move along and out through the bladder, lungs, large intestine, and skin.

Heals wounds Legends have been written around the healing properties of St. John's wort in the battlefield. It has strong antibacterial and anti-viral properties and is a good choice for dirty, septic wounds. It has been helpful for putrid or pus-filled wounds that are stubborn to heal, such as bedsores.

Improves disposition Much time and many dollars have been spent researching the antidepressant qualities of St. John's wort. It is classified as a nervine relaxant, but it can lift the spirits by affecting particular neurotransmitters that affect mood. Combined with other nervine herbs such as passionflower, skullcap, or oatstraw, St. John's wort can contribute to feeling calmer, more in control, and happier.

Contraindications Although research shows that St. John's wort does not act as a monoamine oxidase (MAO) inhibitor, there are many reported cases of adverse effects when St. John's wort is combined with some prescriptions. Consult your doctor before taking it. In addition, some birth control pills contain estrogen, and because St. John's wort may increase the breakdown of estro-gen, taking it while taking birth control might decrease the effectiveness of the pills. St. John's wort also increases photosensitivity.

MEDICINE CABINET

Herbal oil Apply small amounts to affected area as needed, 1 to 3 times per day

Infusion 1 or 2 teaspoons per cup, steep 10 to 12 minutes, 1 or 2 cups per day

Tincture 1 dropperful, 3 times per day

Identification and cultivation

Erect, woody stems are produced in the spring, branched at the top, sometimes with a reddish tinge. Narrow, pale green leaves are arranged oppositely, and translucent oil glands give leaves a perforated appearance when held against the light. Bright yellow, five-petaled flowers grow in dense clusters at the branch tips. Harvest flowers in early to late summer, depending on your altitude. Found in uncultivated ground, woods, hedges, roadsides, and meadows. Perennial. Listed as an invasive or noxious plant in many areas, so check before growing. Grow in slightly acidic soil, full sun to part shade. Zones 3–8.

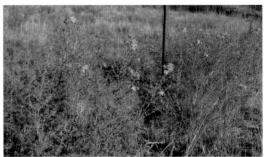

St. John's wort

Sumach

Rhus glabra

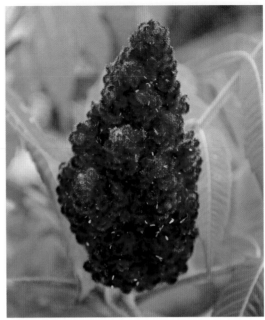
Sumach flower

Also called smooth sumac, scarlet sumach, upland sumach, mountain sumach, dwarf sumach, sleek sumach, staghorn sumach, Pennsylvania sumach **Family** Anacardiaceae **Parts used** Bark, berries

> *Used for all excessive watery states where discharges need to be toned and healed.*

Organs or systems affected Bowels, kidneys, lungs, throat **Therapeutic actions** Astringent, alterative, tonic, vulnerary, antiseptic **Nature** Sour, cold, dry **Plant constituents** Acid, calcium bimalate, oils, resin, gum, starch **Flower essence** Useful for the person who has difficulty connecting to the heart and who feels lonely and separate from others, when it seems that life has passed by

Medicinal uses

Tones the bowels Sumach works on the entire alimentary canal by gently cleansing and working as an astringent. It is particularly helpful in healing internal ulcers and inflammatory sores. The toning action works to pull tissue together and stop excessive discharges, which can have a positive cascading effect, leading to inhibition of any excessive discharge including urine dribbling, leucorrhea (vaginal discharge), diarrhea, night sweats, and internal hemorrhages.

Regulates blood sugar Sumach has an affinity for the kidneys and can be helpful for those with diabetes insipidus, or the excessive wasting of water, perhaps present with Type 1 diabetes. Studies indicate that sumach can help lower blood sugar levels by increasing cellular uptake, but more studies are necessary to substantiate.

Aids with organ prolapse Injections of a sumach decoction have been used to aid prolapsed uterus and bladder.

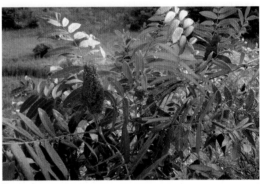
Sumach

Contraindications Generally regarded as safe.

> MEDICINE CABINET
>
> **Decoction** 1 or 2 teaspoons per cup, simmer 12 to 15 minutes covered, 1 to 3 cups per day
> **Mouthwash** 2 teaspoons per cup, steep 1 hour, swish for 2 minutes, 2 times per day
> **Tincture** 1 dropperful, 1 to 3 times per day

Identification and cultivation

Open growing shrub to 10 feet tall, with alternate, lanceolate compound leaves with serrated margins. Leaves turn scarlet in the fall. Tiny green flowers are produced in dense panicles in the spring, followed by large panicles of edible crimson berries in the fall that remain throughout the winter. Grows in thickets, woods, and barren wasteland soil. Harvest berries in the fall, and collect bark in spring. Woody shrub. Sow ripe seed in a cold frame. Grow in rich, moist soil, full sun. Zone 2.

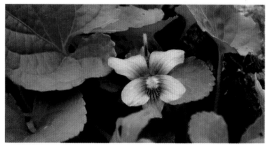

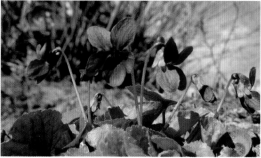

Sweet violet flower

Sweet violet

Viola odorata

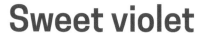

Sweet violet

Also called ordinary violet, common blue violet, garden violet **Family** Violaceae **Parts used** Flowers

> *One of the leading herbs researched for treatment of breast, lung, and intestinal cancers.*

Organs or systems affected Central nervous system, respiratory system **Therapeutic actions** Expectorant, mucolytic **Nature** Sweet, salty, moist **Plant constituents** Saponins, mucilage, salicylic acid, tannin, volatile oil, calcium, magnesium **Flower essence** Helps those who are shy and reserved to open up and share their warmth and sweetness with others

Medicinal uses

Reduces swellings and tumors Traditionally used for swellings and sores of the tongue, sweet violet can also reduce glandular swellings and dissolve tumors and nodules. This herb has been researched in the treatment of cancers, particularly breast, lung, stomach, and intestinal cancers.

Promotes elimination Syrup made from sweet violet is a superb laxative for children.
Moistens dry conditions Sweet violet has a very distinct moistening quality that does not lead to excessive accumulation of fluids. It works well for dry bronchitis conditions and intestinal dryness that leads to constipation or dry stool. It has also been used to help dry skin conditions such as dandruff and eczema.
Calms the nerves My favorite way to use sweet violet is as tea to calm my nerves. The beautiful color and scent are soothing before I even take a sip.
Contraindications Generally regarded as safe.

MEDICINE CABINET

Infusion 1 teaspoon per cup, steep 8 to 10 minutes. For stronger medicinal strength, 4 tablespoons per pint, steep overnight. Never use boiling water, which is too hot for the delicate properties of the flower.
Tincture 5 to 30 drops, 1 to 3 times per day

Identification and cultivation

Small plants, 4 to 6 inches, with dark green, heart-shaped leaves that form a rosette at the base. Deep violet or white aromatic flowers have five petals. Found in fields, hedgerows, and woodlands, especially in calcareous soils. Collect flowers in full bloom, spring to early summer. Perennial. Sow seed in autumn in a cold frame. Grow in well-drained, loamy or sandy soil, full to part shade. Zones 4–9.

Thyme

Thymus vulgaris

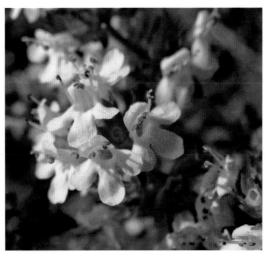
Thyme flowers

Also called garden thyme, whooping cough herb
Family Lamiaceae **Parts used** Leaves, stems

> *This inconspicuous little plant has strong antiseptic and antibacterial properties.*

Organs or systems affected Intestines, uterus, central nervous system, gastrointestinal system, respiratory system **Therapeutic actions** Diaphoretic, tonic, antiseptic, antispasmodic, carminative **Nature** Pungent, dry, bitter, sweet **Plant constituents** Volatile oil, bitter, tannins, flavonoids, saponins, resins **Flower essence** Helps to heighten the senses to be more receptive to the information that that surrounds us

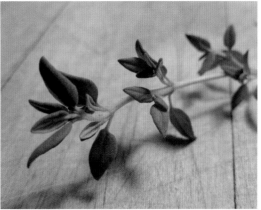
Thyme leaves

Medicinal uses

Soothes respiratory tract and throat Easily obtained by most households, thyme is a healing and antiseptic herb that has been safely used for centuries. As a respiratory tract and throat soother, it is often added to teas for singers and performers to help support their vocal cords. Traditionally used for whooping cough, its fast and effective approach offers babies relief and a good night's sleep.

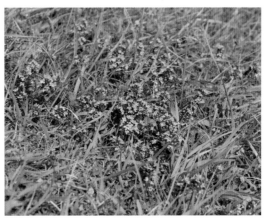
Wild thyme

Calms and relaxes The relaxation application is not only demonstrated in the respiratory tract, but also in the digestion, uterus, bowels, and uniquely the central nervous system. Thyme calms the nerves and sedates the body.

Fights infection Thyme is a good addition to any herb blend for helping rid the body of infection. It has been used with success against virulent bacterial invasion.

Contraindications Should not be taken during pregnancy or by those with a hyperthyroid condition. Thyme essential oil is irritating when applied directly to skin.

MEDICINE CABINET

Infusion 1 teaspoon per cup, steep 8 to 10 minutes covered, 1 to 3 cups per day

Tincture 5 to 30 drops, 1 to 3 times per day

Identification and cultivation

Small, shrubby plants grow 6 to 10 inches tall. Tiny green fragrant leaves arranged oppositely on stems. Delicate purple flowers grow on whorled spikes. Found in herb gardens, but some varieties grow wild in coastal regions. Perennial shrub. Sow seed directly in the garden as soon as the ground is workable. Grow in well-drained soil, full sun. Zones 4–9.

Tormentil

Potentilla erecta

Also called septfoil, cinquefoil, thormantle, flesh and blood, ewe daily, shepherd's knot
Family Rosaceae **Parts used** Roots

> *Tormentil is one of the best plants for toning and soothing the gastrointestinal membranes.*

Organs or systems affected Gastrointestinal tract, skin, respiratory system **Therapeutic actions** Astringent, tonic, hemostatic, nervine, sedative **Nature** Bitter, sweet, cool **Plant constituents** Tannins, acids, glycosides, resin, volatile oils, mucilage **Flower essence** Helps those who feel torment or long-term hopelessness

Medicinal uses

Tones tissues and provides astringent action Tormentil shines in its actions to tone a relaxed bowel and pull tissue back to healthy function. It is often used for acute diarrhea or any abnormal discharge from the body. Although similar to its cousin agrimony, tormentil provides a stronger astringent action with the added benefit of

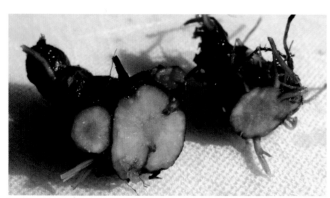

Tormentil roots

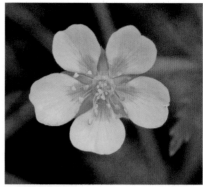

Tormentil flower

producing a bit of mucilage coating, making it helpful for the gastrointestinal tract.

Inhibits excessive bleeding and infection Tormentil is a good choice to slow or attempt to stop any type of bleeding, whether that be excessive menstrual bleeding, bloody stools, or external bleeding. It can clear excessive heat, which often makes such situations worse. It also reduces inflammation and has the potential to stop infection.

Relaxes and clears passageways Tormentil can positively affect areas of restriction, such as the respiratory tract when breathing is difficult, although it does not cure respiratory disease. An infusion sprayed into the nose or used in a neti pot helps open the sinus cavities and dry tissues. It is also recommended for stomach pains or intestinal gripping, releasing the tension and softening the abdomen.

Contraindications Some reports claim that large doses interfere with iron absorption.

MEDICINE CABINET

Decoction 1 or 2 teaspoons per cup, simmer 15 minutes covered, 1 to 3 cups per day, or 6 ounces every 20 minutes until bleeding slows or stops

Powder Externally as an herb cake, or drink 1 or 2 teaspoons in hot water

Tincture 5 to 30 drops, 3 times per day

Identification and cultivation

Low clumping plant with upright stalks, 6 to 12 inches. Glossy leaves are alternate, with three obovate leaflets with serrated margins. Bright yellow flowers with four notched petals bloom from spring to early fall. Grows in dry pastures and meadows. Perennial. Grow in well-drained soil, full to part shade. Zones 5–8, flowers in zones 5–6.

Usnea

Usnea barbata

Also called beard lichen, old man's beard, beard moss, tree moss **Family** Parmeliaceae **Parts used** Entire plant

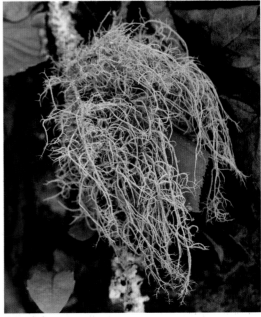

Usnea lichen

This wispy watcher in the trees has strong antibiotic properties.

Organs or systems affected Kidney, lungs, spleen **Therapeutic actions** Antimicrobial, antifungal, immune-modulating, demulcent, laxative, nutritive **Nature** Bitter, sweet, cool, dry **Plant constituents** Lichen acids, polysaccharides, mucilage, anthraquinones, fatty acids, vitamins, carotenoids, essential amino acids **Flower essence** Helps with personal boundaries, for those who believe they are giving away too much of themselves to others

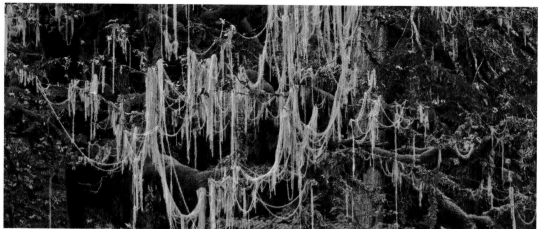
Usnea hanging from forest trees

Medicinal uses

Fights infection This herb is primarily an antibiotic that is especially useful for streptococcus (strep throat), staphylococcus (staph infections), mycobacterium tuberculosis, and other fast-growing organisms. Usnea seems to differentiate good bacteria from bad in the body, sparing the good gut bugs we need to fight infections. Usnea can also be used externally for outbreaks of staph and cellulitis and for infected wounds. It is safe to take with echinacea for a short period of time to boost the white blood cells and give the body a blast of immune support.

Fights viruses Laboratory studies have shown antiviral activity with usnea. It can help fight human papilloma virus (HPV) and cervical dysplasia, and it is a great treatment for systemic and localized yeast infections.

Contraindications Should not be taken during pregnancy. Rare cases of contact dermatitis with topical use.

Identification and cultivation

Shrublike fungus grows symbiotically with a host plant—usually trees, shrubs, or dead wood. Gray-green, round branches resemble hair or Spanish moss. Threads are coarse and dry, with a white elastic inner core (or hyphae). To identify the fungus, pull it apart, and you can feel the slight elastic stretch of the outer layer pull away to reveal an inner white material. Usnea grows in woodlands on branches or trunks of trees or on fallen branches. It tends to absorb pollutants such as heavy metals from the air, so collect it from areas where air pollutants are not present. Best harvested in the wetter times of the year. Almost any walk in the woods will encounter usnea. I recently went for a walk near some waterfalls, and it was like the usnea was throwing itself at me, almost begging me to take it home. Once you find plants in the wild, if there is an abundance, it may be difficult to stop collecting it, particularly if it's practically jumping into your collecting basket.

MEDICINE CABINET

Decoction and infusion 1 tablespoon per cup, lightly simmer 5 minutes covered, steep 10 minutes, 1 to 3 cups per day

Tincture 1 dropperful, 3 times per day

White oak

Quercus alba

Also called English oak, European oak, tanner's oak **Family** Fagaceae **Parts used** Bark

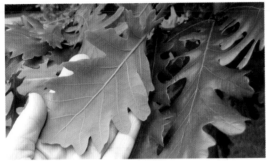

White oak leaves

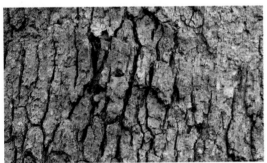

White oak bark

| *White oak is the master astringent.*

Organs or systems affected Bladder, gastrointestinal system **Therapeutic actions** Astringent **Nature** Cool, dry **Plant constituents** Tannic acids **Flower essence** A good choice for one who meets everything head-on and independently, also a healing essence to welcome in graceful surrender and support from others

Medicinal uses

Tones lax and deficient conditions White oak's high calcium and tannin content makes it one of the best examples of a pure astringent that helps tighten body tissues. Wherever there is a deficiency in tone or cellular vitality, white oak is helpful in returning proper structure to enable proper delivery of nutrients. Use for treating diarrhea, when a flaccidity has arisen and bowel health has been decreased; for gum and teeth inflammation and disease; for relief of chronic nasal congestion with post nasal drip; and for poor bladder tone with incontinence or urgency. **Stops hemorrhaging or bleeding** The astringent power of this herb can help stop hemorrhaging or bleeding, including nosebleeds, bloody sputum that is coughed up, and internal bleeding originating from the stomach. **Contraindications** Do not use externally if an extreme skin surface is exposed, such as a severe burn or wound. Baths are contraindicated for those with weakness of the heart muscle.

MEDICINE CABINET

Bath 5 tablespoons per quart, steep at least 1 hour, strain and bathe affected area as needed **Decoction** 1 or 2 teaspoons per cup, simmer 10 to 12 minutes, 1 to 3 cups per day **Fomentation** 3 tablespoons per cup, steep at least 1 hour, strain and apply saturated cloth to area as needed **Gargle or mouthwash** 1 or 2 tablespoons per cup, steep 1 hour, strain and gargle 1 ounce as needed **Tincture** 12 to 60 drops, 1 to 3 times per day

---

Identification and cultivation

Deciduous tree reaches 80 to 100 feet, with scaly, gray bark. Lobed leaves are 4 to 9 inches long with five to nine lobes, bright green on top, whitish below in summer. Acorns are produced in midautumn. Grows in forests with other oaks, but also found along edges of rivers and streams. Collect inner bark in late winter or spring. Deciduous tree. Grow in moist, well-drained, acidic soil, full sun to part shade. Zones 4–9.

Wild carrot

Daucus carota

Also called Queen Anne's lace, bird's nest root, bee's nest **Family** Apiaceae **Parts used** Entire plant

> *A beauty of the summer fields, wild carrot treats incontinence, bladder irritation, and stones and their associated pain.*

Organs or systems affected Bladder, kidneys, stomach, uterus **Therapeutic actions** Stimulant, diuretic, tonic **Nature** Pungent, bitter, sweet, moist **Plant constituents** Volatile oil, alkaloids, asparagine, carotene, glucose, pectin, vitamins E, C, and B **Flower essence** Supports those who want to strengthen intuition or telepathy

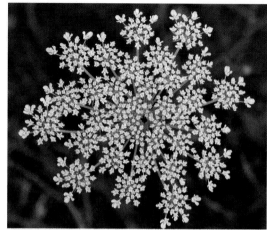
Wild carrot flower

Medicinal uses

Helps eliminate bladder and kidney stones Often used to eliminate all types of stones and gravel in the bladder and kidney, wild carrot is superior to most other herbs, even for stubborn cases. It also opens up urinary blockages.

Eases lower back pain For lower back pain caused by kidney issues, wild carrot may be worth a try if you're having no luck with other healing methods.

Reduces edema and restores bladder A powerful diuretic, wild carrot can decrease swelling in the lower portion of the body. It creates a natural elimination process, resulting in a copious output of urine. Wild carrot is reported to be a bladder restorative, helpful with bladder irritation and incontinence. It may also help to relax an overly stimulated bladder, reducing painful urination.

Stimulates digestion Wild carrot on the tongue can stimulate the gastric juices and digestive fire. It can also help reduce gas and gastric pains. A natural carminative (gas reducer), its volatile oils help move material through the gastrointestinal

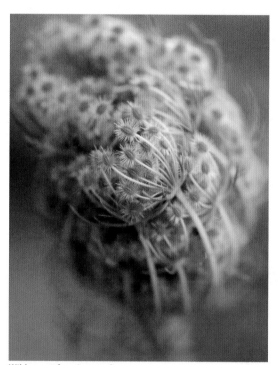
Wild carrot forming seeds

tract with greater ease and reduced flatulence.

Inhibits progesterone production and prevents egg implantation In the late 1980s, studies of wild carrot with mice indicated that it blocked production of progesterone and inhibited fetal and ovarian growth. Some recommend and use it as temporary birth control for humans. Information on wild carrot for implantation prevention has been recorded by ancient physicians Dioscorides, Scribonius Largus, Marcellus Empiricus, and Pliny the Elder. Present-day research suggests that ingesting tincture of wild carrot seed multiple times within 8 hours of conception can stop the process. Traditionally in East Indian culture, women keep a bowl of dried wild carrot seed on hand to inhibit pregnancy.

Contraindications Should not be taken during pregnancy due to uterine stimulant action. Some women experience breast tenderness, bloating, or cramping upon using wild carrot, and research shows this is good cause to seek other contraception methods.

MEDICINE CABINET

Decoction 2 teaspoons root or seed per cup, simmer 8 to 10 minutes covered, 1 or 2 cups per day

Essential oil 1 to 3 drops in capsule, once per day, or 1 or 2 drops topically

Infusion 1 teaspoon of herb per cup, steep 5 to 10 minutes, 1 or 2 cups per day

Tincture 5 to 30 drops, 2 times per day

Identification and cultivation

Herbaceous plant can reach 3 feet tall. Stems are covered in bristly hairs. Slightly hairy tripinnate leaves are finely divided and lacy. White flowers, blooming in early summer to fall, are small and white, clustered in dense umbels, with one central crimson floret. Found in fields, wastelands, and along roadsides. Collect seeds when they are still green. Biennial. Fast growing and an attractant to bees, butterflies, beetles, flies, and wasps. Grow in well-drained, sandy loam in full sun. Zones 3–9.

Wild cherry

Prunus serotina

Also called Virginia prune, choke cherry, rum-cherry, wild black cherry, black cherry, cabinet cherry, whiskey cherry **Family** Rosaceae **Parts used** Dried inner bark

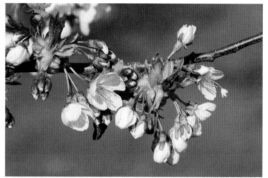

Wild cherry flowers

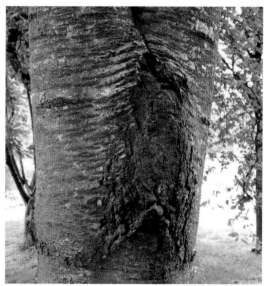

Wild cherry bark

Wild cherry bark is nature's natural cough killer.

Organs or systems affected Heart, lungs, stomach **Therapeutic actions** Sedative, astringent, pectoral **Nature** Bitter, pungent, cool, dry **Plant constituents** Flavonoids, bitter cyanogens, tannins, mucilage, resins, volatile oils, calcium, potassium, iron **Flower essence** Helps those who are feeling gloomy and pessimistic, and who dwell on the negative, to be more optimistic

Medicinal uses

Sedates and cools tissues The overall theme of wild cherry is to sedate and cool tissues in the body to allow organs to function optimally. Two constituents create the dual action of sedating and cooling: cyanogens and flavonoids. Together they work within tissues and organs to reduce heat, inflammation, congestion, and swelling. Wild cherry is effective where there is increased capillary irritation and blood congestion.

Treats wounds and irritations Wild cherry soothes any wound surrounded by redness, which indicates irritation at the cellular level, including external ulcers, punctures, and even pink eye.

Calms the heart Wild cherry is helpful in cases of anxiety and nervous heart palpitations. Taken as tea, it can calm the heart and slow the heart rate.

Stimulates appetite Wild cherry volatile oil is an excellent appetite stimulant and overall digestive tonic, particularly for those who have been ill.

Relieves coughs Cyanogenic glycoside, also known as prunasin, is one of the strongest natural cough relievers. It opens up passageways by

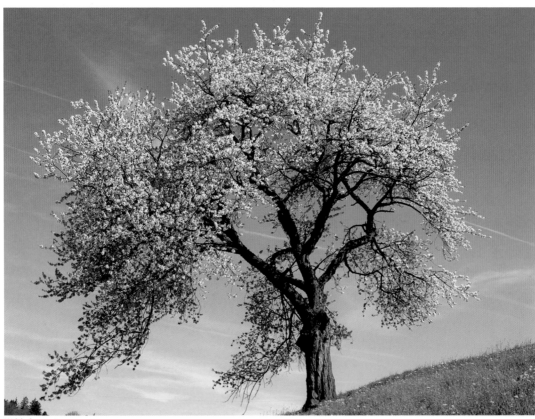

Wild cherry tree

reducing swelling, whether the problem is bronchitis, pleurisy, asthma, or tuberculosis. It helps expel phlegm and release tightness in the chest and throat.

Contraindications Extremely large doses for long periods of time can be toxic due to the cyanogen (cyanide) compounds. Why would we use an herb that is considered toxic? I have personally used wild cherry bark for years and have given recommended doses to others and have experienced no toxicity issues. And I am not alone. Herbalist Michael Tierra of Planetary Herbals has much historical documentation that shows its worth. Perhaps the old adage "the dose makes the poison" is best to keep in mind. Use only the inner bark and never the leaves.

> ——— MEDICINE CABINET ———
> **Decoction** 1 teaspoon per cup, simmer
> 8 to 10 minutes covered, 1 to 3 cups per
> day for acute situations
> **Infusion** 1 teaspoon per cup, steep 15 minutes,
> 1 to 3 cups per day for acute situations
> **Syrup** 1 teaspoon as needed
> **Tincture** 1 dropperful as needed

Identification and cultivation

Wild cherry outer bark is dark gray and heavily ridged on older trees; inner bark is light brown with netted striations. Shiny, bright green, oblong leaves are 2 to 5 inches long, with wavy edges. Small white flowers grow in clusters. Bark can be harvested in fall or late spring. It is important that you harvest bark from fallen branches rather than from a living tree; removing bark from a living tree can kill the tree. Cut a test patch on the wood, removing the outer bark layer to determine whether the inner bark can be easily removed in strips. Young, thin bark is preferred. Deciduous tree. Grow in acidic soil, full sun to part shade. Zones 4–8.

Wild yam

Dioscorea villosa

Also called colic root, China root, yuma, rheumatism root, liver root, devil's bones **Family** Dioscoreaceae **Parts used** Roots, rhizomes

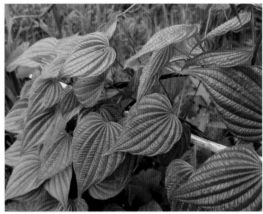

Wild yam leaves

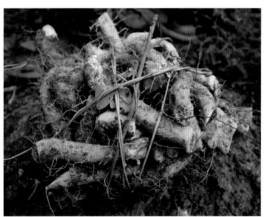

Wild yam roots

Nature's plant-based progesterone, with all the calm that goes with it.

Organs or systems affected Intestines, kidneys, liver, uterus **Therapeutic actions** Antispasmodic, relaxant, stimulant, antibilious, diaphoretic, expectorant, diuretic, hepatic **Nature** Bitter, astringent, oily, cool, dry **Plant constituents** Saponins, alkaloids, tannins, resin, starch **Flower essence** Helps one develop strong will-power to direct life in a positive way

Medicinal uses

Mimics progesterone Japanese scientists in the 1930s studied wild yam and its constituent diosgenin. They found that the diosgenin chemistry was similar to natural progesterone in humans. Wild yam is an excellent herb for balancing hormones and preventing miscarriage, and it can be an effective contraceptive (hence the development of oral birth contraception using progesterone). It can also ease nausea and vomiting in morning sickness with pregnancy.

Relaxes nerves and muscles Wild yam relaxes the central nervous system and smooth muscle tissues. It is used for muscle cramping, colic, gallstones, and intestinal irritation. Its relaxant function also treats over-excitability and nervousness.

Kills fungus One study of the steroidal saponins present in wild yam revealed a strong antifungal action that invades and kills fungus.

Contraindications Taking large amounts can induce vomiting.

MEDICINE CABINET

Decoction 1 to 3 teaspoons per cup, simmer 10 to 12 minutes covered, 1 to 3 cups per day

Tincture 5 to 30 drops, 1 to 3 times per day. To prevent threatened miscarriage, ½ to 1 teaspoon every hour up to 8 hours. For postpartum pain, 1 or 2 dropperfuls in warm water every 30 to 60 minutes.

Identification and cultivation

Slender, reddish brown, wooly vines, up to 9 feet. Cordate leaves, 2 to 4 inches long, have soft hairs underneath. Panicles of small, pale green flowers bloom in the fall. Found in moist woods and forests, often crawling over shrubs and fences and intertwining with thickets and hedges. Perennial climber. Sow indoors and transplant in early summer when in active growing phase. Grow in moist and well-drained soil, full sun. Zones 4–6.

Wood betony

Stachys officinalis

Also called bishop's wort, lousewort, betony, beefsteak plant, high heal-all betonica **Family** Lamiaceae **Parts used** Aerial parts

A nerve tonic, wood betony calms the mind.

Organs or systems affected Bladder, brain, liver, lungs, uterus, central nervous system **Therapeutic actions** Nervine, tonic, carminative, astringent, alterative, stomachic, aperient, antiparasitic **Nature** Bitter, cool, dry **Plant constituents** Alkaloids, glycosides, tannins, bitters, acids, essential oil **Flower essence** Helps those who are unable to ground themselves, and supports the ability to be present, take a breath, and slow down

Medicinal uses

Relieves irritability and stress Wood betony is known for its ability to cure almost any ailment of hysteria or depression, particularly when combined with St. John's wort. Wood betony is a consistent nerve tonic that relieves congestion of tension to move energy and blood and alleviate irritability and stress held within the body.

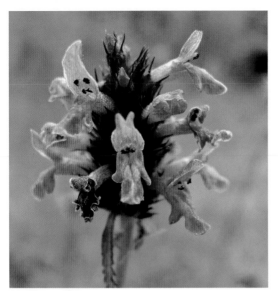
Wood betony flowers

Stimulates digestion The nerves in the stomach also seem to have an affinity for wood betony, which can be taken as a tonic when digestion is slow, with malabsorption of nutrients. Directly stimulating the nerves, it improves the gastrointestinal process.

Contraindications Should not be taken during pregnancy.

MEDICINE CABINET

Infusion 1 or 2 teaspoons per cup, steep 8 to 10 minutes, 1 to 3 cups per day
Tincture 1 or 2 dropperfuls, 1 to 3 times per day

Identification and cultivation

Slender, square, upright stems, 6 to 18 inches. Rough, hairy, lanceolate leaves are 2 to 3 inches long. Purple-red flowers are borne on a terminal spike. Grows in thickets and dry open woods. Perennial. Grow in any soil, sun to part shade. Zones 4–9.

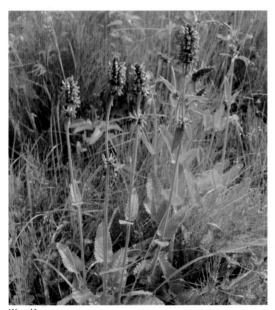
Wood betony

Clears the head It can clear the head of brain fog, dissolve headaches, and end facial twitching with consistent use. It opens and relaxes tissue and is also a good choice for acute head trauma because it increases microcirculation.

Wormwood

Artemisia absinthium

Also called absinthium, old woman, green ginger
Family Asteraceae **Parts used** Leaves, stems

> *Feeling overindulged in the belly? A cup of wormwood tea to the rescue.*

Organs or systems affected Central nervous system, gastrointestinal system, musculoskeletal system **Therapeutic actions** Tonic, antiparasitic, stomachic, stimulant, nervine **Nature** Bitter, pungent **Plant constituents** Volatile oil, bitters, flavonoids, tannins, acids **Flower essence** A shaman's tool that helps one move to the next level, especially during a vision quest

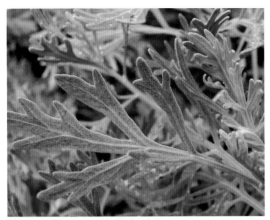
Wormwood leaves covered in fine hairs

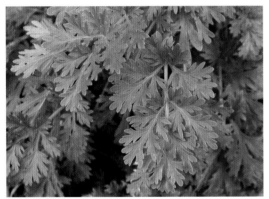
Wormwood leaves

Medicinal uses

Relaxes and stimulates digestion In another life, I worked at a small herb shoppe called Wonderland Tea and Spice in Bellingham, Washington. Every day I felt like I was in an herbal fairyland, blending teas, filling jars, and enjoying the customers who came into the shoppe. One of my regulars, an elderly gentleman, used to visit me every Wednesday. He and his wife had recently moved from Malta to Canada, which was a quick drive from the shoppe. His wife was very particular about what he was and wasn't allowed to eat, but each Wednesday he would come into town, have a hamburger, and then stop by and visit with me. The main purpose of his visit (other than creating the most lovely visuals as he talked about

his homeland) was to have a cup of wormwood tea after his meal. He'd used wormwood in Malta, and he knew it would help him digest the hamburger, rather than pay a terrible digestive price. Wormwood is excellent at removing stagnation from the gastrointestinal tract in a timely fashion.

Eases pain Wormwood liniment is great to get the blood moving where there is stagnation and soreness in the body.

Calms tension Wormwood further assists the digestive process by relaxing tension for expelling gas. Its relaxing quality makes wormwood a popular herb.

Helps with gastrointestinal infections Taken in moderate doses, it can be helpful in moving through episodes of food poisoning or gastrointestinal bacterial infections.

Contraindications Wormwood is very purgative and can induce extreme releasing from the lower bowel, leading to dehydration.

MEDICINE CABINET

Infusion ½ to 1 teaspoon per cup, steep 5 to 10 minutes, drink as needed
Liniment Saturate a cotton ball and apply to area until dry. For infections, use 3 times per day. For sore muscles, use 2 times per day or as needed.
Tincture 1 to 10 drops as needed

Identification and cultivation

Shrub with straight stems, 2 to 3 feet. Grayish, slivery leaves spirally arranged, 1 to 3 inches long, covered with fine hairs on both sides. Small yellow-green flower clusters bloom in spherical heads in early summer to early fall. Collect plants just before flowering, in prairies, dry pastures, light woods, and along footpaths. Perennial. Collect seeds dried directly on the plants; sow indoors before the last frost. Drought tolerant. Grow in well-drained, gravelly soil, full sun. Zones 4–8.

Yarrow

Achillea millefolium

Also called milfoil, thousand leaf, nosebleed, millefolium, ladies' mantle, noble yarrow, thousand seed, old man's pepper, soldier's woundwort, knight's milfoil, devil's needle, devil's plaything **Family** Asteraceae **Parts used** Aerial parts

> *Valued in Chinese medicine and planted around the grave of Confucius, yarrow is a powerful healing herb.*

Organs or systems affected Heart, liver, spleen, cardiovascular system **Therapeutic actions** Diaphoretic, diuretic, stimulant, astringent, tonic, alterative, vulnerary **Nature** Sweet, cool, dry, bitter **Plant constituents** Essential oil, alkaloids, tannins, resin, acids, inulin, glycosides, phytosterols, polysaccharides, lactones, flavonoids, rutin, saponins, potassium, calcium, magnesium, iron, phosphorus, vitamin C **Flower essence** When taken before, after, or during interactions, yarrow helps one acknowledge the necessary boundaries

Medicinal uses

Fights infections Studies show yarrow's antimicrobial and antiviral abilities. In this era when antibiotic resistance is growing, alternatives are necessary, and nature is providing us options. When yarrow was tested against five different types of bacteria (*Staphylococcus aureus*, *Escherichia coli*, *Klebsiella pneumoniae*, *Pseudomonas aeruginosa*, and *Salmonella enteritidis*) and two fungi (*Aspergillus niger* and *Candida albicans*), results indicated that it possessed a broad spectrum of antimicrobial activity against all of them. **Reduces serum lipids** One study showed that yarrow can reduce the levels of serum lipids (the fat that gunks up our blood vessels) and induce an immune response.

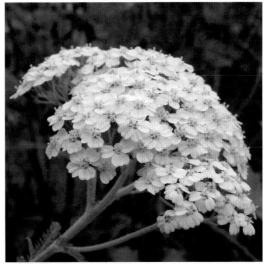
Yarrow flowers

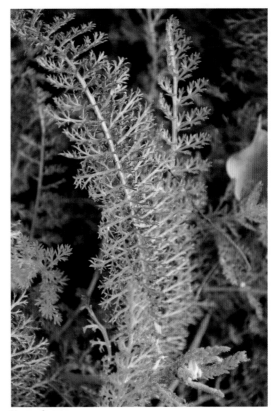
Yarrow leaves

Improves intestinal health Supplementing with yarrow leads to a reduction of pathogenic bacteria in the gastrointestinal tract, which can help to improve intestinal health.

Supports blood circulation Yarrow has a great affinity for the cardiovascular system, moving the blood to support parts of the body as needed. It is excellent for stopping hemorrhages that are bright red in color and for breaking up congested blood such as with bruises and wounds. With symptoms of chills and fever, use yarrow to direct the blood to normalize body temperature. This quality can also be effective in restoring harmony with the reproductive cycle, vitalizing the blood, and moderating menstruation. It's a great choice as a sitz bath for bleeding hemorrhoids and for bringing tone to the entire alimentary canal. Whenever the cardiovascular system is stimulated, typically the lymphatic system is supported as well.

Induces sweating When administered in small amounts, a hot infusion of yarrow will open the skin to induce sweating by gently raising the body temperature, which in turn purifies the blood of bacterial or viral toxins, which cannot survive with the increased temperature. I loved reading an account from herbalist John Christopher (1976) about his administration of yarrow to his daughter, who was sick with influenza. She had gone to their country home for a visit and had fallen ill, with a high fever, restlessness, and a headache. He had noticed yarrow growing nearby, collected it, and gave her hot yarrow tea, despite her initial protests. By the second dosage and within 20 minutes, she was perspiring freely. Within the hour she reported feeling better, and by morning she had recovered. This perfectly demonstrates the ease with which you can help someone with a safe, readily available resource with confidence in the knowledge of plant medicine.

Contraindications Avoid large doses during pregnancy. Allergic reactions in rare cases.

MEDICINE CABINET

Infusion 2 teaspoons per cup, steep 10 minutes, 1 to 3 cups per day, or drink 4 to 6 ounces until perspiration begins
Sitz bath 1 ounce per quart, steep 1 hour, strain and add to hot water in sitz bath basin, soak 20 minutes
Tincture 1 to 2 dropperfuls, 3 to 4 times per day

Identification and cultivation

Erect stems to 3 feet. Feathery leaves are evenly arranged spirally along the stem, slightly hairy, bipinnate or tripinnate. Tiny gray-white or rose-colored flowers bloom in a flat-topped inflorescence. Found along roadsides, in wastelands, pastures, meadows, and dry fields. Perennial. Propagate by seed or division. Grow in sandy, loamy soil, full sun. Zones 3–9.

Yellow dock

Rumex crispus

Also called curly dock, sour dock, garden patience, narrow leaf dock **Family** Polygonaceae **Parts used** Roots

Another liver and skin alterative with the added bonus of reducing bodily heat and increasing energy.

Organs or systems affected Blood, liver, skin, gastrointestinal system **Therapeutic actions** Alterative, tonic, astringent, cathartic **Nature** Bitter, cool **Plant constituents** Anthraquinones, quercitrin, tannins, volatile oils, calcium oxalate, acids, calcium, phosphorus, iron, vitamins A, B, and C **Flower essence** Helps to create powerful centering energy in crisis situations

Medicinal uses

Supports liver and lymphatic function Yellow dock is considered a good choice for liver and skin congestion, as it helps to dissolve hardness in the liver and opens pathways to improve the detoxification process. Acting as an alterative or blood purifier, it sweeps the body of impurities, can often treat difficult skin issues, and supports the lymphatic system.

Assists with mineral absorption Yellow dock helps the body assimilate minerals such as iron, for better absorption and utilization. Many experience more energy and decreased anemia from the use of yellow dock.

Decreases digestive fire Yellow dock is used to treat high digestive fire or excess fire in the middle region of the body, presenting as excess stomach acid, heartburn, belching, and bowel irregularities or pathologies. Chinese medicine refers to this as a damp heat condition.

Contraindications Those with a history of kidney stones (calcium oxalate presence) should avoid using yellow dock. Although it has been shown to aid many cases of diarrhea, it may irritate the situation.

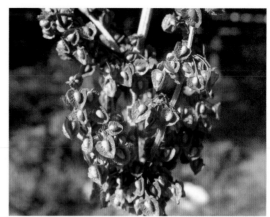
Yellow dock flowers

MEDICINE CABINET

Decoction 1 or 2 teaspoons per cup, simmer 10 to 12 minutes covered, 1 to 3 cups per day

Tincture 10 to 30 drops, 1 to 3 times per day

Identification and cultivation

Erect stems, 1 to 3 feet. Green, smooth leaves with rust-colored spots and wavy edges emerge from a basal rosette. Pale green, drooping flowers grow in clusters. Grows in yards, pastures, abandoned lots, and woods. Harvest roots in the fall, cutting the fresh roots into pieces. Perennial. Plant seeds in early spring. Easily self-pollinates. Grow in moist, rich, sandy loam, part shade. Zones 3–9.

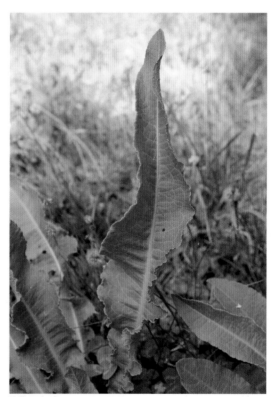
Yellow dock

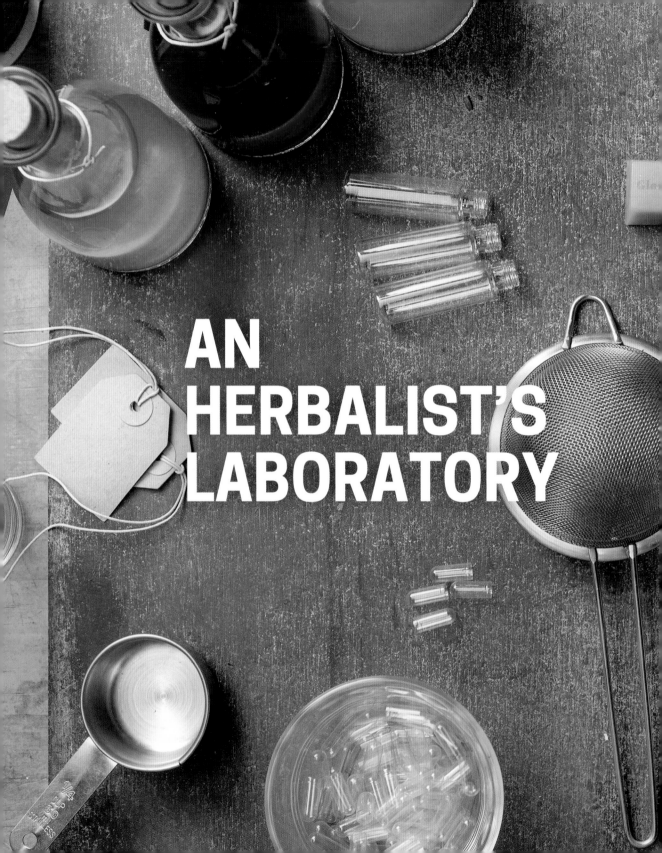

AN HERBALIST'S LABORATORY

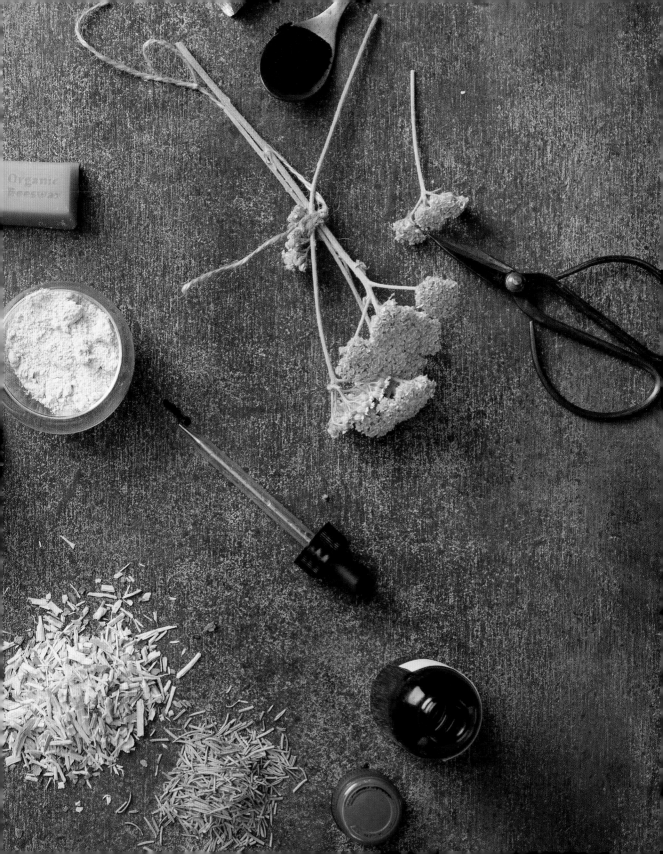

I am often asked which application is stronger in effect—tea, tincture, topical application, or capsule? My usual answer is that they all have the potential to be equally effective. It's all about the situation and how you use the herbs to deal with it. There are countless ways to use herbs for pleasure and as medicine. The good ol' pick, chew, and spit method is very popular around our household, especially with Cordelia, my 3-year-old daughter. She knows that for any kind of bug bite, wild nettle sting, thorn puncture, or other prickly encounter, there's nothing better to soothe the pain than some fresh plantain leaf, chewed up and spit onto the part that hurts. The fact that she can do this herself, and that she gets to spit, is a win-win for everyone.

As you read about different application types, you will likely be drawn toward some and curious about others. As you begin blending herbs, start with what you feel comfortable with, and don't be afraid to experiment. Will things go wrong? Inevitably. But that is part of the learning process for any herbalist. Consider starting with familiar herbal teas before you try a tincture. With time and practice, you will better learn when certain applications target the results you are looking for.

Creating an Herbalist's Kitchen

Imagine your own space, where you can whip up any herbal remedy at a moment's notice. By having some key supplies on hand, you'll be ready to concoct your medicines when you need them. There is nothing worse than thinking you've got everything you need, only to get halfway through a project and find you're missing some important ingredient or gadget. When I created this supplies list, I envisioned all the new and different herbal kitchens that might include these items, and all the wonderful medicines made as a result.

STERILIZE FIRST

Before you begin, sterilize all your cookware and storage containers to reduce the risk of bacterial and fungal contamination. Use the sterile mode in your dishwasher or place the items in boiling water. All your storage containers should be thoroughly dry before use. This little tip will help to ensure that your medicine lasts longer and stays fresher.

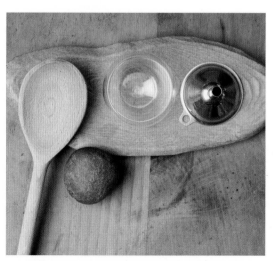

KEY KITCHEN SUPPLIES

Aluminum foil

Baking dish

Calculator

Cheesecloth

Coffee filters

Coffee or nut grinder

Cooking brush or paintbrush

Cooking thermometer

Crockpot

Fine mesh strainers, small, medium, and large

Funnels, small, medium, and large

Glass containers, quart-size with secure lids

Mason jars, pint and quart size

Measuring cups, small, medium, and large

Mixing bowls

Mixing spoons

Muddling bar

Notebook

Packing rod

Pencil

Percolation vessel

Plastic sandwich bags

Rocks or paperweights

Rubber bands

Saucepan, stainless steel or ceramic

Shot glass

Soaking basin

Stockpot, stainless steel or ceramic

Vitamix blender

Waxed paper

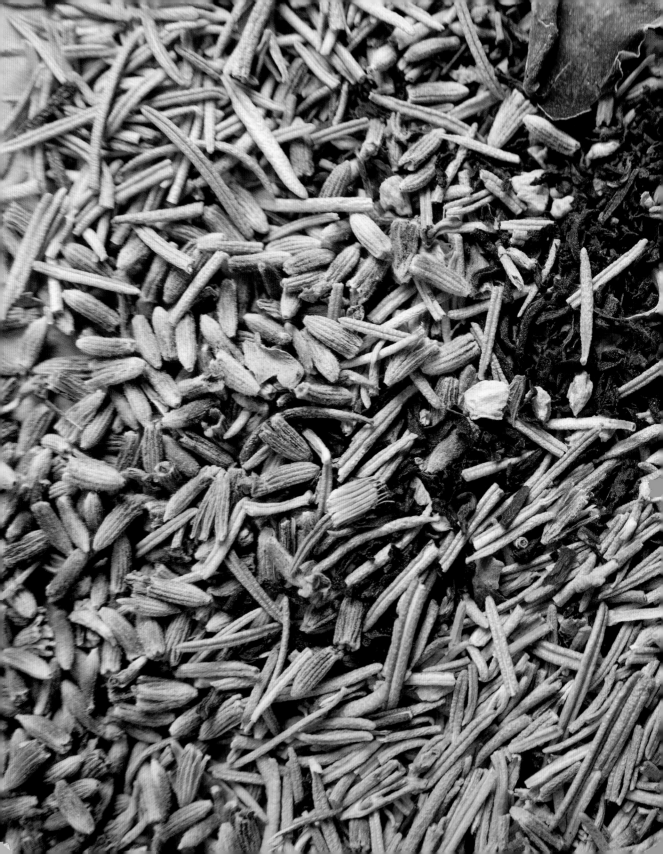

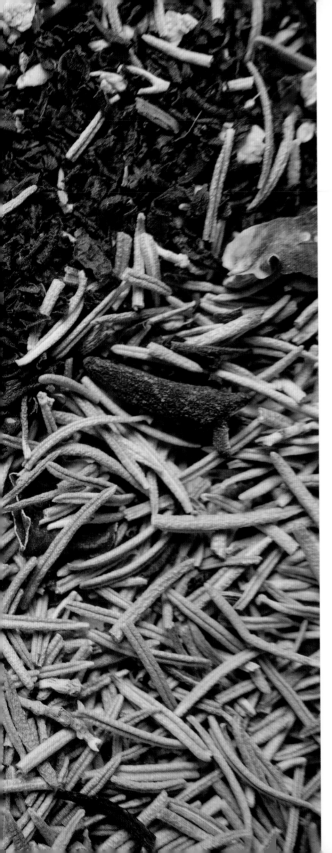

Formulating Herbal Blends

To use herbs to help with day-to-day ailments—
from an upset tummy, to a head cold, to anxiety
—you need to know exactly what it means to create a medicinal herbal blend. What's the difference
between a cup of tea and a draught? How do you
know which herbs to use and how much of any
herb to add to a blend?

Tea blends are a great place to begin, because
bulk herbs are readily accessible and the formulating concepts are easy to grasp initially when you're
working with raw materials. You also get to learn
about herbal flavor combinations and visually
experience what good blends look like. If you've
ever tried Chinese herbs, you know they often
work amazingly well, but they can be quite
challenging to the taste buds. One of the best
things about working with western herbs is that
you can make any tea blend taste good. By adding
herbs such as lemongrass, cinnamon, orange peel,
mint, clove, lavender, red raspberry, fennel, anise,
thyme, and licorice, you can create a real palate
pleaser. The other fun thing about making tea is
you have a little wiggle room to add finishing
touches, such as flowers, to enliven the color or
beauty of the blend.

Learning to make a medicinal tea blend is like
learning to cook. You need to know your ingredients and know which ones work well together in
both flavor and function. Keep in mind that tea
blends are medicinal blends. Even a cup of
chamomile tea has a relaxing effect on the body.
When you're formulating a tea blend, decide what
you want it to do from a medicinal perspective and
think about how you'd like it to taste. Do you want
to relieve the sinus pressure of a head cold or

soothe a tummy ache? Knowing your objective gives the blend purpose and helps you choose herbs appropriately. Blending with focus takes you beyond the basics of your first herbal experiences. With a bit of practice, you'll create some of the yummiest teas on the block.

Basic formulation components

Whether you are making a tea, a tincture, an oil, or a capsule blend, the basic formulation components are the same. Any good herbal blend includes three components: a main action herb or herbs, a nourishing agent, and a stimulating herb or herbs.

The main action herb is the leader, or the focus, of the blend. It directs and facilitates the rest of the herbs to be aimed to the part of the body for which they have an affinity. Many herbs are specifically aligned with certain tissues, organs, or systems and work to improve their overall function. You can choose one main herb, but some blends can have two or three. Typically, the action herb makes up 60 to 75 percent of the total formula. This clearly designates it as the driving force for the blend.

Any time there is disharmony in your health, something in your body is probably not being nourished as it should. Nourishing herbs bring in specific elements such as vitamins, toning minerals, and soothing properties. These herbs can also have an affinity for a particular organ or system. By providing the supporting elements for tissues, organs, or functions, these herbs help the targeted system operate more proficiently. Nourishing herbs can also serve as a buffer from other herbs in a blend. For example, when you use a purgative herb such as cascara sagrada to help eliminate the bowels, it often causes irritation to the mucous membranes in the gut. Adding a nourishing herb such as chickweed to the blend will help to soothe and buffer the irritating action. Usually, one or two nourishing herbs make up 10 to 25 percent of the blend.

The last component to consider is the stimulant herb group. These herbs bring the blend to life by creating an activating, stimulating, or eliminating action to the formula. I like to think of this group as the bus driver who picks up all the other herbs and drives them where they need to go, honking the horn the whole time to wake up the body. Perhaps the bus is also filled with cheerleaders who get everyone all riled up for the big game. These herbs are often classified as herbal stimulants, diaphoretics, diuretics, purgatives, or energizers. One or two stimulants make up 10 to 20 percent of the blend.

Get started with herbal blends

After you choose the herbs, the fun part begins. I suggest you start by choosing herbs you are familiar with in function to encourage your confidence in practicing the art of herbal creations. I always appreciate simple examples when it comes to learning something new, so I've come up with three examples to help you get the ball rolling. Hopefully, these will give you a clearer understanding of how to blend herbs for medicinal purposes. Each formula shows the three components and their percentages in the blend. Don't get hung up on the percentage amounts of each herb. As long as you're within the guidelines of the recommended percentages, you can use whatever amounts you want.

HERBAL BLEND FOR ACNE

Main action herbs Plantain leaf (30 percent) and calendula flower (30 percent). Plantain protects the skin and promotes new skin cell growth, and calendula promotes skin healing. **Nourishing herbs** Nettle leaf (10 percent) and dandelion root (15 percent). Nettles provide a bounty of nourishment for the body, and dandelion root supports liver function, which supports healthy skin. **Stimulating herbs** Licorice (10 percent) and ginger (5 percent). Both herbs are great stimulators that help the body remove waste.

HERBAL BLEND FOR A CHEST COLD WITH COUGH

Main action herbs Horehound (35 percent) and wild cherry bark (30 percent). Horehound is an expectorant that helps discharge congestive materials from the lungs. Wild cherry bark is an expectorant with a slight sedative action that helps move materials up and out of the lungs, while also soothing and calming a repetitive cough. **Nourishing herbs** Elecampane (10 percent) and coltsfoot (5 percent). Elecampane is one of the best herbs for supporting respiratory function and providing overall tone to the lungs. Coltsfoot is not only rich in vitamins A, C, and B, but it also contains the minerals calcium, potassium, and zinc and provides excellent support to respiratory health. **Stimulating herb** Peppermint (20 percent). Peppermint opens up the body and provides cooling to reduce congested heat and release trapped phlegm.

HERBAL BLEND FOR INSOMNIA

Main action herbs Lemon balm (30 percent), chamomile (15 percent), and California poppy (20 percent). All three herbs are premiere sedatives with little or no side effects. They work on the central nervous system to promote relaxation in both mind and body. **Nourishing herbs** Passionflower (10 percent) and schizandra (10 percent). Passionflower is a great nurturer of the central nervous system and helps control overstimulation, which often leads to twitching and restlessness. Schizandra provides nourishment to the adrenal glands, which, when underfunctioning, can cause insomnia. You can also add a bit of skullcap, another nervine, which is an excellent relaxer of what I refer to as "monkey mind"—when you lie in bed and your mind starts jumping all around, reminding you of all the things on your to-do list. **Stimulating herb** Peppermint (15 percent). Peppermint produces both the stimulant action needed and an overall soothing quality to the nerves, making it both a stimulant and relaxant.

Try one of these examples, or open your herbal cabinet and create one on your own. Start with three herbs you currently have and enjoy. Write out the blend and assign each herb its place in the blend: main action, nourishing, or stimulating. Perhaps you already have a favorite blend. Take a look at the ingredients and identify the components. As you create blends, always keep good notes and records of your herbal recipes, because there is nothing worse than formulating the perfect blend and then forgetting what you put in it!

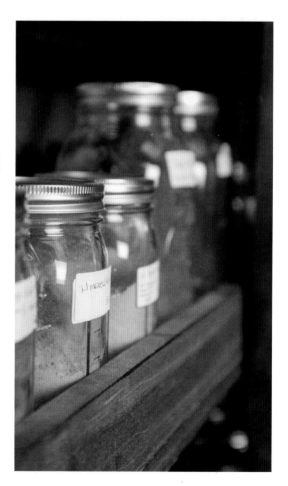

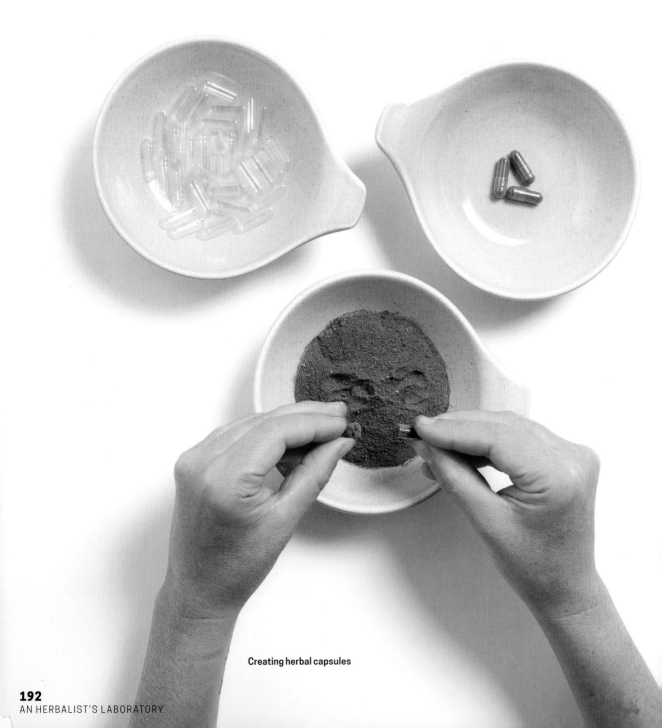

Creating herbal capsules

Delivering the Herbs
Herbal Applications

I have a feeling you are excited and ready to get your hands moving and making some useful and healing herbal medicine. Finally, you get your chance to be creative! Here I provide a list of supplies and instructions on how to make each of the primary herbal application types, from capsules to vinegars. You can make all of these applications at home, and all are appropriate for general consumption to help with day-to-day complaints.

Capsules

Capsules deliver the herbs directly to the stomach. They are convenient and travel well, and they are easy for most people to take—in fact, many prefer taking capsules over herbs in a tea or another formulation, especially when the herbs are not particularly tasty. One caveat regarding capsules, however, is that if malabsorption is an issue for you, capsules may not be the best choice for delivering the benefits of the herbs. If your gastrointestinal system isn't up to par, you'll lose most of the benefits through the elimination system.

Capsules are typically made of gelatin. Everyone has their preference, but I prefer vegetable gelatin capsules over the types processed from animal collagens, because I believe they are easier to absorb and of a cleaner origin. They come in various sizes and types, but the most common sizes are 0 and 00. Capsules come preassembled, so you have to separate the two halves before you can fill them.

You can purchase powdered herbs for making capsules, or you can use a small coffee or nut grinder or a Vitamix to grind herbs into a powder. If you do it yourself, use common sense as to which herbs you'll be able to grind—your grinder won't take kindly to big, knotty roots. Instead, use leaves, flowers, and well-cut sifted roots.

Supplies needed Herb powders, capsules
Kitchenware Grinder or Vitamix, three bowls
Cooking source None

If you are lucky enough to have a local herb shoppe that supplies herbs in powdered form, you can simply purchase the powders and mix them together in a bowl. If you grind the herbs yourself, place them all in a Vitamix or put small amounts into a coffee grinder (preferably not one used for coffee) and grind the herbs to a powder. They may not be super fine, but that's OK, as long as they are small enough to fit into the capsules.

Put the empty capsules in one bowl and the ground herbal mixture in another. Then set up a three-bowl assembly line: capsules, herbs, and an empty bowl. Pull apart a capsule, with a capsule bottom in one hand and a top in the other, and scoop the ground herbs into both; then press the capsule back together. Place each completed capsule in the third bowl. With a little practice and patience, you can become quite efficient, easily creating 500 capsules an hour.

ALLERGY RELIEF CAPSULES

| 1 ounce rosehip seed powder
| ½ ounce nettle leaf powder
| ¼ ounce chrysanthemum flower powder
| ¼ ounce eyebright leaf powder
| ¼ ounce ginkgo leaf powder

Take 2 to 4 capsules as needed.

HEADACHE BE GONE

- 1 ounce white willow bark powder
- 1 ounce wood betony herb powder
- ¼ ounce ginkgo leaf powder
- ¼ ounce valerian root powder

Take 2 or 3 capsules as needed.

MONTEZUMA'S DEFENSE

- 1 ounce goldenseal root powder
- 1 ounce Oregon grape root powder
- ½ ounce myrrh powder
- ¼ ounce charcoal powder

Take 3 capsules as needed every 3 hours for 1 or 2 days.

TUMMY TAMER

- 1 ounce fennel seed powder
- 1 ounce slippery elm bark powder
- ½ ounce catnip leaf powder
- ¼ ounce plantain leaf powder

Take 2 or 3 capsules as needed.

Cordials

Cordials are tonics meant to be taken in small amounts, typically 1 ounce doses, to strengthen the body, mind, and spirit. This comforting and pleasant-tasting medicine can be made with any tonic herbs of your choosing, including herbs to help with digestion, sleep, the heart, or general well-being. Cordials are fun to make with friends, particularly during fruit harvest times, when you can add fresh berries or just-picked cherries to create a dynamic flavor and high nutritional value. Cordials can and should be enjoyed year-round. In the darkest part of winter, I often slowly sip a cordial by the fire. It creates a pleasant warmth in my chest and a peaceful feeling in my heart.

Most cordials range from 17 to 30 percent alcohol by volume, but they can include up to 50 percent alcohol, depending on the alcohol you use. Brandy is traditionally used, because its warm flavor harmonizes with most other flavors. Tequila, vodka, gin, pure grain alcohol, rum, whiskey, wine, and port are also good options. Just keep in mind that the better the quality of the alcohol, the better the end result.

Supplies needed Herbs, brandy (preferably) or wine, fruit (optional)
Kitchenware Quart jar
Cooking source None

For all cordial recipes, place the herbs and fruit in the quart jar and cover with brandy or wine. Let the mixture sit in a cool, dark place, shaking gently each day for 6 weeks. Then strain the mixture well and store in a cool, dark place. Enjoy often.

DIGESTIF CORDIAL

- ¼ ounce fennel seed
- ¼ ounce catnip herb
- ⅛ ounce cardamom pods
- 6 whole cloves
- 8 ounces brandy or wine

LONG LIFE ELIXIR

- ½ ounce agrimony herb
- ½ ounce damiana herb
- ½ ounce hawthorn berry
- ¼ ounce eleuthero root
- ⅛ ounce aniseed
- ⅛ ounce ginger root
- ⅛ ounce licorice root
- 12 fresh or dried cherries
- 32 ounces brandy or wine

WARRIOR HEART

1	ounce blackberries, fresh or dried
1	ounce hawthorn berries, fresh or dried
½	ounce ashwagandha root
½	ounce devil's club root
8	ounces brandy or wine

Draughts

Draughts are small doses of highly concentrated herbal infusions, decoctions, or tinctures that often don't taste good. A draught is typically very strong, and you drink just a small amount quickly—think of it as an herbal shot that you drink in one swig. Draughts are quick and effective medicines, especially in acute pain situations. For example, if you are experiencing kidney stone pain, taking a draught infusion of couchgrass, lobelia, and California poppy would taste intensely bitter, but it could quickly alleviate the pain. If you want to use powdered herbs, they often don't make the most pleasant-tasting drinks, but quickly downing 1 or 2 teaspoons of powdered herbs mixed with 4 ounces of hot water can create potent effects.

Supplies needed Herbal tincture, infusion, or decoction; clothespin for your nose
Kitchenware Shot glass
Cooking source None

Remember that concentrated amounts create strong effects. Draughts are often used in true times of need to relieve great discomfort, or when the body needs to be corrected—with food poisoning, for example.

THE COLD CATCHER
To catch the cold before it begins

1	teaspoon echinacea tincture
1	teaspoon osha root tincture

Add tinctures to 1 ounce water. Drink 1 ounce, 4 times per day for 2 days.

KIDNEY STONE RELIEF TINCTURE BLEND

½	teaspoon California poppy flower tincture
½	teaspoon Jamaican dogwood bark tincture
½	teaspoon marshmallow root tincture
¼	teaspoon juniper berry tincture
⅛	teaspoon dandelion root tincture
⅛	teaspoon turmeric root tincture

Add tinctures to 1 ounce water. Drink 1 ounce every 20 minutes until pain subsides.

WOMEN'S MOON MAGIC TINCTURE BLEND
For menstrual cramp relief

1	teaspoon crampbark bark tincture
1	teaspoon valerian root tincture

Add tinctures to 1 ounce water. Drink 1 ounce, 2 to 6 times per day.

Electuaries

An electuary can be a mother's best friend, a helper to get even the pickiest of young palates to accept herbs. To create an electuary, you mix herbal powders with something that tastes good, such as honey, fruit preserves (my favorite), or syrup, and roll them into a ball, creating an herbal snack or treat. They are a little tricky to make, and you'll need to practice to get the proportions correct, but the final product is well worth the effort. You can even hide cayenne in this application.

Although you can include any herb part, using herb powder or grinding the herb into a powder makes it much easier to mix with the base. Using a demulcent herb (such as slippery elm, marshmallow, or psyllium) powder as part of your blend will help it stick together better and adds a soothing quality to the preparation. Adding coconut can also help stiffen the creation. If you are using fruit preserves as a base, make a small batch to be quickly consumed.

Supplies needed Herbs, honey (or other sweet base), nut butter, coconut oil, demulcent herb (optional), coconut (optional)
Kitchenware Mixing bowl, grinder, storage container
Cooking source Stove

For all electuary recipes, mix together the herbal powders and then add a slightly warmed base—add just enough to create a thick paste. Keep a bit of coconut oil close by and rub some onto your hands to prevent the ingredients from sticking to you too much. Roll the mixture into balls. Some folks prefer a firm mixture, and others like them to be a bit pliable. You can consume them right away, but they tend to harden and become dense in 1 or 2 weeks. Store in a closed container in a cool place to ensure freshness.

I LIKE TO MOVE IT, MOVE IT
For cardiovascular support

- 1 ounce ginkgo leaf powder
- 1 ounce horse chestnut powder
- ⅛ ounce cayenne powder
- ¼–½ cup nut butter
- ¼–½ cup honey
- ¼–½ cup coconut

Mix herbs together in a bowl. Add equal amounts of nut butter, honey, and coconut, starting with ¼ cup of each and adding more until you reach the desired consistency. Pinch off 1½ teaspoon amounts and roll into smooth balls. Eat 2 per day for tonic effects.

NOT THE SOUVENIR I ASKED FOR
For eliminating parasites

- 1 ounce wormwood powder
- ½ ounce black walnut powder
- ¼ ounce slippery elm powder
- Honey

Mix herbs together in a bowl. Add enough honey to reach desired consistency. Pinch off 1 teaspoon amounts and roll into smooth balls. Eat 1 ball, 4 times per day for 5 to 10 days.

THROAT SOOTHER

- ½ ounce thyme leaf powder
- ¼ ounce rose petal powder
- 1 ounce slippery elm bark powder
- Honey

Place herbs in a bowl and add just enough warm (not hot!) honey to create a thick, syrupy consistency, like sticky dough or putty. Pinch off ¼ teaspoon amounts and roll into smooth balls. Eat as desired.

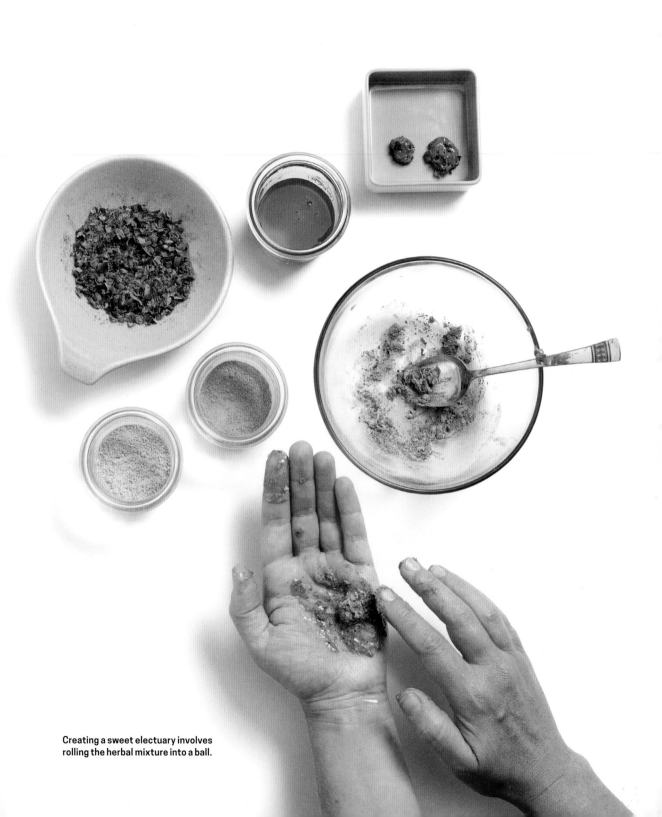

Creating a sweet electuary involves rolling the herbal mixture into a ball.

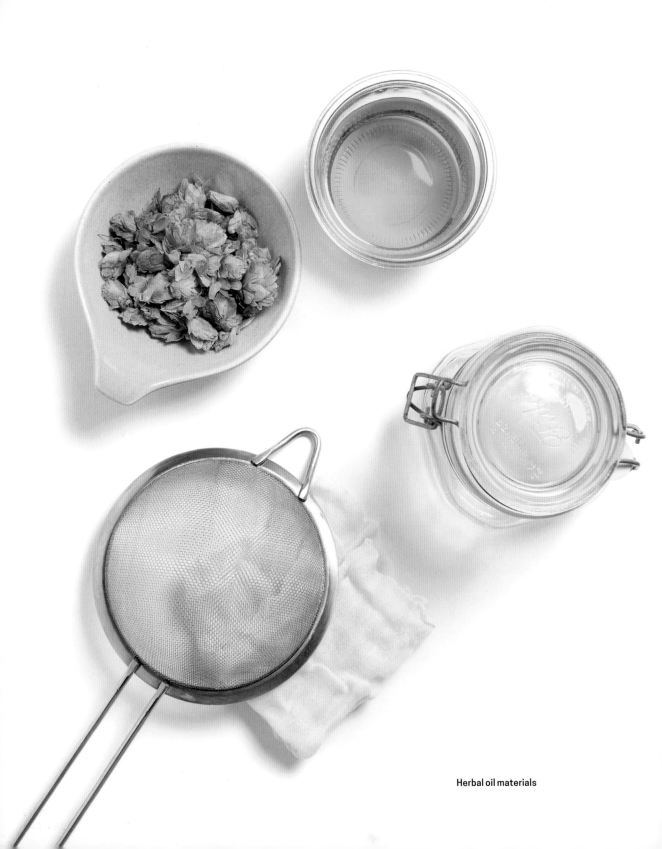

Herbal oil materials

Herbal oils

I love making herbal oils. When infused in oil, herbs create the most lovely colors and scents, and there are so many ways to use them. Herbal oils are made of herbs infused into a base such as olive, almond, avocado, jojoba, grapeseed, apricot, or castor oil. Not to be confused with essential oils, which are made through a distillation process that captures the volatile oils of an herb, medicinal herbal oils extract all the physical constituents of a plant into the oil medium.

Essential oils tend to be absorbed and then affect the body systemically as well as locally. When applied topically, a medicinal herbal oil penetrates deeper and focuses on the area in which it is applied. For example, a simple poke root oil massaged into the skin around the lymph glands is wonderful for helping to release blocked glands. At the first hint of a sore throat, I've noticed that my neck glands swell. If I catch it in time and slow down long enough to care for myself, just a couple of applications of poke root oil massaged into my neck can often nip a cold before it begins. Tattoo artists recommend herbal oils to customers to prevent skin infections and help healing. Massage therapists use them to promote anti-inflammatory actions and muscle relaxation. I often use herbal oils in place of lotions because they are readily absorbed, and bases such as grapeseed oil include natural antioxidants that protect the skin. Herbal oils are often used as the base of other herbal creations such as salves, creams, scrubs, and lotions. They are perfect to use on babies and kids, because they are often made with kid-friendly herbs and are a comforting application.

Although many dried herbs can be used in an herbal oil recipe, a handful must be processed fresh, including St. John's wort, arnica, California poppy, garlic, and mullein flower, because the medicinal constituents are depleted when the herbs are dried. You can use many types of oils as a base, but olive oil is the most common. Herbalists have varying opinions about the best methods for creating herbal oils, but in my experience, three methods work best and produce good results: the oven or crockpot method, the solar infused method, and the folk method. For all of the listed recipes, use the method you prefer unless directed otherwise. Because these methods involve using lower heat temperatures, any of the base oils are viable options. With a little research, you can choose oils according to their particular qualities for more specific results.

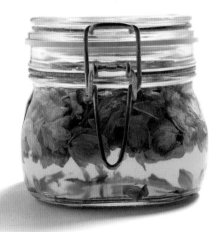

Hop strobiles being infused in oil

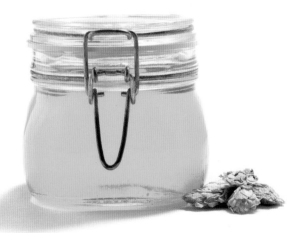

Finished herbal oil after hops have been removed

Like medicinal herbal oils, essential oils are therapeutic grade oils for the intended use of health and healing. Essential oils are created through a distillation process that separates the hydrosol (plant water) from the essential oil of the plant. The essential oil rises to the surface of the hydrosol and is then removed in its pure, unadulterated form—at least this should be the case. Be wary, however, of the essential oils you use and be sure to do your research, because some are better than others.

You can use essential oils in many ways, but I typically don't recommend applying them directly to the skin, because many are quite caustic. Although you may not feel anything negative after applying an essential oil full strength, microscopic evaluation has shown minute cellular damage from such application. If you want to use an essential oil topically, first dilute it with olive, apricot, or coconut oil. Some essential oils such as oregano, however, should never be used in contact with the skin. They are best added to a vaporizer or essential oil diffuser so you can simply breathe in very small amounts. You can also add a few drops to a bath or place a drop or two on your pillow. Many folks make tiny pillows to carry in a briefcase or purse, adding a few drops of essential oil to the pillow so it's ready for inhalation therapy as needed.

Oven and crockpot methods

The oven method requires higher heat and a shorter infusion time. Many believe you should grind dried herbs first to help break apart the cellular structure for easier extraction, but I don't think that is necessary. You should, however, ensure that the herbs are oil soluble. As the herbs are being heated in the oil, the aroma is intoxicating and creates a peaceful ambiance within your home.

Supplies needed Herbs, oil of choice
Kitchenware Deep glass baking dish or crockpot, kitchen towel, cheesecloth, quart mason jar
Cooking source Oven or crockpot

For the oven method, place the herbs in a deep glass baking dish and pour in enough oil to cover the herbs by 1 or 2 inches. If you like to be more precise, use a 1 to 10 ratio of herbs to oil. Stir the mixture well and place the dish in the oven at 150–170°F (65–75°C) for 4 to 6 hours, stirring every hour or so. Remove the dish from the oven, stir the mixture again, cover it with a kitchen towel, and let it sit overnight. In the morning, strain the mixture through the cheesecloth. Pour the herbal oil into a clean, dry jar, and store it in a cool, dark place.

For the crockpot method, place herbs in the crockpot and pour in enough oil to cover the herbs by 1 or 2 inches. The depth may be difficult to determine because you cannot see it, but you can stick your clean finger or a wooden spoon in to the bottom of the pot to get a good idea of the oil level. Set the crockpot on the lowest possible heat setting. Most crockpots get too hot, so make sure you use one with a very low setting, and leave the lid off or ajar. Heat the oil for 4 hours, stirring occasionally. Strain the mixture through the cheesecloth. Pour the herbal oil into a clean, dry jar, and store it in a cool, dark place.

Solar infused method

With this method, the sun heats the mixture to pull the herbs' medicinal qualities into the oil. Use only fresh herbs. After you hand-pick the desired herbs, let them wilt for 8 to 12 hours, making sure they do not dry completely.

Supplies needed Herbs, oil of choice
Kitchenware Two 1-quart mason jars, cheesecloth, rubber band, basting syringe (optional)
Cooking source Sun

Place wilted herbs directly into the jar. Fill the jar with oil in a 1 to 5 ratio of herbs to oil. Place a piece of cheesecloth over the mouth of the jar and secure it with a rubber band; do not put a top on the jar. Set in a sunny window sill for 2 or 3 weeks, shaking the mixture every day. After a couple of days, you may notice some gunk in the bottom of the jar; this is the remaining water from the herbs that has escaped into the oil. You can either decant the oil into another vessel or use a basting syringe to pull the gunk out. Check the oil every few days and repeat this process as necessary. When the oil is ready, strain it twice through cheesecloth. Pour it into a clean, dry jar, and store it in a cool, dark place.

Folk method

This is the easiest method by far. Instead of using a heat source, you place the herbal oil mixture into a paper bag, which raises the temperature a bit.

Supplies needed Herbs, oil of choice
Kitchenware Grinder (if using whole herbs), two 1-quart mason jars with lids, paper bag, cheesecloth
Cooking source None

Fill a mason jar halfway with dried, coarsely ground herb(s). Add oil to reach the top of the jar and close the lid tightly. Place the jar in a paper bag and set it in a warm place. Shake the jar several times per day for 1 or 2 weeks. Then strain the oil into another jar, secure the lid, and let it sit for a few more days. Strain the oil again with fine cheesecloth. Pour the herbal oil into a clean, dry jar, and store it in a cool, dark place.

CALENDULA FLOWER OIL

This antibacterial oil is good for cuts, scrapes, and wounds.

- 1 ounce dried calendula flowers
- 16 ounces olive oil

PHYTOLACCA (POKE ROOT) OIL

This oil relieves swollen or congested lymph glands.

- 1 ounce of poke root, coarsely ground
- 8 ounces olive oil

FRESH ST. JOHN'S WORT OIL

- Fresh flowering tops of St. John's wort
- Olive oil

Fill a quart mason jar three-quarters full with St. John's wort. Fill to the top with olive oil. Place cheesecloth over the top and secure with a rubber band. Set the jar in the warm sun for 14 days. Decant the oil every 3 or 4 days to remove accumulated gunk.

The castor bean (*Ricinus communis*) is known principally as a cathartic (strong laxative). A gentler use is in the form of an oil pack, placed over the abdomen, usually with heat applied. The gentle heat opens up the pores and pulls the castor oil into the body. The oil decreases inflammation, binds toxins or excess hormones for elimination, and stimulates the immune system. It is also absorbed into the lymphatic system, providing a soothing, cleansing, and nutritive treatment.

A castor oil pack has many applications, especially for headaches, liver disorders, constipation, intestinal disorders, gallbladder inflammation or stones, uterine fibroids and ovarian cysts, PMS, conditions with poor elimination, nighttime urinary frequency, and inflamed joints. It should not be used during pregnancy or menstruation, or if the person is bleeding.

Supplies needed Castor oil, white cotton or wool flannel pack material, hand towel, heating pad or hot water bottle

Cooking source Stove, if using hot water bottle Apply 1 or 2 tablespoons of castor oil either to a specific body part or the entire abdomen. If you are treating the abdomen, spread the castor oil from beneath the ribs to the pubic bone and across the chest. Next, place the pack material over the oil. Layer a towel on top of that (castor oil stains anything it touches, so choose a towel that you are donating to the cause). Fill a hot water bottle with hot water, or warm a heating pad to medium heat, and place it on top of the towel. Relax for 30 to 45 minutes.

Rather than using a hot water bottle or heating pad, you can sit in a hot bath after applying the castor oil to your body. Castor oil's high viscosity keeps it from washing off.

Liniments

Liniments are topical applications that can increase blood circulation and stimulate healing. Liniments are great for cuts, scrapes, boils, acne, sprains, strains, arthritis, bruises, and cardiovascular complaints. For external use only, they stimulate tissues in the promotion of relaxing, drawing, cooling, warming, cleansing, moving, and relieving pain. The results depend on which herbs you use and the goal you have in mind.

Supplies needed Herbs, menstruum (the substance, or solvent, that dissolves the herbs)
Kitchenware Glass container, fine mesh strainer or cheesecloth
Cooking source None

Many liniments use isopropyl (rubbing) alcohol as a menstruum, but witch hazel, grain alcohol, or vinegar can also be used. To make a liniment, place the herbs in a clean glass jar, and then add the menstruum. Close the jar tightly and let it sit in a cool, dark place for 2 weeks, shaking it once

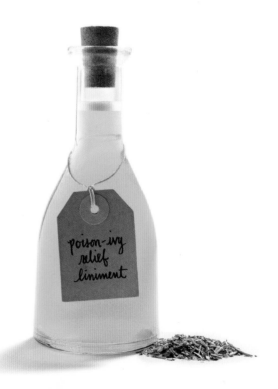

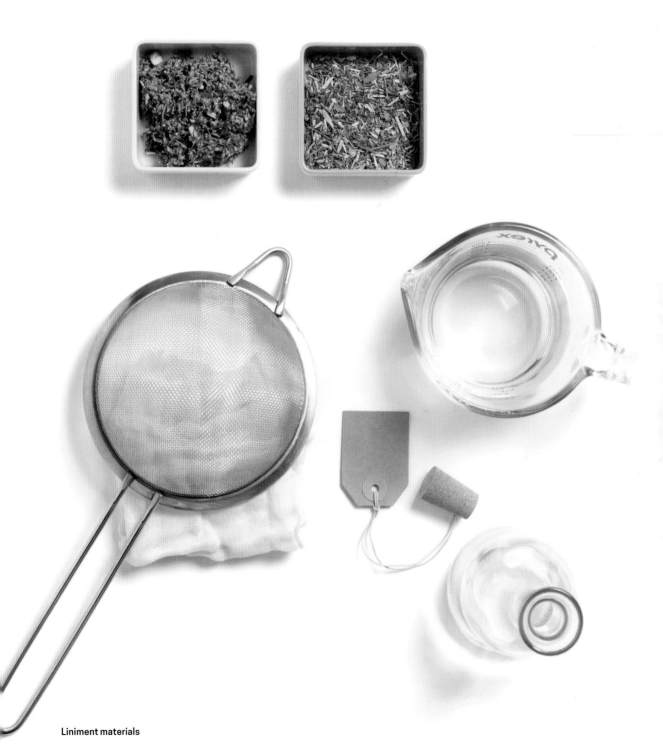

Liniment materials

per day. Then strain out the herbs with a fine mesh strainer or cheesecloth, and store the liniment in a clean, dry, glass container in a cool, dark place. Apply externally as appropriate.

KLOSS'S HERBAL LINIMENT

Jethro Kloss's herbal liniment from his 1939 book, Back to Eden, *is probably one of the best and most well-known examples of this application. A medicine cabinet must at our house, this simple liniment has antibacterial, anti-inflammatory, and antifungal properties, with both drawing and pain-relieving actions. It's also wonderful for treating fungal infections, boils, carbuncles, and scrapes, and we use it diluted for any wounds our animals might acquire.*

    1   ounce myrrh powder
    ½   ounce goldenseal powder
    ¼   ounce cayenne powder
    16   ounces rubbing alcohol

SORE MUSCLE LINIMENT

This liniment will greatly excite the skin and tissues to release muscle tension and move blood stagnation that is causing pain.

    ½   teaspoon cayenne powder
    1   tablespoon ginger root
    2   tablespoons poplar buds
    1   tablespoon peppermint leaf
    8   ounces rubbing alcohol
    8   ounces apple cider vinegar

ANTISEPTIC LINIMENT

    ½   ounce lavender flowers
    ½   ounce rosemary leaf
    ½   ounce chamomile flowers
    ¼   ounce calendula flowers
    16   ounces menstruum

Poultices and fomentations

Poultices and fomentations are two externally applied applications that help to alleviate pain, infection, swelling, and inflammation. There is nothing I like better than plucking an herb from my yard and using it immediately for medicine. Poultices are that easy—a direct application of the plant onto the body. You can use fresh plants, dried herbs, or powders in poultices. Chew up the plant and apply it directly, or mash it up in a bowl and add hot water to create a damp cake or paste. I call them herb cakes. Fomentations are strong infused herbal formulas made with water or vinegar. After saturating a cloth with the fomentation, you apply it externally where needed.

Supplies needed Herbs, hot water
Kitchenware Bowl, crushing tool such as a muddling bar, muslin gauze or cheesecloth, heating pad or hot water bottle (optional)
Cooking source Stove (if using hot water bottle)

Poultices and fomentations are suitable for strains, sprains, cuts, stings, burns, skin conditions, abscesses, and pain. Depending on the problem, I typically recommend using one or the other for 10 to 30 minutes at a time. I've found it helpful in some cases to apply gentle heat over the herbs or saturated cloth. When possible, combining an external treatment such as these with an internal treatment is your best approach to healing.

SPRAINED ANKLE POULTICE

    ½   ounce witch hazel leaf
    ½   ounce ginger root powder
    ½   ounce comfrey leaf
    ¼   ounce bay laurel leaf
         hot water

Add herbs and hot water to a bowl. Crush the mixture with a muddling rod and add tiny amounts of hot water as needed to create a thick mass of herbs. It should

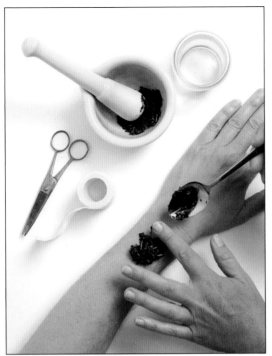

Applying a poultice for wrist pain

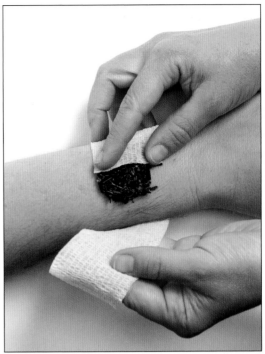

Gently wrapping with gauze

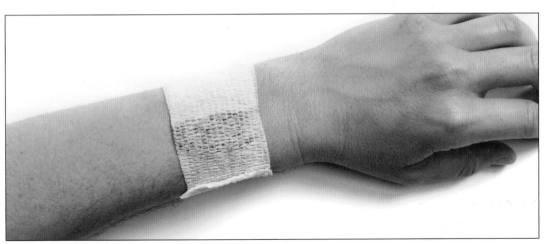

A wrapped poultice application

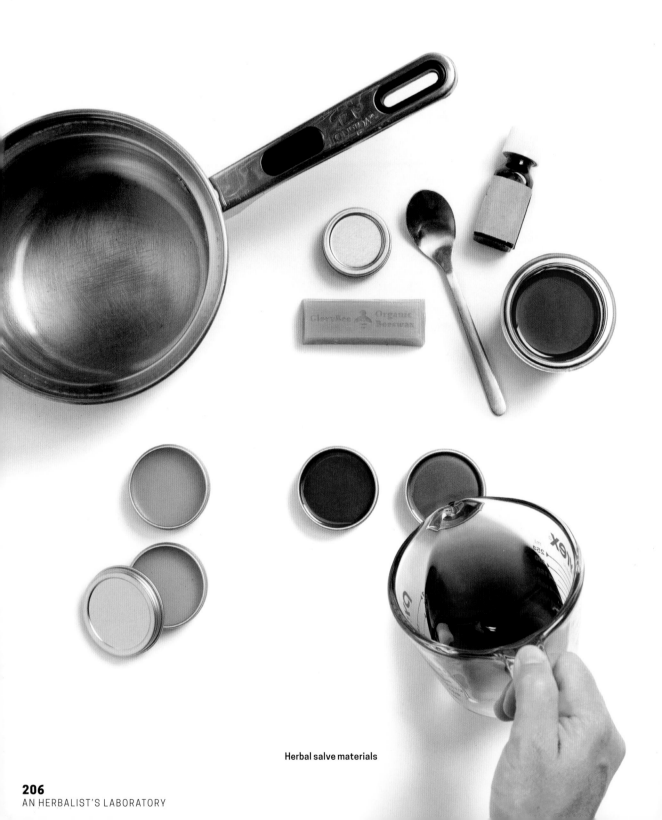

Herbal salve materials

not be runny, but thick like paste. It doesn't need to be pretty, and, yes, it is messy. After the mixture is the desired consistency and after checking that the temperature is suitable for topical application, apply a thick mass directly to the affected area. Cover with muslin gauze or cheesecloth for 30 minutes.

STINGERS STING AWAY

| 1 or 2 fresh plantain leaves

Chew up the leaves and spit the pulpy mixture onto the affected area. Keep it on for 10 minutes, and then reapply freshly chewed plantain as needed.

ABSCESS POULTICE

I use this often for my cat, who seems compelled to defend our territory from all other creatures. But it works great with the people folk, too. I sometimes place a slightly warm heating pad over the area to help draw out the abscess. In my experience, the abscess opens, and you can lightly press the area to drain the fluid. You don't want to allow it to close again until it is fully drained, so do not apply herbs such as calendula flowers or comfrey leaf afterward, because they will close up the tissue and trap the infection.

| ½ ounce mullein leaf
| ½ ounce plantain leaf
| ⅛ ounce lobelia leaf
| Hot water

Mix all herbs in a bowl and add just enough hot water to soften the herbs and thicken the mixture. Let cool to comfortable temperature and apply directly to the abscess, leaving it in place for 10 to 20 minutes if possible.

Multiple applications are usually necessary. Apply twice daily with gentle heat for 3 days.

Salves

Salves are basically herbal oils remade into a convenient, nonliquid form. They are a great way to deliver herbs deep into tissues. Although rubbing a salve onto affected tissue is recommended, I often use them for cuts and scrapes and leave a bit unabsorbed on top to create a protective layer—sort of a natural bandage.

Salves can be used for almost any problem and are safe for all ages. I can get really creative when making salves. My Boo Boo salve has special fairy sparkle dust on the top that my little girl loves. And I've created a stress-free salve that I use at work. When I'm feeling tense and overwhelmed, I rub a little into the back of my neck and on my temples to help bring things quickly back into perspective. I use my Calm Tummy salve when I've overindulged in my not-so-good-for-me favorite foods. Salves can be used for much of the same things as teas, tinctures, and capsules—they are simply a different mode of application.

Salve consistency is based on preference and consideration of use. Using an herbal oil as a base, you can add a little or a lot of beeswax to create a soft and greasy or a hard salve. In general, use ¾ to 1 ounce of beeswax to every cup of oil. This is the best starting point for consistency, and you can add more or less beeswax depending on your preference. Sometimes you'll hear the word "balm" interchanged with the term "salve." A balm contains a high amount of essential oils, often delivering a perfumelike aroma when applied to the skin.

Supplies needed Herbal oil, olive oil, beeswax, essential oils (optional)
Kitchenware Saucepan, stirring spoon, stainless steel teaspoon, refrigerator, glass measuring cup with pour spout, several 1 ounce glass or metal containers with caps, thin cotton kitchen towel
Cooking source Stove or oven

For each salve recipe, place herbal oil in a small saucepan and heat on low. Temperature is a very important consideration here, because if the oil gets too hot, it will burn and be useless. It should be just warm enough to melt the beeswax slowly. Use 1 part beeswax to 4 parts oil. Add the beeswax and stir continuously until it's completely melted. Remove the pan from the heat and dip a stainless steel teaspoon into the pan to collect a bit of oil. Place the spoon in the refrigerator for 5 minutes, and then check the consistency of the salve on the spoon. If the consistency is too firm, add ¼ cup of oil to the pan mixture and reheat. If it isn't firm enough, add ¼ ounce of beeswax to the pan and reheat. Perform the spoon test again until you reach the desired consistency.

After the salve reaches the desired consistency and temperature, remove the pan from the heat and pour the mixture into a measuring cup for easy dispensing into containers. This needs to be completed relatively quickly because the beeswax will begin to harden as soon as it is removed from the heat. Add any desired essential oils to the measuring cup and stir quickly. Pour immediately into small containers. Some say that if you are using essential oils, you should cap the containers right away to avoid losing the essential oil aroma through heat evaporation. I find, however, that if the jars are capped while the salve is still warm, the center of the salve collapses like a soufflé pulled from the oven too soon. I place a thin cotton kitchen towel over the jars to cool overnight, and then cap them in the morning.

BONK AND BOO BOO SALVE

Use the herbal oil you create in this recipe to make the salve.

- ¼ ounce calendula flowers
- ¼ ounce lavender flowers
- ¼ ounce chickweed herb
- ½ teaspoon bilberries
- ½ teaspoon comfrey leaf
- ½ teaspoon plantain leaf
- 1½ cups olive oil
- 1½ ounces beeswax
- 30 drops lemon essential oil

CALM TUMMY SALVE

Use the herbal oil you create in this recipe to make the salve.

- 1 ounce fennel seed
- ¼ ounce catnip herb
- ¼ ounce chamomile flowers
- ½ cup olive oil
- ½ cup jojoba oil
- ¾ ounces beeswax
- 30 drops lavender essential oil

BARKING DOGS SALVE
For tired feet

Use the herbal oil you create in this recipe to make the salve.

- ½ ounce fresh St. John's Wort
- ½ ounce valerian root
- ¼ ounce fresh California poppy leaf
- ¼ ounce black cohosh root
- 1 cup olive oil
- ¾ ounce beeswax
- 30 drops peppermint essential oil

Massage into feet for 5 minutes. Better yet, have someone else do it for you.

BABY SLEEP SALVE

Use the herbal oil you create in this recipe to make the salve.

- ½ ounce chamomile flowers
- ½ ounce lavender flowers
- ¾ cup olive oil
- ½ ounce beeswax
- 15 drops lavender essential oil

Rub pea-sized amount onto baby's head or body before bedtime.

Sitz baths

Sitz baths are a wonderful topical application that help to heal tissues, calm inflammation, reduce pain, and improve blood circulation. They involve the cardiovascular system to help carry away waste matter and bring in fresh new blood and its vital healing components. Sitz baths involve submerging the lower pelvis and buttocks in warm water and an herbal infusion for 15 to 20 minutes. They are best used multiple times per day for healing hemorrhoids, post labor soreness, a cold uterus, boils, urinary infections, or discharges. You can purchase sitz baths that fit into your toilet for comfortable support or purchase a basin from a pharmacy or drug store.

Supplies needed Herbs, water
Kitchenware Quart jar, cheesecloth, soaking basin
Cooking source Stove

Some recommend combining sitz baths with hydrotherapy, which requires alternating hot and cold baths to create a vasodilation and vasoconstriction action that helps moves blood, lymphatic congestion, and white blood cells to promote healing and regulate body temperature. In this application, you would sit in the hot sitz bath for 3 to 6 minutes, and then switch to a cold sitz bath for 1 minute, for 3 to 6 rounds.

For all sitz bath recipes, infuse the herbs in 1 quart of water for 4 hours. Strain the infusion through a cheesecloth and pour the liquid to the sitz basin with 1 cup of hot water. Submerge and relax for 15 to 20 minutes.

BOIL ON THE BUM

- 2 tablespoons comfrey leaf
- 2 tablespoons plantain leaf
- 1 teaspoon myrrh powder
- 1 teaspoon goldenseal root powder

URINARY TRACT SUPPORT
For occasional bladder irritation

- 2 tablespoons uva ursi leaf
- 1 tablespoon nettle leaf
- 1 tablespoon goldenrod flower
- 1 tablespoon pipsissewa leaf
- 1 teaspoon goldenseal root powder

MENSTRUAL MOON CRAMPING

- 2 tablespoons crampbark bark
- 1 tablespoon silk tassel herb
- 1 tablespoon black cohosh root
- 1 tablespoon valerian root

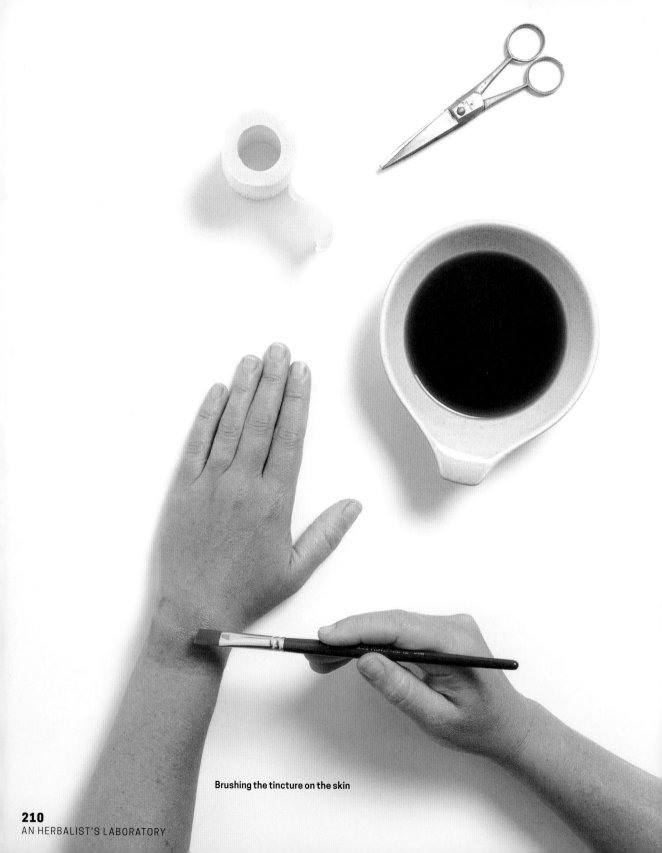

Brushing the tincture on the skin

Soft casts

A soft cast is an application of an herbal tincture painted directly onto the skin in several layers, to create a shellacked appearance. They are best used when the skin is intact, and they are not recommended for wounds that need to drain. Soft casts are recommended for poor circulation and for fractures when modern casting is not possible or desirable. Appropriate applications include broken bones (using comfrey leaf tincture), torn ligaments, inflammation, and vascular complaints such as varicose veins and spider veins.

Supplies needed Herbal tincture, cotton gauze
Kitchenware Bowl, cooking brush or paintbrush
Cooking source none

Pour the tincture into a bowl. Dip a brush into the tincture and brush a thin layer onto the affected area of the body. Let dry completely. Apply more tincture, layer-by-layer, allowing each layer to dry completely before applying the next. Continue applying layers of tincture until a veneer or sheen is present. Wrap the area lightly with cotton gauze to cover and secure the cast. Leave the cast on until the tincture is completely absorbed into the skin—note that this can take weeks.

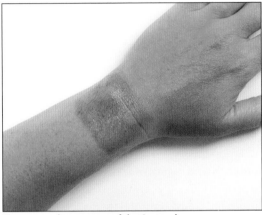
The veneered appearance of the tincture layers

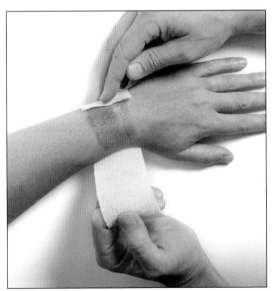
Wrapping the area with gauze

VARICOSE VEIN SOFT CAST
Use an equal blend of the following:

Horse chestnut tincture

Yarrow flower tincture

Gotu kola herb tincture

Witch hazel bark tincture

PLANTAR FASCIITIS AND LIGAMENT HEALER
Use an equal blend of the following:

Yucca root tincture

Turmeric root tincture

Devil's claw root tincture

Garlic tincture

Ginkgo herb tincture

Succuses

A succus is the result of grinding, squeezing, or mashing a plant to extract the fresh herb juice. This power-packed medicine delivers incredible healing potential, releasing the raw vitamins and minerals of the plant in their most vital forms when you drink the juice or apply it topically. It is a great option for those who want to avoid the alcohol content in tinctures, because it can be used fresh or with just a touch of alcohol added strictly for preservation purposes. On the downside, the herb choices are limited, because few herbs produce enough juice for this application.

Several succuses are worth particular mention. Calendula succus is a wonderful post-surgical site topical application that reduces the risk of infection, encourages tissue healing, and reduces potential scarring. Nettle and watercress juices are packed with minerals and are readily absorbed by the body when consumed, offering quick regenerating nutrition when needed.

Supplies needed Herbs, grain alcohol (such as brandy)
Kitchenware Food processor, Vitamix, blender, or wheatgrass grinder; herb press, pressing cloth, or muslin cloth; measuring cup; glass container; fine cheesecloth; bottle; label
Cooking source None

NETTLE SUCCUS

A great deliverer of nutrients with a powerful amount of B vitamins and trace minerals, nettle succus is helpful for those trying to gain strength after an illness or surgery.

Fresh nettle leaves

Brandy

Grind up the nettle to a mush, being sure to collect all juice produced during the process. Place the mush and juice in an herb press, pressing cloth, or muslin cloth, and using light pressure initially that increases with time, press the mixture through the cloth for up to several hours, depending on the herb and its quality.

Collect the rendered juice and measure it. Divide this volume by 3 to determine the appropriate amount of brandy to add for preservation (add brandy to equal one-third of the juice volume). Add the brandy and agitate the mixture well to mix. Pour into a jar, seal, and let sit for 4 days. Then strain with very fine cheesecloth—succus can produce excessive amounts of sludge after settling. Pour the succus into a bottle, add a label, and store it in a cool, dark place. Can be stored for several years.

Suppositories

Herbal suppositories are easy to make. They are helpful in providing direct application of herbs exactly where they are needed and in supplying herbal medicine to those who are unable to take nourishment through regular means. Use suppositories to target day-to-day problems that occur in the lower body, such as in the rectum, lower intestines, and vagina, or in the upper body, such as in the nasal cavity. Anyone who has suffered from hemorrhoids can attest to the severe pain they can cause. A soothing, direct herbal application will provide a welcome relief. Suppositories can also be useful for the ill or elderly who aren't able to obtain enough nutrients by eating. A nutrient-packed suppository can deliver vital food through direct absorption in the lower colon. In my office, I see a lot of middle-aged women suffering from irritation and lack of moisture in the vaginal canal. I prescribe an herb-rich, cocoa butter–based suppository to heal the tissues and cool inflammation. For men, a suppository inserted into the rectal canal can help soothe a swollen and painful prostate. For children, an appropriate herbal suppository can quickly reduce high fever and calm anxiety.

The herbs you choose depend on the need at hand. For example, astringent herbs can be used to tone and contract tissues when trying to reduce hemorrhoids or discharges. Herbs high in vitamins and minerals can provide easily absorbed

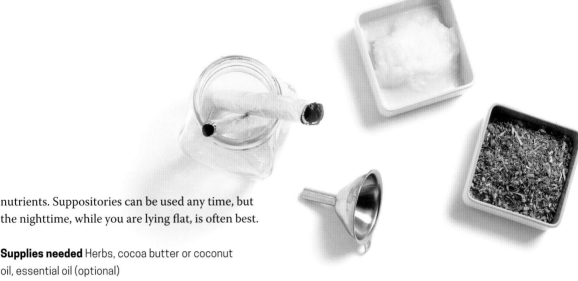

nutrients. Suppositories can be used any time, but the nighttime, while you are lying flat, is often best.

Supplies needed Herbs, cocoa butter or coconut oil, essential oil (optional)
Kitchenware Pencil or premade mold, aluminum foil, bowl, double boiler, kitchen thermometer, small funnel, freezer, glass storage jar and lid, putty knife, waxed paper
Cooking source Stove

Make suppositories using either a warm process or a cold process. The warm process involves melting oil, adding the herbs, and pouring the mixture directly into molds. The cold process involves kneading and hand mixing the herbs and oil together and rolling the mixture into appropriate-sized suppositories.

Warm process

First prepare the mold. Wrap two or three layers of aluminum foil around a pencil, leaving 1 or 2 inches of the pencil uncovered. Gently slide the foil off the pencil, close off one end, and stand each mold upright in a glass or jar, open end up.

Shave the cocoa butter or break it into small pieces and place in the top of a double boiler. Add the powdered herbs and a kitchen thermometer. Heat on low, slowly, to a temperature of 92°F (33°C). Remove the top portion of the double boiler and continue stirring the herbs and cocoa butter until they are well interlaced and all the butter is melted.

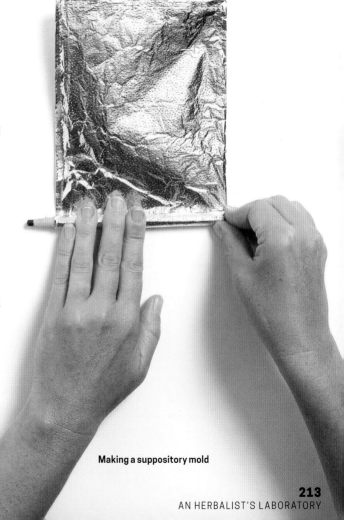

Making a suppository mold

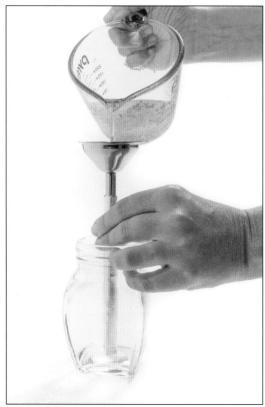
Pouring oil into the mold

Pour the mixture through a funnel into a mold. Hold the mold completely upright for a couple of minutes to let the mixture firm a bit, and then put it in the freezer for a few minutes. Remove the molds from the freezer and cut the suppositories into 1- to 1½–inch pieces, shaping them a bit to your preference. Remove the foil and store the suppositories in a sealed and labeled glass jar in the refrigerator.

Cold process

Mix the coconut oil and powdered herbs in a bowl. Use your hands or a putty knife to fold the mixture into itself. Add essential oil (optional) and mix again. Place the entire mixture in the center of a large piece of waxed paper. Roll it into a long roll, like a Tootsie roll. When it is rolled to the correct width appropriate for your use, place the roll in the freezer for 5 minutes. Remove and cut into 1- to 1½–inch pieces. Store in a sealed and labeled glass jar in the refrigerator.

BUM BUM RELIEF SUPPOSITORY
For hemorrhoids, warm method

- 2 tablespoons yarrow flower powder
- 2 tablespoons plantain leaf powder
- 2 tablespoons comfrey leaf powder
- 1 tablespoon turmeric powder
- 1 tablespoon calendula flower powder
- 1 cup cocoa butter

DRY NOSE SUPPOSITORY
Cold method

- 2 tablespoons comfrey leaf powder
- ½ cup coconut oil, room temperature
- 15 drops peppermint essential oil

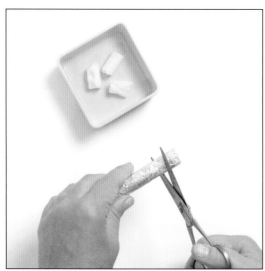
Cutting the suppositories into pieces

PROSTATE RELIEF SUPPOSITORY

- 2 tablespoons saw palmetto berry powder
- 1 tablespoon thyme leaf powder
- 1 tablespoon myrrh powder
- 1 tablespoon nettle seed powder
- 1 cup coconut oil

GET 'ER GOING SUPPOSITORY
For constipation relief

- 1 tablespoon peppermint leaf powder
- 1 tablespoon cascara sagrada bark powder
- 1 tablespoon slippery elm bark powder
- ½ cup coconut oil

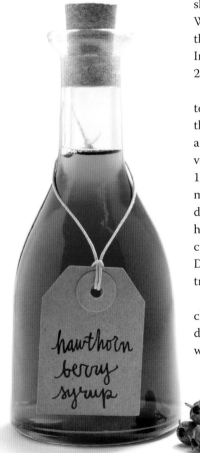

Syrups

A sweet syrup is an easy way to dispense good-tasting herbal medicine. I often recall Mary Poppins and her "spoonful of sugar" when I think of herbal syrups, especially when my daughter demands a second teaspoon of medicine. They take little effort to make, and the only tricky part is ensuring that your proportions are correct to create a stable, nonfermenting end result.

Honey is a relatively new ingredient for herbal syrups. Because many folks are avoiding white sugar these days, they often use honey or raw sugar as an alternative. Although I also try to avoid white sugar, I think its preservative properties are far greater than those of honey or other types of sugars. If you want to use raw, brown, or unrefined sugar for syrup, you must simmer the syrup and skim off the impurities before you store it. Whether you use honey or sugar, it's important that you add the appropriate amount to the recipe. In general, use a ratio of 1 part herbs and water to 2 parts honey or sugar.

You also need to keep in mind the herb-to-water ratio: 1 part herb to 5 parts water. Remember that weight ounces are different from fluid ounces, and don't confuse weight measurements with volume measurements. For example, if you weigh 1 ounce of horehound leaf, you must put it into a measuring cup and measure the volume to determine how much water to add. So if the horehound measures 6 ounces in the measuring cup, you'll add 30 ounces of water ($6 \times 5 = 30$). Distilled water is best, because it does not contain trace minerals that can contaminate the syrup.

It's also important to strain the syrup with cheesecloth before you store it to ensure that all dust or fine particles that can cause problems are withdrawn. You can also add vegetable glycerin,

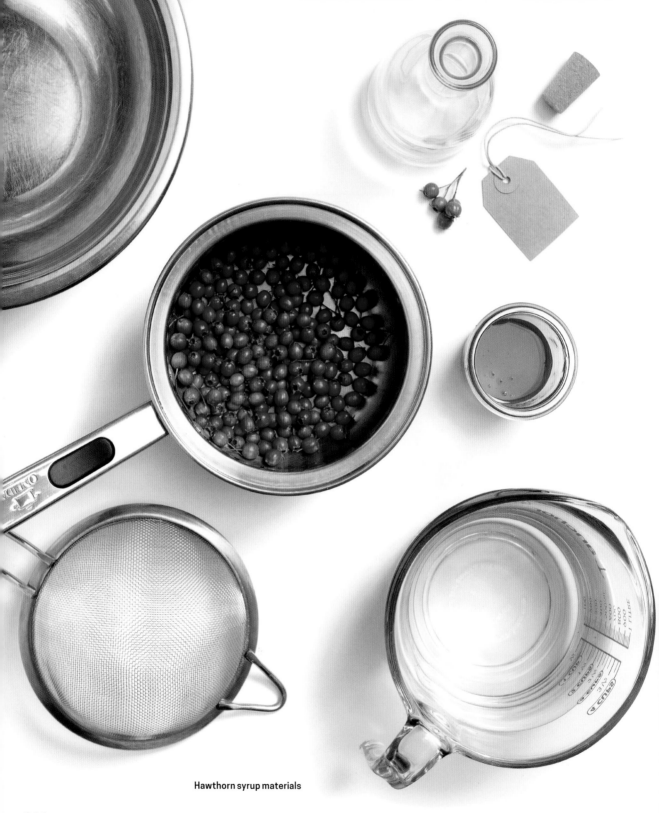

Hawthorn syrup materials

essential oils, apple cider vinegar, or brandy to a syrup to help improve its shelf life. A syrup can last a very long time if it is made properly. I currently have a bottle of my bilberry eye syrup in the cupboard that's as fresh as the day I made it, with honey, 14 months ago.

Supplies needed Herbs, distilled water, honey, vinegar (optional), vegetable glycerin (optional), brandy (optional)
Kitchenware Stockpot and lid, stirring spoon, strainer, cheesecloth, sterile bottles with caps
Cooking source Stove

To make syrup, add the herbs to the water in a stockpot and simmer the mixture on low for 1 hour, with lid ajar, stirring occasionally. Pour the mixture through a strainer, and then measure the total volume. Return it to the pot and add twice as much honey, based on the amount you just measured. Stir until the honey dissolves. At this point you can add ingredients such as vegetable glycerin to help retard fermentation. Add enough glycerin to equate a 30 percent volume of the total syrup. For example, if you measure 24 ounces of syrup, add 8 ounces of vegetable glycerin. If you want to add brandy, add about 10 percent of the total syrup volume (for 24 ounces syrup, about 2½ ounces brandy). Apple cider vinegar gives any syrup a unique flavor and preservation power; add it to taste.

Strain the syrup through a fine cotton cheesecloth and pour into sterile bottles with tight-fitting caps. Air and heat are the two worst enemies of a syrup. Store well-sealed bottles in a cool, dark cupboard to ensure a long shelf life.

WILD CHERRY COUGH SYRUP

- 9 cups distilled water
- 1 ounce wild cherry bark
- 1 ounce horehound leaf
- ½ ounce mullein leaf
- ½ ounce marshmallow root
- Honey

NERVOUS HEART SYRUP
For anxiety and stress

- 1 ounce hawthorn berries
- 1 ounce vervain leaf
- ½ ounce linden leaf
- ½ ounce kava root
- 2 pints distilled water
- Honey

DREAMING SYRUP
To encourage the dreaming cycle during sleep

- 1 ounce mugwort leaf
- ½ ounce hop flowers
- ½ ounce rosemary leaf
- ½ ounce devil's claw root
- 2 pints distilled water
- Honey

EVERYONE'S FAVORITE ELDERBERRY IMMUNE SYRUP

- ½ cup elderberries
- ¼ cup ashwagandha root
- ¼ ounce ginger root
- 1 teaspoon cinnamon chips
- Pinch of whole clove
- 3 cups distilled water
- Honey

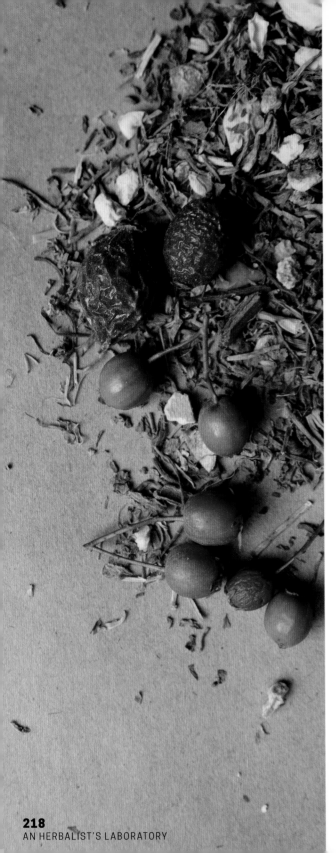

Teas

I love teas and recommend them often. They are a great way to get actively involved in the process of caring for yourself, because you can see, touch, and taste the herbs as you take them. I find this a great healing approach. Teas are also great when you need to take a long-term remedy, such as a tonic to produce a restorative action in the body.

Teas are typically tolerated well by most people, and they have one distinct advantage over some other applications: they are absorbed and processed through the gastrointestinal system. Therefore, if you want to treat problems with the mouth, stomach, small or large intestines, kidneys, or bladder, drinking herbal tea will move the herbs directly to the affected tissues. For stomach upsets or bladder infections, for example, herbal tea will pass through the affected organs to support them as needed.

You can make medicinal teas as infusions and decoctions. An infusion pulls the active principles from the herbs into water, typically hot water poured over the herbs. An infusion is used with the more delicate parts of herbs such as flowers, leaves, and stems. You can use fresh or dried plant material for tea infusions and steep by the cup, usually for 8 to 10 minutes—or, for a stronger medicinal effect, steep 4 hours or overnight. Dosage depends on the condition being addressed, but a typical medicinal brew is made with 4 or 5 tablespoons of herbs in 1 quart of water, infused overnight, strained the next morning, and consumed that day. In contrast, bitter herbs, such as hops, are best steeped for a shorter amount of time to limit their bitter taste. A little practice will go a long way here.

A decoction is similar in goal to an infusion, but decoctions are created from herb roots and bark, either fresh or dried. Simply infusing roots and barks typically won't pull out the medicinal qualities unless they are left to infuse for at least 4 hours, so a low boil is necessary. To make a decoction, simmer 1 to 3 teaspoons of the herb per

10 ounces of water, or 1 ounce of herb to 3 cups water, on low, covered, for 10 to 15 minutes. Strain out the herbs and drink as needed. Decoctions will keep for 2 or 3 days in the refrigerator, but if the liquid appears milky or foggy, throw it out and make a new batch.

Most of the medicinal tea recipes in this book create 1 quart of tea, which is the amount you'll consume each day. You can use mason jars or old spaghetti jars—any clean jar will do. The ideal water temperature for tea is a little less than boiling (212°F, or 100°C). Pour the water over 4 or 5 tablespoons of herbs, cover the jar, and let it steep overnight. In the morning, strain to remove the herbs.

As for dosage, drink the quart of strained tea each day, hot or cold, for a sustained physiological effect. Divide it into 3 cups to drink that day or put it in a water bottle and sip it all day long. If you are aiming for a tonic effect, drink 1 quart each day for 8 to 12 weeks. I don't recommend drinking the same formula longer than that without a break, because sometimes after consuming the same herbs for a long time, your body will react to them differently. Long-term consumption of the same herbs can also reduce their medicinal effectiveness.

MEDICINAL STRENGTH TEA

4 or 5 tablespoons herbs

1 quart water

Place herbs in a quart jar. Pour almost boiling water over the herbs and fill to the top. Tighten the lid on the jar and steep overnight. Strain in the morning. Drink hot or cold throughout the day, or divide into 3 or 4 cups.

LOOSE LEAF HERBAL TEA

1 to 3 teaspoons herbs

1 cup water

Steep herbs in 1 cup hot water, covered, for 5 to 10 minutes. Strain and enjoy.

HERBAL TEA WITH ROOTS

1 to 3 teaspoons herbs

1 cup water

Simmer herbs in 1 cup water, covered, for 15 minutes on low heat. Remove from heat and steep for 10 minutes. Strain and drink.

Tinctures

Medicinal tinctures have been used for as long as distilled alcohol has been available. They were the primary form of medicine administration until the development of pharmacology and its (and most patients') preference for pills. When a tincture is made, the herbs' medicinal constituents are extracted into a liquid medium called a menstruum, often alcohol and water, which is strong enough to break down the plants' cell walls and pull out the medicinal constituents.

I often think of the movie *Willy Wonka and the Chocolate Factory* when I think of the tincture-creation process. In the movie, character Mike Teavee tries to use Willy's teleport machine, which separates whatever enters it into individual molecules. You can see them floating along the ceiling as they make their way to the other end of

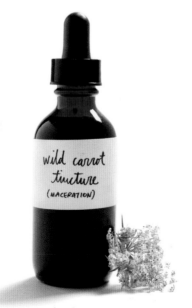

the factory. Like the process that occurs in Willy's machine, in the tincturing process, the plant changes from solid plant material to a dynamic medicinal liquid state.

Tinctures can be created from fresh or dried herbs.

- When creating tinctures with fresh herbs, use 1 part herbs to 2 parts menstruum.
- When using dried herbs, use 1 part herbs to 5 parts menstruum.

For some plants, wine, vinegar, and vegetable glycerin can also work as a menstruum.

HERBS THAT CAN BE EXTRACTED WITH WINE, VINEGAR, OR GLYCERIN

Burdock root
Chamomile flower
Cleavers herb
Dandelion leaf and root
Echinacea root
Elderberries and elder flower
Fennel seed
Ginger root
Goldenseal root
Hawthorn berries, leaf, and flower
Mugwort herb
Mullein herb
Nettle herb and seed
Oat tops and herb
Peppermint herb
Siberian ginseng root
Skullcap herb
Uva ursi herb
Valerian root
Vitex berries

After the herbal constituents are extracted, you take the herbal tincture sublingually, or under the tongue. Here the alcohol menstruum offers another advantage: alcohol and alcohol-based products diffuse directly through tissues and into the bloodstream. This is handy when you need a

remedy to work quickly, such as to relieve a headache or stop bleeding. Tinctures are also good options for those with underfunctioning intestinal absorption, because the herbal medicine bypasses the gastrointestinal system and goes straight into the bloodstream, and no ingredients are eliminated.

In apothecary measurements, a 1 ounce tincture is equal to 8 drams, or 30 milliliters (ml). For tincture ingredients, herbal books often refer to the amounts as "parts" rather than listing each ingredient amount in ounces or milliliters, for example. Each part is equal in volume. Because each ounce of tincture equals 8 drams, when we list the herbal ingredients for 1 ounce of tincture, we divide the ingredients into 8 equal parts.

To ensure that tincture ingredients add up to 100 percent, you can use percentages and a little math to measure the exact amount of each herb in a recipe to equal 1 fluid ounce. To determine the volume, in milliliters, of each of the 8 parts in an ounce of tincture, use this formula: 30 ml ÷ 8 = 3.75 ml. If an ingredient calls for 2 parts, multiply 3.75 by 2 (7.5 ml); if 3 parts, multiply by 3 (11.25 ml). You get the picture.

Consider an example of a 1 ounce tincture recipe for liver support. This tincture formula adds up to 8 parts, 100 percent, 30 ml.

2 parts, 25 percent, or 7.5 ml (3.75 ml × 2 parts) milk thistle seed

2 parts, 25 percent, or 7.5 ml (3.75 ml × 2 parts) Oregon grape root

2 parts, 25 percent, or 7.5 ml (3.75 ml × 2 parts) dandelion root

2 parts, 25 percent, or 7.5 ml (3.75 ml × 2 parts) burdock root

Using a little more math, you know that a 2-ounce tincture would use 16 parts (2 ounces × 8 parts). A 4 ounce tincture would use 32 parts, and an 8 ounce tincture would use 64 parts.

As for dosages, drop dosing works extremely well for some conditions and for sensitive patients.

Tincture dosages can vary, but with most herbal tinctures, the traditional dosage amounts are fine. You might consider starting with less, however, if tinctures contain more potent or stimulating herbs with specific actions.

- For acute issues: 2 dropperfuls every 2 to 3 hours for 1 or 2 days, and then 2 dropperfuls 2 or 3 times per day for 5 days
- For chronic issues or used as tonic: 2 dropperfuls, 3 times per day, for 8 to 12 weeks

Supplies needed Herbs, alcohol, vinegar, glycerin, distilled water

Kitchenware for maceration Jar, blender, measuring cup, waxed paper, rubber band, calculator

Kitchenware for percolation Percolator, jar, grinder, measuring cup, calculator, packing rod, coffee filters, rock weight, Pyrex bowl with lid, mixing spoon, rubber band, plastic baggies

Cooking source None

SOLVENT RANGES FOR ALCOHOL-CREATED HERBAL TINCTURES USING DRY HERBS

Every herb has an ideal solvent range—the most optimal alcohol percentage in which the plant constituents will extract. If you use a lower percentage of alcohol than the herbal extraction requires, you may not extract the herb's full medicinal properties. If you use a higher percentage of alcohol, it can destroy the herbs' efficacy. It is important to use the appropriate alcohol solvent ranges for the herbs you want to extract. In the first column, "herb" denotes any part of the plant that grows above ground, including the stem, leaf, and flower.

COMMON NAME	BOTANICAL NAME	SOLVENT PERCENTAGE
alfalfa leaf	Medicago sativa	40 to 50
angelica root	Angelica archangelica	70 to 75
arnica flower	Arnica montana	50 to 70
ashwagandha root	Withania somnifera	50 to 55
aspen bark	Populus tremuloides	60 to 70
astragalus root	Astragalus membranaceus	30 to 45
barberry root	Berberis vulgaris	50 to 70
bayberry bark	Myrica pensylvanica	35 to 60
bearberry	Arctostaphylos uva-ursi	45 to 65
benzoin gum	Styrax benzoin	95
betony leaf	Stachys officinalis	35 to 50
bistort herb	Polygonum bistorta	35 to 50
black cohosh root	Actaea racemosa	60 to 80
black walnut hull	Juglans nigra	40 to 50
bladderwrack	Fucus vesiculosus	25 to 50
blessed thistle herb	Cnicus benedictus	45 to 60
bloodroot root	Sanguinaria canadensis	55 to 70

COMMON NAME	BOTANICAL NAME	SOLVENT PERCENTAGE
blue cohosh root	*Caulophyllum thalictroides*	40 to 70
blue flag root	*Iris versicolor*	65 to 90
blue vervain herb	*Verbena officinalis*	40 to 50
buchu leaf	*Agathosma betulina*	50 to 65
burdock root	*Arctium lappa*	40 to 60
calamus root	*Acorus calamus*	50 to 65
calendula flower	*Calendula officinalis*	50 to 80
cascara sagrada	*Rhamnus purshiana*	20 to 25
catnip leaf	*Nepeta cataria*	50 to 60
cayenne fruit	*Capsicum frutescens*	80 to 95
cedar berry or leaf	*Thuja occidentalis*	65 to 75
chamomile flower	*Matricaria recutita*	45 to 65
chaparral herb	*Larrea divaricata*	65 to 75
chaste berry	*Vitex agnus-castus*	40 to 60
chickweed herb	*Stellaria media*	35 to 65
cleavers herb	*Galium aparine*	32 to 65
collinsonia	*Collinsonia canadensis*	40 to 75
coltsfoot	*Tussilago farfara*	30 to 40
comfrey leaf	*Symphytum officinale*	50 to 65
comfrey root	*Symphytum officinale*	24 to 50
corn silk	*Zea mays*	35 to 65
cow parsnip seed or bark	*Heracleum lanatum*	65 to 70
crampbark	*Viburnum opulus*	50 to 60
dandelion root	*Taraxacum officinale*	35 to 65
devil's claw	*Harpagophytum procumbens*	50 to 75
devil's club	*Oplopanax horridus*	50 to 70
dong quai	*Angelica sinensis*	20 to 65
echinacea root	*Echinacea purpurea*	45 to 75
elderberries	*Sambucus nigra*	40 to 50
elder flower	*Sambucus nigra*	35 to 60
elecampane	*Inula helenium*	45 to 70
eleuthero	*Eleutherococcus senticosus*	60
eyebright	*Euphrasia officinalis*	35 to 50
false unicorn root	*Chamaelirium luteum*	45 to 70
fennel seed	*Foeniculum vulgare*	60 to 70
feverfew leaf and flower	*Tanacetum parthenium*	50 to 75
figwort leaf and flower	*Scrophularia nodosa*	50 to 60
fringe tree bark	*Chionanthus virginicus*	55 to 70

COMMON NAME	BOTANICAL NAME	SOLVENT PERCENTAGE
garlic bulb	*Allium sativum*	65
gentian root	*Gentiana lutea*	35 to 60
ginger	*Zingiber officinale*	75 to 80
ginkgo leaf	*Ginkgo biloba*	55 to 75
ginseng root	*Panax quinquefolius*	30 to 70
goldenrod	*Solidago canadensis*	45 to 60
goldenseal root	*Hydrastis canadensis*	55 to 70
gotu kola herb	*Centella asiatica*	25 to 60
grindelia buds and flowers	*Grindelia robusta*	65 to 70
hawthorn berry	*Crataegus oxycantha*	40 to 70
hops strobile	*Humulus lupus*	50 to 75
horehound herb	*Marrubium vulgare*	35 to 65
horseradish root	*Cochlearia armoracia*	40 to 55
horsetail herb	*Equisetum arvense*	35 to 65
hydrangea root	*Hydrangea arborescens*	30 to 50
hyssop herb	*Hyssopus officinalis*	35 to 60
immortal root	*Asclepias asperula*	35 to 50
juniper berry	*Juniperus communis*	60 to 75
kava kava root	*Piper methysticum*	60 to 75
licorice root	*Glycyrrhiza glabra*	20 to 65
lobelia herb	*Lobelia inflata*	40 to 70
lomatium root	*Lomatium dissectum*	65 to 70
ma huang herb	*Astragalus membranaceus*	20 to 65
maidenhair fern	*Adiantum aethiopicum*	60
marshmallow root	*Althea officinalis*	20 to 65
milk thistle seed	*Silybum marianum*	70 to 95
motherwort herb	*Leonurus cardiaca*	45 to 70
mugwort	*Artemisia vulgaris*	40 to 55
mullein flower	*Verbascum thapsus*	35 to 70
mullein leaf	*Verbascum thapsus*	50 to 60
myrrh gum	*Commiphora myrrha*	85 to 95
nettle leaf	*Urtica dioica*	35 to 50
oatstraw	*Avena sativa*	40 to 65
Oregon grape root	*Mahonia aquifolium*	45 to 70
osha root	*Ligusticum porteri*	60 to 75
passionflower	*Passiflora incarnata*	40 to 65
pau d'arco	*Tabebuia impetiginosa*	45 to 50
peppermint leaf	*Mentha piperita*	45 to 60

COMMON NAME	BOTANICAL NAME	SOLVENT PERCENTAGE
periwinkle	*Vinca minor*	35 to 50
pipsissewa herb	*Chimaphila umbellata*	35 to 60
plantain leaf	*Plantago major*	35 to 50
pleurisy root	*Asclepias tuberosa*	40 to 50
poke root	*Phytolacca americana*	40 to 65
prickly ash bark	*Zanthoxylum clava-herculis*	55 to 70
propolis		65 to 95
pulsatilla	*Anemone tuberosa*	70
red clover flower and herb	*Trifolium pratense*	40 to 65
red raspberry leaf	*Rubus idaeus*	35 to 50
red root	*Ceanothus americanus*	32 to 37
sage	*Salvia officinalis*	50 to 75
sarsaparilla (Mexican)	*Smilax medica*	40 to 45
saw palmetto berry	*Serenoa repens*	50 to 80
shepherd's purse	*Capsella bursa-pastoris*	40 to 65
skullcap herb	*Scutellaria lateriflora*	45 to 65
spikenard	*Aralia racemosa*	50 to 60
squaw vine herb	*Mitchella repens*	35 to 65
St. John's wort flower	*Hypericum perforatum*	55 to 65
turkey rhubarb	*Rheum palmatum*	35 to 50
usnea	*Usnea barbata*	70 to 95
valerian root	*Valeriana officinalis*	55 to 65
white oak bark	*Quercus alba*	15 to 50
white pine bark	*Pinus strobus*	60
white willow bark	*Salix alba*	35 to 50
wild geranium root	*Geranium maculatum*	35 to 55
wild indigo root	*Baptisia tinctoria*	50 to 65
wild yam root	*Dioscorea villosa*	55 to 65
witch hazel bark	*Hamamelis virginiana*	40 to 65
yarrow flower	*Achillea millefolium*	35 to 60
yellow dock root	*Rumex crispus*	40 to 50
yerba manza root	*Anemopsis californica*	40 to 65
yerba santa	*Eriodictyon californicum*	60 to 74
yucca root	*Yucca species*	65

You can make tinctures in either of two ways: using the maceration method or the percolation method. Just to complicate things, the maceration method itself has two approaches: the folk way and the standard way.

The maceration method

The basic steps of the folk maceration method are simple. Place the herbs in a jar, pour alcohol over them, seal the jar, and let it sit for 2 to 4 weeks, shaking it daily. During maceration, the liquid surrounding the herbs softens or separates the herbs into parts and draws out their active medicinal elements.

Letting the liquid sit is just one aspect of the tincture maceration process. The other and almost more important step is shaking the jar every day. To break down the plants' cell walls and draw out all of the medicinal goodness, you need to shake the jar for a minute or two every day. If the jar leaks when you shake it, remove the lid and place a square piece of waxed paper over the mouth of the jar to act as a gasket before returning the lid. Or wrap a rubber band snuggly under the lid before replacing it.

I am often asked, "What if I steep it longer than 4 weeks?" I've never seen a tincture turn ineffectual if it is steeped longer. When all the constituents are extracted from the plant, steeping it longer will not create a stronger effect. If you want to create a more potent tincture, perform a second or third round of maceration, adding new material each time: strain and remove the original marc (the herbal waste produced during the tincturing process), add new herbs to the already created tincture, secure the lid, and store it for 2 to 4 weeks, again shaking it every day.

Vodka is the most commonly used menstruum for the maceration tincturing method. If you are using vodka, you do not need to add water, because most vodkas are 80 proof, or 40 percent alcohol and 40 percent water. The other option is to use 190-proof ethanol, grain alcohol, if you want to get specific with your alcohol percentages and solvent ranges. Grain alcohol is obtainable in many states but is usually kept behind the counter, so you need to ask for it. If you are using grain alcohol, use these alcohol-to-water ratio guidelines for your menstruum:

- When creating tinctures with fresh herbs, use 75 percent grain alcohol and 25 percent water.
- When creating tinctures with dried herbs, use 50 percent grain alcohol and 50 percent water.

FOLK MACERATION USING DRIED HERBS

Herbs

Vodka

Fill approximately one-fifth of a quart jar with coarsely chopped or ground dried herbs. Add vodka to cover 1 or 2 inches above the herbs. Secure the lid and shake the jar. In a day or two, check to determine if more vodka is needed to maintain that 1 or 2 inches of liquid above the herbs. Store in a cool, dark place for 2 to 4 weeks, shaking every day. Then strain the mixture through cheesecloth and squeeze the excess liquid from the marc (the herbal waste). Store the tincture in a tightly sealed, labeled bottle in a cool cupboard.

FOLK MACERATION USING FRESH HERBS

This is one of my favorite ways to make a tincture.

Fresh herbs

Grain alcohol or vodka

Water

Fill a quart jar to the top with fresh herbs. If you're using grain alcohol, mix together 3 parts grain alcohol (24 ounces) and 1 part water (8 ounces), or use vodka and no water, and pour it into a blender along with the herbs. Give it a few whorls to mix it all together before pouring it back in the jar and securing the lid. Store in cool, dark place for 2 to 4 weeks, shaking every day.

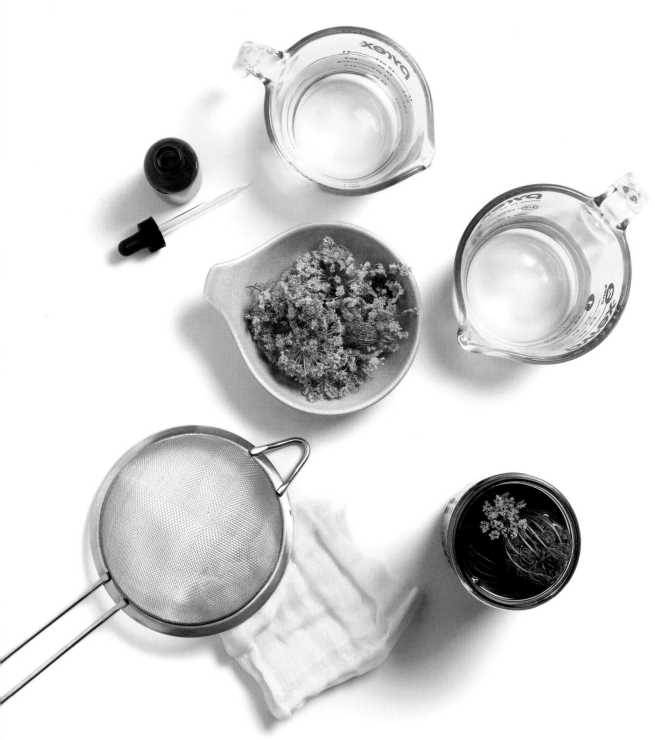

Materials for a tincture using the maceration method

STANDARDIZED MACERATION METHOD

Every time I teach this subject, my students' eyes glaze over. The standardized method is based on math and calculations. But don't worry—we'll get through this together. I have never been good at math. I like it and find it fascinating, but I rarely got the answer correct in math class. The thing is, the standardized method enables you to have a consistent outcome when you make the same tincture over and over. This is accomplished by using several equations. It is best to use the metric system when measuring ingredients for a standardized tincture, because you will be working with both liquids and solids (powdered herbs), and you need a precise and uniform measuring system for both.

STANDARDIZED MACERATION USING POWDERED ECHINACEA

You may begin with any amount of powdered herbs. In this example, however, I use 1 ounce of dried echinacea root to yield a small amount of tincture, and to keep it simple.

1 ounce echinacea root powder

Vodka

1. Convert 1 ounce dried echinacea root powder to grams: 1 ounce = 28.3 grams.

2. Multiply 28.3 (grams) × 5 (dried herb to menstruum ratio is 1 part herb to 5 parts menstruum): 28.3 × 5 = 141.5 ml, the total amount of menstruum (vodka in this case) required for macerating the dried herb. (If you are new to the metric measurements, you may be scratching your head, thinking, "I thought we were just in grams?" And

this is true, but grams and milliliters are equal in the metric system, which makes it easy to work with both solids and liquids.)

3. Place the herbs and vodka in a jar, secure the lid, and shake it. Store in a cool, dark place for 2 to 4 weeks, shaking it every day.

STANDARDIZED MACERATION USING FRESH CALIFORNIA POPPY FLOWERS

As with the dried herb standardized recipe, you may begin with whatever amount of herb you want as long as you use the calculations to determine the amount of alcohol and water used.

300 grams fresh California poppy flowers

Grain alcohol

Distilled water

1. Multiply 300 (grams) × 2 (fresh herb to menstruum ratio is 1 part herbs to 2 parts menstruum): 300 × 2 = 600 ml.

2. Multiply 600 × 0.75 to determine the total grain alcohol amount (with fresh herbs, the total menstruum ratio is 3 parts alcohol, or 75 percent, to 1 part water, or 25 percent): 600 × 0.75 = 450 ml. Pour 450 ml of alcohol into a glass jar.

3. Multiply 600 × 0.25 for the total water amount (fresh herbs menstruum is 25 percent water): 600 × 0.25 = 150 ml. Pour 150 ml of water into the jar.

4. Pour the jar of menstruum and herbs into a blender and blend for a few seconds.

5. Place the herbs and menstruum back into the jar and secure the lid. Store in cool, dark place for 2 to 4 weeks, shaking every day.

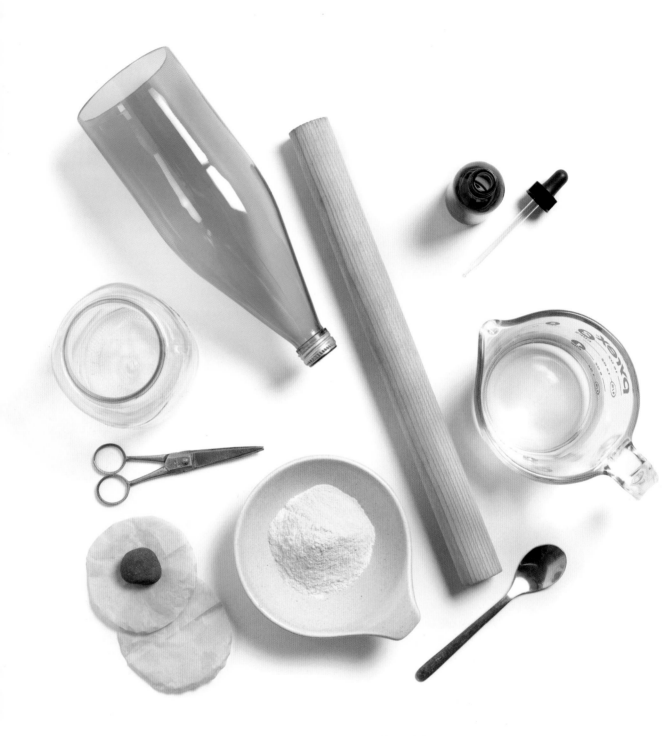

Materials for a tincture using the percolation method

Percolation Method

I love making tinctures using the percolation method. I have found an art in this process that is like few others in the practice of herbal medicine. Nevertheless, herbalists seem to have widely varying opinions on just about everything, and the tincture percolation method is a hotly debated topic. Go to any herbal gathering and ask, "Do you think the percolation process creates a valid and worthwhile medicine?" and you'll see what I mean. In my opinion, the percolation method is an example of how biochemistry is used to create herbal medicine. In biochemistry, the purpose is to titrate substances to obtain accurate and precise results. Although I cried each week in my college biochemistry class because I could never quite reach that result, I see the beauty of what we were trying to accomplish in the percolation method.

This process extracts the herbal components from dried herbal powders through a slow saturation and drip (percolation) process. It uses gravity to draw down the menstruum through the herbs, pulling out the medicinal constituents as it goes. The biggest advantage in this method is that you can prepare a tincture in as few as 3 days, versus the 2 to 4 weeks that maceration requires. And no pressing or straining of the herbs is required, because the act of percolating draws out all of the important constituents from the herbs within the percolation apparatus.

The percolation apparatus is a glass cylinder-shaped bottle or cone. Purchase one from a lab equipment supplier or create one from a glass Perrier water bottle.

MAKE A PERCOLATOR FROM A PERRIER BOTTLE

To make your own percolation apparatus, you can cut the bottle yourself, or, easier yet, take it to a professional glass cutter and let an expert cut the bottle for you.

Empty Perrier bottle and cap

Glass cutter (look for one at a hardware store or craft supplier)

String

Rubbing alcohol

Matches

Bowl of ice water

1. Place the bottle on its side on a flat surface, and use the glass cutter to score around the bottom, staying as close to the bottom of the bottle as you can. Hold the bottle in one hand and carefully score it with the cutter using moderate pressure, being careful not to press too hard or you'll crack the glass. Keep the score on a consistent plane as you slowly rotate the bottle—you must score it only once around to avoid cracking the bottle or ruining the edge.

2. Soak a piece of cotton string in rubbing alcohol and tie it around the score line.

3. Light the string on fire, and count to 7. Then immediately dunk the entire bottle in a bowl of ice water, the colder the better. At this point, the bottom will pop off.

When you begin the percolation process, you'll place the sterilized percolation bottle, with the cap screwed on, upside down in a sterilized quart mason jar. The cap is very important. You use it to control the rate of percolation and maintain pressure within the percolation bottle.

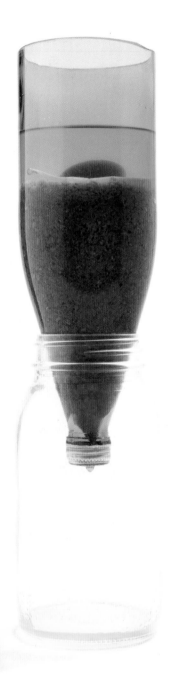

What cannot be percolated? Any herbs with a high gum content or resinous nature, such as myrrh, marshmallow, and frankincense, must be macerated, because the gum or resin is too sticky to pass through the percolator. Percolations also demand the use of a correct solvent range based on the plant you are tincturing. Therefore, you need to use 190-proof alcohol for this preparation.

What I can say about tincture percolations is that in my clinical practice, the medicinal qualities have proven their effectiveness. As a bonus, the flavors are amazing. When you taste the first couple of drops in the recipe, notice the aroma and flavor. Both are often diminished in macerations. Herbalist James Green once suggested that you start practicing percolations using herbs and water. This is a cost-efficient way to practice, troubleshoot, and develop your skills without breaking the bank.

PERCOLATION METHOD USING DRIED BURDOCK ROOT

You may begin with whatever amount of herb you want as long as you use the calculations to determine the amount of alcohol and water used.

4 ounces ground burdock root

Grain, grape, corn, or cane alcohol

Distilled water

Unbleached coffee filter

Packing rod

Rock or crystal (to use as a weight)

1. Weigh the herbs and convert to grams (1 ounce = 28.3 grams): 4 (ounces) × 28.3 = 113.2 grams.

2. Multiply 113.2 grams × 5 (dried herb to menstruum ratio is 1 part herb to 5 parts menstruum): 113.2 × 5 = 566 ml, the total amount menstruum required.

3. Place the ground burdock root in a measuring cup to determine the volume in milliliters. This determines the approximate volume of the marc (the herbal waste), which will be discarded. Later, we'll add in more menstruum to make up for what was lost in the percolation process. In this example, the burdock volume is 295.75 ml.

4. Add the marc volume to the total menstruum volume to determine true total menstruum volume: 295.75 (ml) + 566 (ml) = 861.75 ml of true total menstruum volume. Again, we need to add extra for what will be left behind in the discarded marc.

5. Determine the preferred solvent range for burdock root. Based on the solvent range chart, it is 40 to 60 percent. We will use 60 percent alcohol. When making your tinctures, you can determine how much solvent you want to use within that range. With practice and good note-taking, you'll find the percentage you like best for taste and effectiveness.

6. Prepare 861.75 ml of menstruum, with 60 percent grain, grape, corn, or cane alcohol and 40 percent distilled water (861.75 × 0.60 = 517.05 ml alcohol; 861.75 × 0.40 = 344.7 ml water). Add the alcohol and water to a glass container, close tightly, and set aside.

7. Place the ground burdock root in an airtight container and moisten it with the menstruum to begin breaking down the herbs. Add just enough menstruum to achieve a dry, crumbly consistency and a slight change in the herbs' color. If you need a place to begin, add approximately two-thirds of the total marc volume (not the total menstruum volume). For this example, you would add 197 ml of menstruum (two-thirds of 295.75 = 197). After a bit of practice, you'll easily be able to determine how much menstruum to add. Less is better; if you add too much to begin with, your percolation material will be too damp, and the best thing to do is change course and turn it into a maceration. This step also causes the herb powder to swell in preparation for the packing of the percolator.

8. Close the container and set it aside for 12 to 24 hours.

9. Secure the cap on the percolation bottle. Then grab an unbleached coffee filter, and cut two circular pieces the same size as the largest opening of your bottle. Fold one of the filter circles in half and then in half again. Slide your finger down into one side and open to create a little cone-shaped filter.

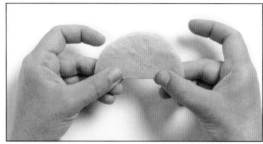

Fold the filter piece in half.

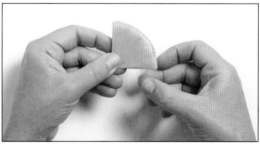

Fold it in half again.

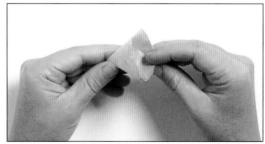

Slide in your finger to open the filter cone.

10. Place the little cone, entering from widest end (bottom) of the percolation bottle, into the narrow neck, pointed side toward the cap end. It might help to run a little distilled water through the bottle to help the cone filter stick to the sides. The cone should be smooth, flush on all sides, pointed directly down, and centered.

11. Open the container of moistened herbs and divide it into three parts. You will add the herbs to the percolation bottle in three phases. Spoon in a third of the moistened burdock root powder, being careful that the cone filter is making contact on all sides of the bottle so that powder isn't slipping past. Check as you work to ensure that the cone filter's tip stays pointed straight down and is not tipped to the side. Gently pack the first addition of herbs using a packing rod. Then add the next third, and then the last third, packing after each addition.

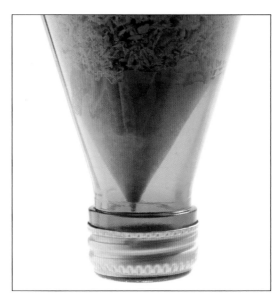

A perfectly packed percolation bottle

- Packing the herbs with a packing rod is a delicate process. If you don't tamp it enough, the herb will loosen when you add the menstruum and will not percolate efficiently. If you tamp too much, the percolation will either take days to finish or it won't happen at all because the menstruum cannot get through. In general, you should tamp it extremely lightly with the first third, and then tamp a little more each time.

- Ideally at the end you will not see the different layers or cracks or rivers in the powered pack when you look at it through the glass bottle. You are never pressing the herb down, just light tamping to create an even layering.

12. Add the second, unfolded, tiny filter on top of the packed herb. Place a rock in the middle of the filter to hold it in place so that when the menstruum is poured in, the filter stays put.

13. Set the capped percolation bottle inside a mason jar, with the cap at the bottom. I like to use a narrow mouthed jar because it allows the percolator to sit up higher so I can watch the process. Work on a flat, even surface.

14. Open the cap at the bottom of the percolation bottle halfway. If you don't do this and then pour your menstruum in, air and pressure will disrupt the pack, quickly turning your hard work into a maceration tincture. After the cap is open, begin slowly pouring in some of the menstruum. This is when you get to see how well you've performed each step as you watch the menstruum slowly saturate and make its way through the herbs. Maintain 1 or 2 inches of menstruum above the packed herbs.

15. Once the tincture begins to drip out of the bottom—and this will be determined by your pack job—taste a drop or two. Then close off the cap tightly. Lift the bottle very gently, because once the menstruum is added, the percolation does not like to be moved. If you still have some menstruum left at this point; secure the lid and set it aside.

16. Place a plastic bag over the top of the percolator, securing it with a rubber band. Let it sit undisturbed for 12 to 24 hours, checking from time to time to make sure no drips have escaped from the cap.

17. The next day, remove the plastic bag and open the cap one-quarter of a turn to begin the dripping, or percolation, process. The dripping rate should be about 1 drop per second. You must stay with your percolator throughout this process, because as the menstruum moves through, you'll slowly add the rest of the liquid to the top, until all menstruum has been added. At that point, you can walk away for a bit to let it complete. This can take 2 hours or more, depending on the many variables of packing, alcohol type, herb consistency, and other factors.

18. When the dripping stops, carefully remove the percolator bottle, stir up the percolate in the mason jar, and bottle it up.

Vinegars

Herbal vinegars are a wonderful addition to any kitchen. Many herbalists' refrigerators store salad dressings made with nettles, comfrey, alfalfa, and chickweed. Herbal vinegars offer an abundance of nutrients in a tasty, positive base, but they are not only for the tasting. Using a vinegar foundation, you can also make wonderful herbal cleaning products and superior topical treatments. Although vinegars cannot extract all medicinal elements from every herb, they do seem to have an affinity for herbs that are high in trace minerals and vitamins. Vinegar tones and aids in regulating the digestive function and was once used in most facial toners and beauty products as a key ingredient to keep the face fresh and the hair shiny. And vinegar is easily tolerated and has virtually no toxicity potential.

Supplies needed Herbs, apple cider vinegar
Kitchenware Quart jar with lid, strainer
Cooking source None

Many believe that herbal vinegars have a short shelf life, but I'm of the opposite camp. Some of my herbal vinegars stay vibrant and potent for many years when they are sealed well and stored in a dark, cool cabinet. You can use fresh or dried herbs in vinegars, but keep in mind that fresh herbs will add some water content to the vinegar, which can create a muddy effect.

Not all vinegars are the same. Choose high quality types such as apple cider vinegar, which is high in nutritional value and complements the healing actions of the herbs. You can get as creative as you'd like with your choices, however, because there are many different types of vinegars available, including some that are flavored. These can add real pizzazz to your next herbal experience.

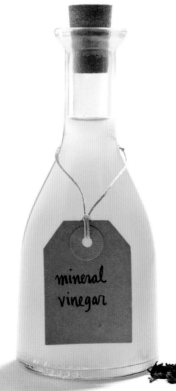

mineral vinegar

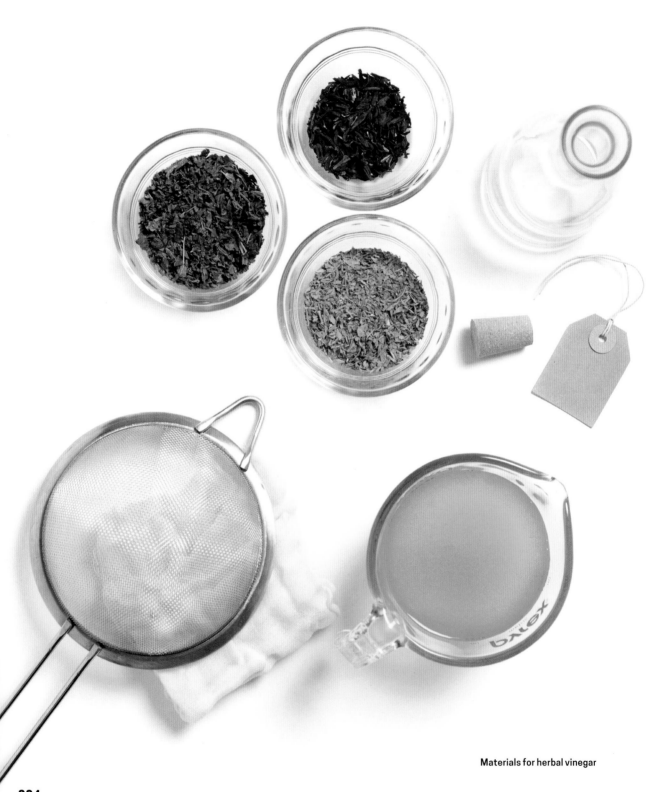

Materials for herbal vinegar

VINEGAR OF THE FOUR THIEVES
To ward off cold and flu

This is an old eclectic recipe (one of many versions) once used to ward off the plague.

- 1 pint apple cider vinegar
- Big pinch of wormwood herb
- Big pinch of meadowsweet herb
- Big pinch of wild marjoram
- Big pinch of sage
- A few juniper berries
- 15 cloves
- ½ ounce elecampane root
- ½ ounce angelica root
- ½ ounce rosemary leaf
- ½ ounce of horehound herb

Place all ingredients into a mason jar, seal tightly, and store the mixture for 2 weeks in a cool, dark place, shaking each day. Then strain the mixture well and bottle it up. Store it in a cool, dark place. Take 1 teaspoon of vinegar orally to prevent illness. You can also use it externally, rubbing it on hands, face, and neck.

POISON OAK AND IVY RELIEF
Topical treatment

- 1 pint apple cider vinegar
- ¼ ounce plantain leaf
- ¼ ounce sage leaf
- ¼ ounce mugwort herb
- ¼ ounce horsetail herb

Fill the jar three-quarters full with herbs and add vinegar to the top. Set in a partially sunny window for 2 weeks, shaking every day. Strain, bottle, and store in cool, dry place. Apply several times per day onto weepy, itchy blisters.

BONE-UP HERBAL VINEGAR
For bone mineral health

This is a good tonic to take every day, on its own or poured onto salads.

- 1 pint apple cider vinegar
- ⅛ ounce nettle leaf
- ⅛ ounce alfalfa leaf
- ⅛ ounce chickweed herb
- ⅛ ounce comfrey leaf
- ⅛ ounce horsetail herb
- 3 sprigs of rosemary (optional)
- 2 garlic cloves (optional)

Fill the jar three-quarters full with herbs and add vinegar to the top. Set in partially sunny window for 2 weeks, shaking every day. Strain, bottle, and store in cool, dry place or in the refrigerator.

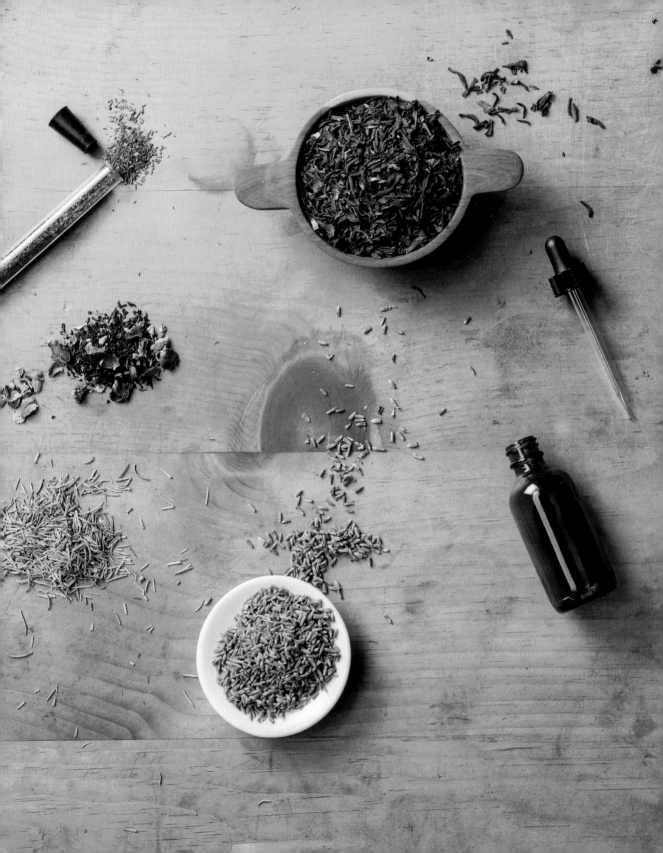

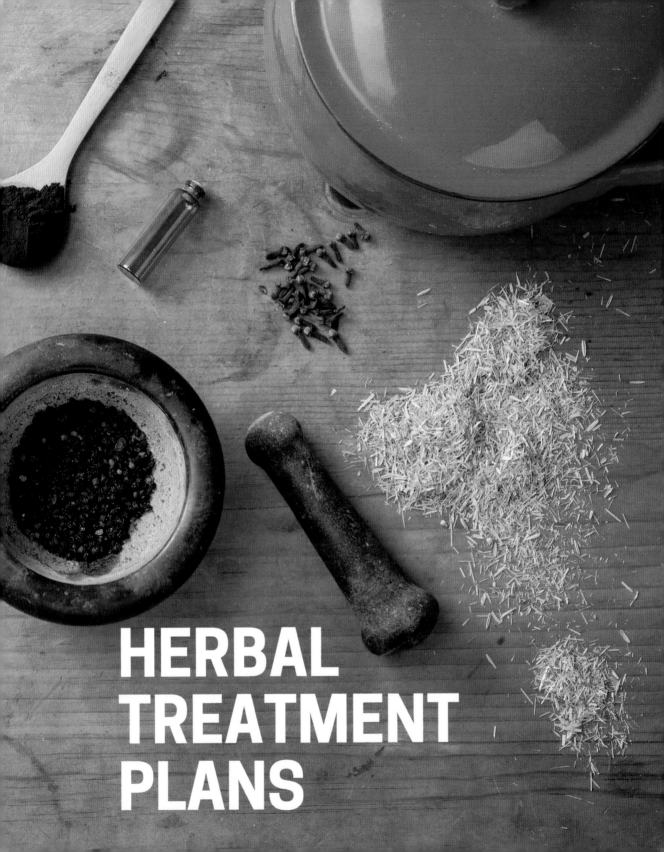

HERBAL
TREATMENT
PLANS

These guiding treatment plans cover some of the most common conditions I see in my practice and shoppe. Use them as is or as a foundation to build upon as you begin experimenting with new herbs you have studied. You should be able to find the ingredients used in these recipes at either a local or online medicinal herb supplier. Near the end of the book you'll find a list of suppliers that sell reliable, high quality, vibrant herbs. You can also find many herbs growing in your garden or neighborhood.

- Unless noted, dried herbs should be used in recipes.
- If an ingredient includes the word "herb," use any part of the plant that grows above ground, including the stem, leaf, and flower. Otherwise, the ingredient will note root, flower, stem, or leaf.
- Herbal ingredients for teas, washes, and salves are listed in ounces, teaspoons, and tablespoons.
- Herbal ingredients for tinctures are usually listed in parts, or drams.
- Unless noted otherwise, to make the teas in these recipes, add 4 or 5 tablespoons of herbs to 1 quart of almost boiling water.
- For dosages, see "Adult Dosing Basics."
- For recipes that do not include instructions, see "An Herbalist's Laboratory" for information regarding how to create and use them.

ADULT DOSING BASICS

Dosages are offered as a simple guideline. Remember that herbs are best used in frequent smaller doses throughout the day. Larger quantities are not better in most cases. For children's dosages, see the section "Bumps, Bruises, and Other Childhood Conditions."

APPLICATION	CHRONIC OR TONIC DOSAGE	ACUTE DOSAGE
Capsule	2 capsules 1 or 2 times per day	2 or 3 capsules, 3 or 4 times per day
Poultice and compress	Typically used for acute conditions	Apply 2 times per day, 20 minutes with gentle heat
Syrup	1 teaspoon 3 times per day	1 teaspoon, 4 to 6 times per day
Tea	3 cups per day, or 1 quart throughout the day	2 to 4 cups per day
Tincture	1 dropperful 3 or 4 times per day	2 dropperfuls every 2 or 3 hours for 1 or 2 days; then 2 dropperfuls 2 or 3 times per day for 5 days

Acne

Acne is one of the most common patient complaints in my practice. Acne can appear at any time on anyone, youngster or adult, as small pimples, painful lumps, or generalized redness. Most commonly acne indicates the presence of inflammation in the body, presented on the skin as pimples. They may or may not have a cystic quality, which is the inclusion of a generally viscous, yellowish white fluid in tissue that is often swollen and tender.

The origins of acne can be direct cause and effect, or they can be elusive and challenging to treat. The first things to investigate are skin cleanliness, liver function efficiency, hormonal imbalance, bowel toxicity, lymphatic congestion, and nutrient insufficiencies. I also consider the emotional well-being of the person suffering from acne. Highly stressful times can lead to chronic inflammation and acne. From the emotional energetic perspective, low self-esteem can also increase acne.

Supporting liver function can help clear toxins from the body and blood and help balance the hormones, which all can cause an over-accumulation of wastes in the body if they are underfunctioning. As a result, the skin's cleansing capabilities are recruited to draw out impurities through the surface. It's all about alterative herbs here. You can start by choosing a strong formula to help clean the liver and blood, to lessen blood toxicity, and to improve overall bodily function.

The skin's condition is a true reflection of gastrointestinal health. Skin is clear of acne when the gastrointestinal tract is functioning optimally. Bowel toxicity results from improper diet choices as well as stress or chronic inflammation in the gastrointestinal tract. I prescribe healing demulcents (such as marshmallow, licorice, fennel, and slippery elm) and carminatives (such as wintergreen, cumin, and ginger) to calm irritated tissues and help improve overall absorption. If you suffer from acne, consider examining your diet and using the anti-inflammatory dietary guidelines in this book for a comprehensive approach to dealing with the problem.

Teas are a great treatment option because they help soothe tissues as they pass through the gastrointestinal system. Tinctures can be more convenient, however. An herbal wash is similar to a tea, but it is stronger and used topically. It is made like a fomentation, but instead of soaking a cloth and placing it where needed, you soak or splash the wash directly on the body.

TEA OR TINCTURE BLEND FOR ACNE

If the acne is related to hormones, add ¼ ounce each of sassafras and sarsaparilla. If the acne sufferer is female, include 1 ounce of dried chaste berry. All three herbs work in the body to balance hormones such as testosterone and precursor hormones to estrogens. An imbalance of these hormones can result in acne.

If you're making tea, use herbs in the amounts listed. If you're making a tincture blend, each of these ingredients is in a tincture form; use the listed amounts and mix all the tinctures together in one bottle.

- 1 ounce burdock root
- 1 ounce dandelion root
- 1 ounce Oregon grape root
- 1 ounce lemon peel
- ½ ounce orange peel
- ½ ounce red clover herb
- ½ ounce yellow dock root
- ¼ ounce calendula flower
- ¼ ounce licorice root
- Tiny pinch of cayenne
- 1 ounce dried chaste berry (optional)
- ½ ounce each sassafras and sarsaparilla (optional)

TEA OR TINCTURE BLEND FOR BOWEL TOXICITY

This tea is best made and consumed immediately, rather than steeping it overnight. If you're making tea, use herbs in the amounts listed. If you're making a tincture blend, each of these ingredients is in a tincture form; use the listed amounts and mix all the tinctures together in one bottle.

- 1 ounce slippery elm bark
- 1 ounce plantain leaf
- 1 ounce Oregon grape root
- ½ ounce fennel seed
- ¼ ounce ginger root

Tea: 2 teaspoons per cup, simmer 10 minutes covered.

Reducing lymph congestion can be very helpful in reducing acne. Lymph glands are the body's waste collectors. When systemic toxicity is high, the lymph glands must work overtime. If there is too much waste in the body and the lymph system cannot keep up, the skin attempts to cleanse the body by pushing materials up and out to the surface.

LYMPHATIC TEA OR TINCTURE BLEND
For a gentle, long-term approach

If you're making tea, use herbs in the amounts listed. If you're making a tincture blend, each of these ingredients is in a tincture form; use the listed amounts and mix all the tinctures together in one bottle.

- 1 ounce cleavers herb
- 1 ounce calendula flowers
- ¾ ounce ginger root
- ½ ounce fenugreek seed

TEA BLEND FOR ZINC DEFICIENCY

Zinc deficiency is another common cause of acne. A zinc-packed tea formula can help raise the amount of zinc in the body.

- 1 ounce thyme leaf
- ½ ounce sage leaf
- ½ ounce cardamom pods
- ¼ ounce licorice root

Tea: 1 teaspoon per cup, steep 5 minutes.

PLANTAIN LEAF SPOT TREATMENT

This is one of my favorite topical treatments.

- Plantain leaf powder
- Warm water

Mix a small amount of plantain powder with warm water, apply to acne spots, and let sit for 10 minutes. Then rinse. Use every day.

ACNE WASH
To tone inflamed areas

- 1 pint water
- Equal amounts of the following ingredients:
- Lavender flowers
- Rose petals
- Chickweed herb

Add 4 tablespoons of combined blend to 1 pint water, steep 1 hour. Bathe affected area in wash for 20 minutes. Alternatively, splash the herbal wash onto your face repeatedly for about 2 minutes, or douse the area with a saturated cotton ball.

HELPFUL TOOLS FOR TREATING ACNE

Hydration contributes to many health conditions, including acne. Without proper water intake, your body cannot properly flush wastes. For proper hydration, drink half of your body weight in ounces each day. For example, if you weigh 140 pounds, drink 70 ounces of water each day.

Exercise regularly. Although you may think sweating worsens acne, it is important for cleansing the blood and opening up channels to release toxicity.

Follow the anti-inflammatory dietary guidelines to reduce overall inflammation.

Vitamin D deficiency is a common cause of acne. Take 2000 to 4000 IUs per day for 2 months.

Topically apply poke root oil to improve overall lymphatic function. Apply 1 teaspoon to congested lymph areas once per day for 2 weeks.

Topically apply juniper essential oil in an olive oil base to trouble spots.

Take crabapple flower essence, 4 drops, 4 times per day.

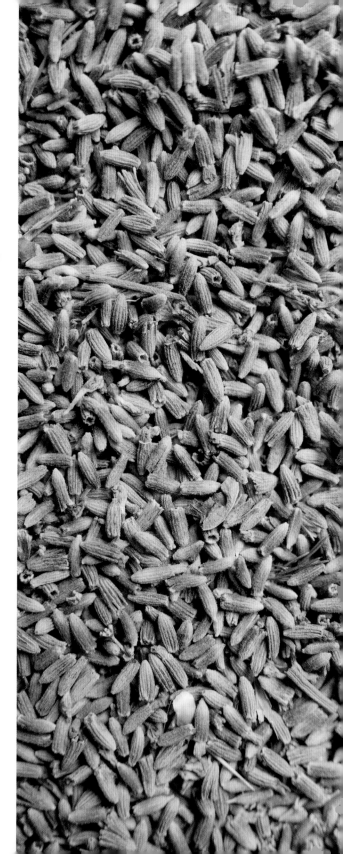

Bumps, Bruises, and Other Childhood Conditions

There are few things I am more passionate about than the use of herbs with children. Throughout the plant kingdom, there are many medicinal plants that work in gentle and safe ways, making them wonderful helpers when our little ones are not at their best. Children respond very quickly and effectively to herbal medicine, mainly because of the efficacy of the plants, but also perhaps because the little patients are nonbiased toward herbal medicine.

DOSAGE GUIDELINES FOR CHILDREN

Any parent who is just learning about herbs needs some guidance to determine the appropriate amounts of herbs for children. The two most important factors are making sure to use a safe amount of herbs, but also using enough to be effective. Use these dosage tables to determine the appropriate amount of herbs to give a child.

TEA DOSAGES FOR CHILDREN
(if adult dosage is 1 cup, or 8 ounces)

Younger than 1 year	½ to 3 teaspoons
2 to 4 years	1 to 4 ounces
4 to 7 years	2 to 4 ounces
7 to 11 years	4 to 6 ounces

CHILD DOSAGES, AGE 12 OR OLDER

APPLICATION	DOSAGE
Glycerite tinctures	1 dropperful, 3 or 4 times per day
Syrups	1 teaspoon, 3 to 6 times per day, depending on case

TINCTURE DOSAGES FOR CHILDREN
(if adult dosage is 2 dropperfuls, or 60 drops)

Younger than 3 months	2 drops
3 to 6 months	3 drops
6 to 9 months	4 drops
9 to 12 months	5 drops
12 to 18 months	7 drops
18 to 24 months	8 drops
2 to 3 years	10 drops
3 to 4 years	12 drops
4 to 6 years	15 drops
6 to 9 years	24 drops
9 to 12 years	30 drops (1 dropperful)

You can also use two equations to determine dosage of any herbal medicine to achieve the percentage of the adult dosage appropriate for a child:

Young's Rule Add 12 to the child's age, and divide the child's age by this total. For example, to determine the dosage for a 4-year-old: $4 + 12 = 16$. Then $4 \div 16 = 0.25$, or one-fourth of the adult dosage.

Cowling's Rule Divide the child's age at his or her next birthday by 24. For example, the dosage for a child who is 3, turning 4 at his next birthday, would be $4 \div 24 = 0.16$, or about one-sixth of the adult dosage.

ELDERBERRY SYRUP

For colds and immune health

This syrup is not recommended for children under 18 months.

- 2 ounces elderberries
- ½ ounce rosehips seeds
- ½ ounce boneset herb
- ½ ounce chamomile flowers
- ½ ounce yarrow flowers
- ¼ ounce rose petals

Refer to dosage guidelines for children.

BUMPS AND BRUISES SALVE

For scratches, scrapes, stings, bumps, and burns

- ¼ ounce lavender flowers
- ¼ ounce calendula flowers
- ¼ ounce chickweed herb
- ¼ ounce plantain leaf
- 5 homeopathic Arnica pellets

Refer to dosage guidelines for children.

PRESCHOOL BARRICADE TEA OR SYRUP

To protect your child from preschool germs

- 1 cup elderberries
- ½ ounce rosehip seeds
- ¼ ounce reishi mushroom pieces
- ¼ ounce rosemary leaves
  - Honey to taste (for syrup)

Tea: Add 4 or 5 tablespoons to 1 quart of hot water. Refer to dosage guidelines for children.

CALM CHILD TEA OR SYRUP

Use this tea or syrup before dinner or bed to help your child wind down.

- 1 ounce rose petals
- 1 ounce hawthorn berries

- ½ ounce chamomile flowers
- ¼ ounce lavender flowers
  - Honey (for syrup)

Refer to dosage guidelines for children.

TUMMY TEA

- ½ teaspoon catnip herb
- ¼ teaspoon ginger root
- ⅛ teaspoon cinnamon chips
  - Small amount of dried peach, cranberry, or blueberry pieces

Use 1 or 2 teaspoons per cup. Steep 2 to 5 minutes covered. Refer to dosage guidelines for children.

BABY BATH FOR COLD OR TEETHING

- ¼ ounce yarrow flowers
- ¼ ounce catnip herb
- ¼ ounce chamomile flowers

Place herbs in a muslin bag and add to a warm bath. Place baby in bath, and soak for 10 to 15 minutes, ensuring that the baby stays warm.

HELPFUL TOOLS FOR TREATING BUMPS, BRUISES, AND OTHER CHILDHOOD CONDITIONS

Essential oils are great in the diffuser—lavender to help with sleep, rosemary for a cold, fennel for an upset tummy.

Place aromatic plants, such as lavender, rosemary, thyme, and lemon balm, along your walkway. These are all naturally antiseptic and help clear away germs as you and your kids enter your home. Kids love to brush their hands along the herbs as they walk to the door.

Fatigue and Brain Function

When fatigue is holding you back from getting the most of your day, it's time to investigate where all your energy is going. Some causes are more obvious than others, such as lack of sleep and overwork, but others, such as malabsorption, dehydration, stress, and inflammation, may not quickly come to mind. All of these are huge energy suckers, and as long as they play a part in your daily life, your energy is going to be low. A few herbal recipes can help you jump start your energy and get your brain firing on all cylinders.

Unless noted otherwise, to make the teas in these recipes, add 4 or 5 tablespoons of herbs to 1 quart of almost boiling water. Then drink 3 cups per day or 1 quart throughout the day, hot or cold. With tinctures, for chronic complaints, take 1 dropperful 3 times per day. For acute issues, take 2 dropperfuls every 2 or 3 hours for 1 or 2 days, and then 2 dropperfuls 2 or 3 times per day for 5 days. For recipes that do not include instructions, see "An Herbalist's Laboratory" for information regarding how to create and use them.

WAKE UP TEA

- 1 ounce yerba mate leaf
- ½ ounce spearmint leaf
- ½ ounce agrimony herb
- ¼ ounce hibiscus flower

1 or 2 teaspoons per cup, steep 8 to 10 minutes. Drink as desired.

ENERGY NOW TINCTURE

- 3 parts eleuthero root
- 3 parts ginkgo leaf
- 1 part guarana seed
- 1 part peppermint leaf

1 or 2 dropperfuls as needed.

AFTERNOON PICK ME UP TEA

- 1 ounce orange peel
- ½ ounce lavender flowers
- ½ ounce ginger root
- ¼ ounce lemongrass herb
- ¹⁄₁₆ ounce cayenne powder

1 or 2 teaspoons per cup, steep 8 to 10 minutes. Drink as desired.

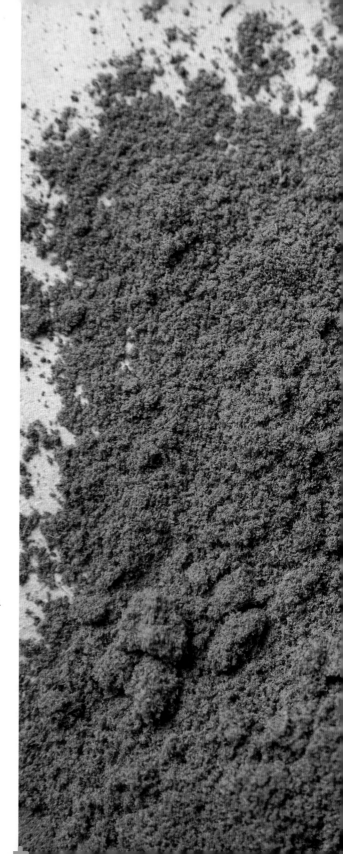

ENERGY BALLS

This is a great snack to help you get over that afternoon slump.

2	cups nut butter
1	cup honey
6	tablespoons Siberian ginseng powder
1	tablespoon guarana powder
1	tablespoon nettle leaf powder
1	tablespoon spirulina powder
1	tablespoon kola nut powder
1	tablespoon cinnamon powder
½	teaspoon sea salt
¼	teaspoon cardamom powder
1	cup shredded coconut
1	cup carob or chocolate chips

Mix together the nut butter and honey until smooth and set aside. In a separate bowl, mix all of the herbal powders together and then add the remaining ingredients. Fold the herbal mix into the nut butter and honey. Mix and knead well. Pinch off enough dough to make 1-inch round balls. Store in an airtight container for 1 or 2 weeks. Eat 1 or 2 to get going.

Female Complaints

A woman's body is as beautiful as it is dynamically complex. Contained within it are the mysteries of conception and the rhythms of the moon. Unfortunately, our modern times have not necessarily helped promote a healthy perception or hormonal function of the female body. As a result, many woman suffer emotionally and physically from a malfunctioning endocrine system, leading to monthly uterine pain, irregular menses, infertility, emotional instability, cysts, fibroids, and other problems. Thankfully, many herbs tone, regulate, and nourish the female endocrine system in a gentle and safe way. I often think about the uterus and its support system of thirty ligaments. If only we as women had that kind of support in our day-to-day lives! The ligament closest to the uterus is the suspensory ligament, which cradles the uterus like a mother cradles a baby. Herbs act similarly when it comes to the female body—gently, with wise care.

The ovaries make reproductive hormones, primarily estrogen and progesterone. Estrogens direct cells to grow and multiply, while progesterone directs them to slow their growth and mature normally. Estrogen creation relies on other hormones in the surrounding tissues, such as fat, skin, and muscle, whereas progesterone is produced after the ovum (the egg) is released. If regular ovulation is not occurring, these hormones are most likely out of balance.

Another tricky aspect of the female endocrine system is that these hormones are present in our bodies to varying degrees at all times. During premenopause and perimenopause, each and every day, a woman's hormone levels change and adjust based on the menses cycle. Estrogen tends to be higher in the first half of the cycle and progesterone in the latter, but excessive estrogens and shorter progesterone cycles are quite common.

Stress, a common factor these days, can also cause an imbalance of estrogen and progesterone. Progesterone is the loving, gentle hormone. The female body, by design, would have ample progesterone to provide support throughout menses. When progesterone is low or absent, menstrual cycles can be shorter, heavy uterine bleeding may occur, or conception can be difficult or impossible. In addition, when a woman is under stress, her adrenal glands tend to work very hard and cortisol (the stress hormone that keeps us going) is produced. To meet the demands of stress, her body gives up the available progesterone and converts it to cortisol. To restore progesterone levels, lowering overall stress and supporting the adrenal glands is necessary.

Hormone levels do not shift quickly. They take time, nourishment, and gentle coaxing to re-regulate. Therefore, consistency and a sufficient amount of time is necessary to create physiological change.

Unless noted otherwise, to make the teas in these recipes, add 4 or 5 tablespoons of herbs to 1 quart of almost boiling water. Then drink 3 cups per day or 1 quart throughout the day, hot or cold. With tinctures, for chronic complaints, take 1 dropperful 3 times per day. For acute issues, take 2 dropperfuls every 2 or 3 hours for 1 or 2 days, and then 2 dropperfuls 2 or 3 times per day for 5 days. For recipes that do not include instructions, see "An Herbalist's Laboratory" for information regarding how to create and use them.

ENDOCRINE TEA TONIC
For balancing hormones

- 1 ounce bupleurum root
- 1 ounce chaste berry
- ½ ounce wild yam root
- ½ ounce lemongrass leaf
- ¼ ounce licorice root
- ¼ ounce ginger root

Drink 3 cups per day for 12 weeks.

ENDOCRINE TINCTURE
For regulating menses

- 4 parts chaste berry
- 3 parts dong quai root
- 1 part ginger root

1 dropperful 3 times per day for 12 weeks.

UTERINE FIBROIDS TEA OR TINCTURE BLEND

This is just one aspect of the treatment of uterine fibroids. See a certified practitioner to discuss a thorough and well-rounded approach. Although I've had success using teas and tinctures to treat fibroids, it takes a lot of commitment on the behalf of the patient.

If you're making tea, use herbs in the amounts listed. If you're making a tincture blend, each of these ingredients is in a tincture form; use the listed amounts and mix all the tinctures together in one bottle.

- 2 ounces burdock root
- 1 ounce dandelion root
- 1 ounce Oregon grape root
- 1 ounce wild yam root
- 1 ounce orange peel
- ¾ ounce yellow dock root
- ¾ ounce fennel seed
- ¼ ounce ginger root

Tea: Drink 3 cups per day for 12 weeks. Tincture: 2 dropperfuls, 3 times per day for 12 weeks.

MENSTRUAL CRAMPING TINCTURE

3 parts crampbark

2 parts California poppy herb and flower

1 part black cohosh root

1 part blue cohosh root

½ part burdock root

½ part Jamaican dogwood bark

1 or 2 dropperfuls at onset of discomfort.

FERTILITY TEA

I give credit to Rosemary Gladstar for this recipe, and in jest I have often warned women of its effectiveness—many women who use this tea have returned to my shoppe with big, beautiful, baby-filled bellies.

4 ounces sassafras root

3 ounces wild yam root

2 ounces licorice root

1 ounce chaste berry

1 ounce cinnamon chips

1 ounce ginger root

½ ounce dong quai root

¼ ounce orange peel

Pinch of stevia

Drink 3 cups per day for 12 weeks or until conception occurs.

HELPFUL TOOLS FOR TREATING FEMALE COMPLAINTS

I've had success supporting menses with this simple recommendation: From day 1 of menses to day 15, drink 2 cups of peppermint tea per day. From day 15 to day 1, drink 2 cups of chamomile tea per day.

Use Magnesia Phosphorica (Mag Phos) cell salts for menstrual cramping. Take six pellets under the tongue every 20 minutes until cramping subsides.

An Arvigo abdominal massage, a technique created by naprapath Rosita Arvigo, is a wonderful external abdominal massage that realigns the uterus and ensures that blood vessels are not constricted or constrained, which is often a cause of pain. Look for an Arvigo certified practitioner in your area.

Lavender, clary sage, sweet fennel, and geranium essential oils can be helpful.

Place castor oil packs on the abdomen.

Chamomile

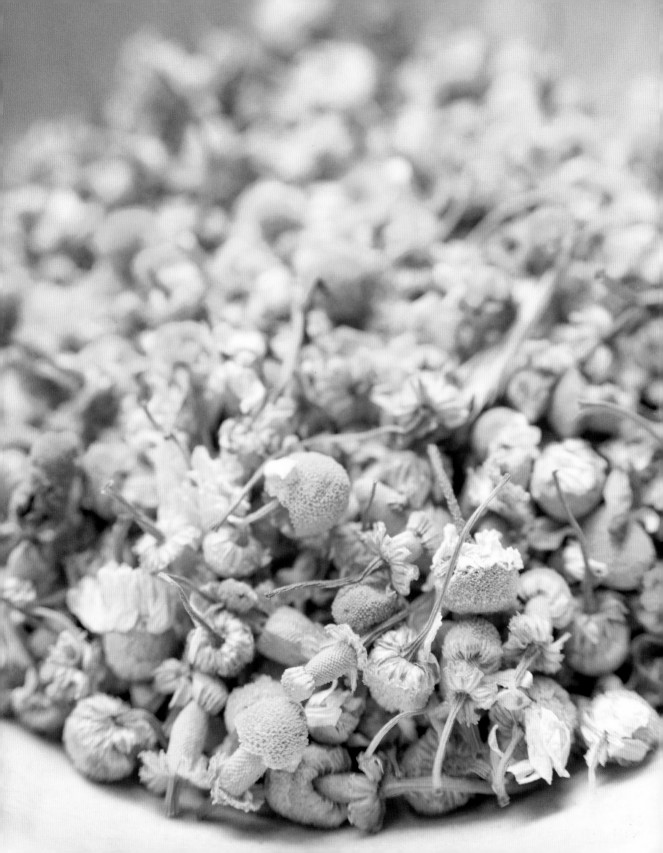

Inflammation and Pain

Inflammation can include a wide range of symptoms from myriad causes. Some are obvious, such as a sprain to the wrist, but others are silent and slow to see or feel, creating flare-ups that seem to come out of the blue. In either case, learning to recognize your body's signals and which herbs will turn down the inflammation burner will prove helpful.

Unless noted otherwise, to make the teas in these recipes, add 4 or 5 tablespoons of herbs to 1 quart of almost boiling water. Then drink 3 cups per day or 1 quart throughout the day, hot or cold. With tinctures, for chronic complaints, take 1 dropperful 3 times per day. For acute issues, take 2 dropperfuls every 2 or 3 hours for 1 or 2 days, and then 2 dropperfuls 2 or 3 times per day for 5 days. For recipes that do not include instructions, see "An Herbalist's Laboratory" for information regarding how to create and use them.

SPRAIN SUPPORT OIL

Equal amounts of the following ingredients:

- Wormwood herb
- Witch hazel leaf or bark
- Bay laurel leaf
- Poplar bud

Apply liberally and frequently.

ANTI-INFLAMMATORY TEA

- 1 ounce cat's claw bark
- ½ ounce marshmallow root
- ½ ounce turmeric powder
- ½ ounce yucca root
- ¼ ounce ginger root
- ⅛ ounce licorice root

Use 2 teaspoons per cup, simmer 10 minutes covered. Drink 2 cups per day.

PAIN-FREE TINCTURE

Because willow bark contains salicin, those who are allergic or sensitive to aspirin or who are taking blood thinner medication should not take this tincture.

- 3 parts white willow bark
- 2 parts valerian root
- 1 part Jamaican dogwood bark
- 1 part kava kava root
- 1 part black cohosh root

1 to 2 dropperfuls as needed, not to exceed 6 doses per day.

HELPFUL TOOLS FOR TREATING INFLAMMATION AND PAIN

Use essential oils, such as frankincense, camphor, fennel, bergamot, and thyme.

Apply castor oil packs topically to the affected area or to the abdomen for intestinal inflammation.

Eat only organically grown foods. They reportedly have two to five times more nutrients than nonorganic foods, and eating organic will decrease your exposure to pesticides, which increase inflammation.

Do not eat any single food more than three or four times per week. Plan your meals ahead and try to find at least ten recipes you enjoy.

ANTI-INFLAMMATORY GUIDELINES

FOOD CATEGORY	FOODS TO EAT	FOODS TO AVOID
Beverages	Minimum of half your weight in ounces per day of filtered water; small amounts of rice, oat, almond, or soy milk; herbal teas	Coffee, soda, juice, caffeinated teas, alcohol
Butter and oil Mix 1 lb. organic butter with 1 cup extra virgin olive oil to use as a spread. Store in refrigerator.	Olive oil for cooking, coconut oil only for baking, and nut or seed oils for salads	
Dairy	Small amount of organic butter and organic eggs	Cheese, animal milk, and commercial eggs
Fruit Eat only one or two pieces of fruit per day. If possible, bake the fruit before eating (such as a baked apple or pear). Eat mostly fruit from the 3 and 6 percent categories.	**3 percent** Cantaloupe, rhubarb, melon, strawberries **6 percent** Apricot, blackberries, cranberries, papaya, peach, plum, raspberries, kiwi **15 percent** Apple, blueberries, cherries, grapes, pear, pineapple, pomegranate **20 percent** Banana, fig, prune	Citrus fruits except lemon
Grains Avoid if sensitive to grains.	Amaranth, barley, buckwheat, millet, quinoa, basmati rice, brown rice, rye, teff, rice crackers, wheat-free crackers	All wheat products—breads, cereals, white flour, wheat pasta—and all corn products
Legumes Soak legumes overnight and cook them slowly the next day.	Split peas, lentils, kidney beans, pinto beans, black beans, garbanzo beans, mung beans, adzuki beans	
Meat Eat protein with every meal to regulate and maintain steady blood sugar and energy. Eat only meat, not skin, of organic or free-range chicken and turkey.	Organic or free-range chicken and turkey, wild game, lamb	Beef, pork
Nuts and seeds Grind seeds and add to steamed vegetables.	Ground flax, pumpkin, sesame, sunflower seeds; cooked grains; nuts and seeds, including nut butters	Peanuts and peanut butter

FOOD CATEGORY	FOODS TO EAT	FOODS TO AVOID
Seafood Ocean fish are an excellent source of essential fatty acids and should be eaten two or three times per week. Poach, bake, or broil wild (not farmed) cold water fish.	Wild salmon, cod, haddock, halibut, mackerel, sardines, tuna, trout, summer flounder	Shellfish: shrimp, crab, lobster, clams
Soy	Fermented soy (tempeh or miso)	Tofu can cause reactions in some people. Eliminate if necessary.
Spices	Most spices	Cayenne and pepper flakes
Sweeteners Avoid	Pure maple syrup, brown rice syrup, raw honey, stevia	Sugar or any processed sweetener
Vegetables Mostly lower carbohydrate vegetables in the 3 to 6 percent category. Steaming vegetables improves the use or availability of the food nutrients, enabling the intestinal mucosa to repair itself. Use minimal raw vegetables except as a salad. Eat at least one or two green vegetables each day.	**3 percent** Asparagus, bean sprouts, beet greens, broccoli, red and green cabbage, cauliflower, celery, Swiss chard, cucumber, endive, lettuce (green, red, romaine, mixed greens), mustard and dandelion greens, radishes, spinach, watercress **6 percent** String beans, beets, bok choy, brussels sprouts, chives, collards, kale, kohlrabi, leeks, onion, parsley, red pepper, pumpkin, rutabaga, turnip, zucchini **15 percent** Artichoke, parsnip, green peas, squash, carrot **20+ percent** Yam, sweet potato	Tomato, potato, pepper, eggplant

Insomnia

It seems everyone has experienced a bout of insomnia at one point or another. Some are not so fortunate, and the lack of sleep is an ongoing concern. Lack of sleep can wreak havoc on your life. Your brain loses function and your emotions become unbalanced. Sleep is also necessary for cellular regeneration and detoxification. During sleep, the body shifts its blood balance from alkaline to acidic to pull together all of the day's accumulated toxins and prepare them for elimination. Because all of this is going on while you sleep, it's important that you not redirect your body's focus to digestion, for example, by eating before you go to bed.

Those who suffer from insomnia have varying degrees of sleepless nights and patterns. Some have no problem falling asleep, but then wake up and are not able to return to sleep. Some lie in bed for hours, waiting for sleep to come. Others are startled awake in the middle of the night and their brains immediately begin chattering away, what I call the "monkey mind."

Stress, overwork, and emotional upset seem to be common causes for insomnia. Stress and overwork take a toll on the adrenal glands, which can result in insomnia. Emotional upset is more directly correlated to the heart energetic system of Chinese medicine theory. At night, the Yang energy, the soul's vibrant energetic moving aspect, should be quiet and contained within the Yin, the slow and still energy of the soul. When emotions are high, whether this results from grief, joy, fear, or anger, it is difficult for the Yin to contain the Yang because the energy is moving too much and is too big.

The first goal in treatment is to find a way to get to sleep. Then you can identify what is causing the insomnia. Is it stress, overwork, or emotional issues? Pain, breathing issues, medications, late intake of caffeine or food, or poor sleep habits? Spend some time examining these aspects and choose the most appropriate herbs to treat the underlying causes driving the insomnia.

Unless noted otherwise, to make the teas in these recipes, add 4 or 5 tablespoons of herbs to 1 quart of almost boiling water. Then drink 3 cups per day or 1 quart throughout the day, hot or cold. For recipes that do not include instructions, see "An Herbalist's Laboratory" for information regarding how to create and use them.

KNOCKOUT TINCTURE

- 2 parts California poppy herb and flowers
- 2 parts hawthorn berries
- 2 parts hops flowers
- 1 part passionflower herb
- 1 part agrimony herb

2 dropperfuls 30 minutes before bed and then 2 more dropperfuls at bedtime.

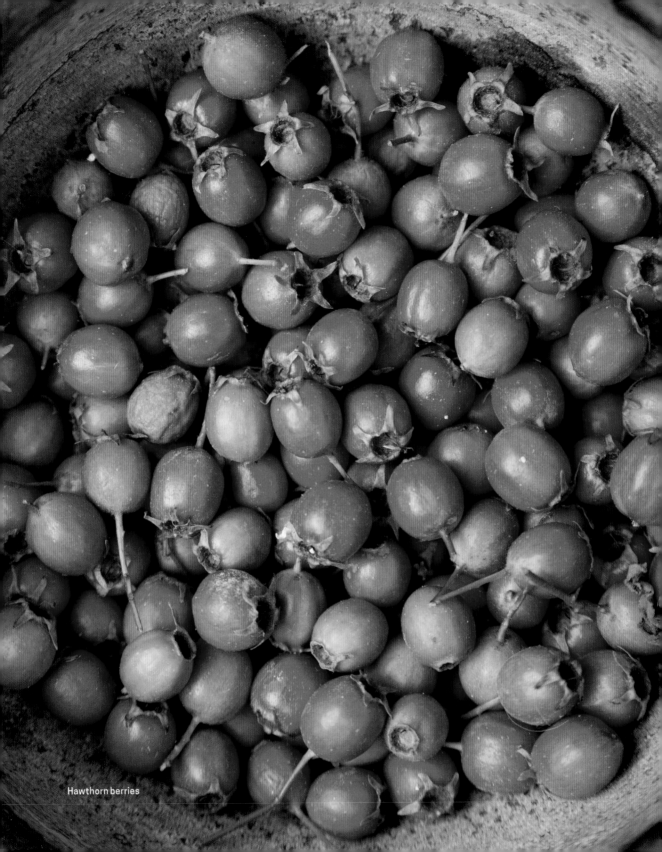
Hawthorn berries

SLEEP TEA

- 1 ounce catnip herb
- 1 ounce skullcap herb
- 1 ounce passionflower herb
- ½ ounce chamomile flowers
- ½ ounce rose petals
- ½ ounce lavender flowers
- ¼ ounce hops flowers

Use 2 teaspoons per cup, steep 5 to 8 minutes covered. Drink 1 hour before bedtime.

For a muscle relaxant component, add 1 ounce crampbark, valerian root, or black cohosh root.

SLEEP PILLOW

Equal amounts of the following ingredients:

- Lavender flowers
- Rose petals
- Chamomile flowers

Fill a small (such as 4-by-4-inch) pillow with herbs and sleep with it.

SLEEP SALVE

Keep this salve at your bedside.
Equal amounts of the following ingredients:

- Chamomile flowers
- Valerian root
- Lavender flowers
- Hops flowers

Apply to the temple region of the forehead, as needed.

SLEEP CAPSULES

- 1 ounce valerian root powder
- 1 ounce skullcap herb powder
- 1 ounce hops flower powder

Take 2 to 4 capsules, 1 hour before bedtime.

HOT BATH WITH RELAXING BATH SALTS

- 1 ounce lavender
- 1 ounce mugwort
- 1 ounce rose petal powder
- 8 ounces Epsom salts

Place herbs in a muslin bag. Pour salts directly in hot bath along with bag of herbs.

HELPFUL TOOLS FOR TREATING INSOMNIA

Use an essential oil diffuser or place a couple drops onto your pillow: catnip, ylang ylang, clary sage, lavender, and marjoram.

Establish a sleep routine. Give your body cues that it is time to slow down and prepare for sleep, just as we do with babies.

Avoid computers and TV 30 minutes before bedtime.

Increase your calcium and magnesium intake.

Menopause

Menopause occurs when the ovaries stop releasing eggs and menstruation ceases. The period called premenopause, or perimenopause, when the monthly cycle of ovulation and menstruation becomes less regular, can begin 8 to 10 years before menopause. This entire period of transition is also known as the climacteric phase, because the reproductive phase of life is reaching its climax.

The most common signs and symptoms of menopause are hot flashes, vaginal dryness, vaginal thinning and irritation, inability to climax, decreased sex drive, and disturbances in emotional health.

Most research says that the cure for difficulties with sex in menopause is more sex, but it is difficult to have good sex when it doesn't feel good. Many herbs can heal, tonify, and calm inflamed vaginal tissues; lubricate the vaginal walls; and relax tight muscles. Herbs can be particularly beneficial if pain is caused by dryness, infection, or irritation. At the same time, herbal remedies can restore normal, helpful bacterial flora to the mucous membranes lining the vagina. Many of these plants contain protective essential oils or other biochemicals that reduce inappropriate microbes.

Unless noted otherwise, to make the teas in these recipes, add 4 or 5 tablespoons of herbs to 1 quart of almost boiling water. Then drink 3 cups per day or 1 quart throughout the day, hot or cold. With tinctures, for chronic complaints, take 1 dropperful 3 times per day. For acute issues, take 2 dropperfuls every 2 or 3 hours for 1 or 2 days, and then 2 dropperfuls 2 or 3 times per day for 5 days.

For recipes that do not include instructions, see "An Herbalist's Laboratory" for information regarding how to create and use them.

HERB TEA FOR LIBIDO

- 3½ ounces of shatavari root
- 1 ounce maca root
- ½ ounce tribulus fruit
- ½ ounce licorice root
- ½ ounce rose petals

Use 1 tablespoon per cup, steep for 20 minutes covered, and strain. Drink 1 cup, hot or cold, 3 times per day.

VAGINAL TISSUE HEALER

Use as a sitz bath, tea, or salve.

- ¼ ounce chamomile flowers
- ¼ ounce calendula flowers
- ¼ ounce elder flowers
- ¼ ounce comfrey leaf
- ¼ ounce yarrow flowers

HORMONE BALANCE TINCTURE

- 3 parts maca root
- 3 parts nettle leaf
- 1 part dong quai root
- 1 part sage leaf

1 dropperful 3 times per day.

OSTEOPOROSIS HERBAL VINEGAR OR TINCTURE BLEND

If you're making vinegar, use herbs in the amounts listed. If you're making a tincture blend, each of these ingredients is in a tincture form; use the listed amounts and mix all the tinctures together in one bottle.

- ½ ounce St. John's wort herb
- ¼ ounce hawthorn berry
- ¼ ounce black cohosh root
- ¼ ounce nettle leaf
- ¼ ounce alfalfa herb
- 1 pint apple cider vinegar

Vinegar: 1 teaspoon, 2 times per day. Tincture: 1 dropperful, 2 times per day.

HOT FLASH TINCTURE

- 3 parts sage leaf
- 3 parts peppermint leaf
- 2 parts black cohosh root

1 or 2 dropperfuls, 2 or 3 times per day.

TEA FOR KEEPING THINGS COOL

- 2 ounces linden flowers
- 2 ounces chickweed leaf
- 2 ounces hibiscus flowers
- 1 ounce marshmallow root
- 1 ounce chamomile flowers

1 or 2 teaspoons per cup, steep for 15 minutes. Drink at room temperature as often as needed.

TEA FOR MEMORY AND CEREBRAL CIRCULATION

- 3 ounces gotu kola leaf
- 2 ounces skullcap herb
- 2 ounces linden leaf
- 2 ounces rooibos tea
- ½ ounce rosemary leaf
- ½ ounce sage leaf

2 teaspoons per cup, steep 5 to 10 minutes covered. Drink hot or cold, 2 cups per day.

HELPFUL TOOLS FOR TREATING MENOPAUSE

Use essential oil blend for vaginal dryness: ylang ylang and helichrysum in a base of jojoba oil applied topically twice per day.

Ancient cultures have been documented to have used plants such as maca, kudzu, and dong quai to treat vaginal dryness, and these herbs have again proven their worth in modern scientific studies.

Exercise liberates the stored estrogen and is very important!

Take vitamin D internally and apply vitamin E topically.

Respiratory Ailments

Head congestion, runny nose, or cough—none of them is any fun. But armed with a little herbal knowledge, you can combat the cold blues and get back to your regular routine. Herbs high in volatile oils are great for the respiratory system because they penetrate on contact and begin alleviating symptoms right away. Herbs such as reishi and echinacea root are designed to stimulate the fighter cells that can give you a big hand up to avoid going down. Astragalus is a wonderful herb for strengthening the overall immune system in the prevention of colds and flus. One word to the wise: you should understand how best to use the two most common cold herbs—astragalus and echinacea.

Imagine a giant fortress. Atop the fortress is a handful of guards who walk and patrol to safeguard against invasion. Taking astragalus is like asking the reserve guards to step up to the wall to patrol. With a guard at every post, nothing can come in. Unfortunately, it works the other way around, too. If one little sneaker cold somehow makes its way in, and you continue to take astragalus, you've sealed the exits and the enemy cold becomes trapped inside the body. My advice, then, is to take astragalus before cold and flu season or before you get on a plane to arm your body with strong forces, but always discontinue its use if you happen to catch a sneaker.

Echinacea was probably the first herbal medicine to make it big in the common marketplace. It was marketed heavily as an herb that could stimulate the immune system, shorten the duration of a cold, and build up long-term immunity protection for the body. But only one of these claims is true. Echinacea does stimulate the immune system, but only for a short duration—a protective blast, so to speak. It gives you a sudden, quick blast of fighter cells to nip the very beginnings of a cold or flu. So, for example, if your officemate has been coughing and sneezing, take the echinacea, and take it often, for a day or two. Is the hint of a sore throat signaling that you're about to get a cold? Take the echinacea. But if the cold isn't nipped, and two days later it's still there, no matter how big or small, put the echinacea down and choose more appropriate herbs for treating a cold. Colds and flus rarely enter the body and hover—they come in, go deeper, and blossom.

Unless noted otherwise, to make the teas in these recipes, add 4 or 5 tablespoons of herbs to 1 quart of almost boiling water. Then drink 3 cups per day or 1 quart throughout the day, hot or cold. With tinctures, for chronic complaints, take 1 dropperful 3 times per day. For acute issues, take 2 dropperfuls every 2 or 3 hours for 1 or 2 days, and then 2 dropperfuls 2 or 3 times per day for 5 days. For recipes that do not include instructions, see "An Herbalist's Laboratory" for information regarding how to create and use them.

HEAD COLD OR FLU TEA

- 1 ounce peppermint leaf
- 1 ounce spearmint leaf
- 1 ounce yarrow flowers
- ½ ounce aniseed
- ½ ounce boneset herb
- ½ ounce ginger root

Use 2 teaspoons per cup. Steep 10 minutes covered. Drink as hot as possible, 3 cups per day.

CHEST COLD TINCTURE

- 3 parts usnea
- 2 part mullein leaf
- 1 part horehound leaf
- 1 part coltsfoot leaf
- 1 part wild cherry bark

Take 2 dropperfuls every 2 hours for 24 hours, and then 2 dropperfuls every 3 hours for 5 days or until systems subside.

BUILD MY IMMUNE RESERVES TEA OR TINCTURE BLEND

If you're making tea, use herbs in the amounts listed. If you're making a tincture blend, each of these ingredients is in a tincture form; use the listed amounts and mix all the tinctures together in one bottle.

- 2 ounces elderberries
- ¾ ounce rosehips
- ½ ounce astragalus root
- ¼ ounce ashwagandha root
- ¼ ounce licorice root

Tea: Drink 1 to 3 cups per day. Tincture: Take 1 dropperful, 1 to 3 times per day.

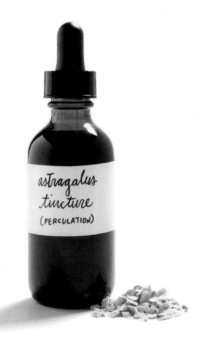

HERBAL INHALATION

- 1 ounce thyme leaf
- 1 ounce wild cherry bark
- 1 ounce marshmallow root
- 1 ounce eucalyptus leaf

Fill a large stockpot with water and bring to a boil. Turn off the heat and add the herbs. Cover and let steep 5 minutes. Uncover and let heavy steam roll off the top to prevent burning your face. Cover your head with a towel, lean over the pot, and breathe as deeply as you can for five breaths. Take a break and repeat as often as desired. Heat and reuse this pot of herbs for 1 or 2 days.

HERBAL BATH FOR COLD AND FLU

- 2 ounces chamomile flowers
- 2 ounces rosemary leaf
- 2 ounces eucalyptus leaf

Put herbs into a large muslin bag and add to a hot bath. Soak 20 to 30 minutes while drinking ginger root or yarrow tea.

GINGER ROOT OR YARROW TEA

Drink this tea while soaking in the bath.

- 1 teaspoon elder flowers
- ½ teaspoon yarrow flowers
- ½ teaspoon ginger root
- 1 hop strobile

Add herbs to 1 cup hot water. Steep 8 minutes covered. Drink hot while taking an herbal bath.

HELPFUL TOOLS FOR TREATING RESPIRATORY AILMENTS

Try the warm sock treatment.

Use essential oils in a room diffuser: rosemary, lavender, eucalyptus, pine, fir, and thyme.

WARMING SOCK TREATMENT

Warming socks are a warm and cozy treatment for any condition that involves congestion. They can also help increase circulation and stimulate the immune system.

Most people report a significant decrease in congestion after using this treatment, which is particularly helpful for several other conditions as well:

- Sprains, strains, pain, and inflammation of feet or ankles
- Fevers
- Headaches or migraines
- Ear infections
- Sore throats
- Upper respiratory infections
- Coughs and colds
- Bronchitis
- Sinus infections

The warming sock treatment works in several ways. First, it sends a clear message to the brain: "Oh my! I've got cold, wet feet! You need to warm them up." The brain reacts by slightly increasing the overall body temperature and increasing blood circulation in an attempt to warm the feet. The increase in body temperature creates an inhospitable environment for bacteria and viruses, and the increased circulation mobilizes immune cells to fight infection, reduce congestion, and remove blood stagnation if an injury is present.

Here's what you'll need:

Pair of medium-weight 100-percent cotton socks

Pair of thick, 100-percent wool socks

A warm bath or footbath

Towel

Rosemary essential oil (optional)

Ice water

Make sure your feet are warm. Soak them in warm water, or take a warm bath, for at least 5 to 10 minutes. Then dry your feet. Optionally, rub rosemary essential oil into your feet for additional immune support. Next, soak the cotton socks in ice water. Wring them out well and put them on. Put on heavy wool socks over the wet cotton socks, being sure that the dry wool socks cover all the wet cotton socks. Immediately go to bed, snuggling in tight with adequate blankets. Leave the socks on overnight. This treatment works best if repeated for three nights in a row, to ensure resolution. Warming socks are also effective and easy for treating children during naptime.

Skin Conditions

I've said it once and I'll say it again: the condition of the skin is often a direct reflection of what is happening inside your body. If your insides are working well, are nourished, and are in good health, your skin is clear. We often look to the liver when skin disorders are present, but we should also examine the gastrointestinal and central nervous systems to ensure they are in balance as well. Mineral-rich herbs such as nettle, alfalfa, horsetail, comfrey, and kelp are powerhouses for the body and enliven the skin to look its best.

In my practice, I have noticed that eczema seems to be more deficiency-related and psoriasis is often attributed to genetics. In other words, eczema seems to come on when a physical deficiency occurs from either lack of certain nutrients or decreased function in one or more bodily systems. A good example would be an eczema outbreak after a stressful week at work. This implies that the central nervous system is unable to handle the stress, leading to the eczema. Eczema is easier to treat with herbs after you identify the source of the outbreak. Another example is an insufficiently functioning gastrointestinal system that is accumulating inflammation and waste. These irritants cause eczema in some of my patients, and once the gastrointestinal tract is soothed and treated, the eczema calms down.

Another skin ailment, contact dermatitis, is an allergic reaction that produces a rash, sometimes with discomfort. It can result from a wide range of sources, including contact with harsh cleaning products, poison ivy, or another irritant. After the irritant is touched, inflammatory cells respond.

The reaction often looks like a burn or has raised, blisterlike welts. The goal is to calm the skin and attempt to clear the toxins from the body.

Fungal skin infections such as ringworm are contagious and quite common. They are typically spread through skin-to-skin contact or contact with contaminated items. Although they rarely cause serious problems, they should be treated, and herbs offer a competent approach.

Unless noted otherwise, to make the teas in these recipes, add 4 or 5 tablespoons of herbs to 1 quart of almost boiling water. Then drink 3 cups per day or 1 quart throughout the day, hot or cold. With tinctures, for chronic complaints, take 1 dropperful 3 times per day. For acute issues, take 2 dropperfuls every 2 or 3 hours for 1 or 2 days, and then 2 dropperfuls 2 or 3 times per day for 5 days. For recipes that do not include instructions, see "An Herbalist's Laboratory" for information regarding how to create and use them.

ECZEMA TINCTURE

- 2 parts chickweed herb
- 1½ parts yellow dock root
- 1½ parts red clover herb
- 1½ parts nettle leaf
- ¾ part elecampane root
- ½ part calendula flowers
- ¼ part marshmallow root

Use 1 or 2 dropperfuls, 3 times per day.

ECZEMA WASH

- 1 ounce chickweed herb
- 1 ounce plantain leaf
- 1 ounce elder flowers
- 1 ounce chamomile flowers
- ½ ounce marshmallow root

Steep 6 tablespoons per quart hot water, covered, for 2 hours. Put into a basin and soak affected area for 20 to 30 minutes, twice per day.

POISON IVY LINIMENT

For contact dermatitis

Equal amounts of the following ingredients:

- Mugwort herb
- White oak bark
- Plantain leaf
- Echinacea root
- Chickweed herb

Soak herbs completely covered in isopropyl alcohol for 4 weeks. Strain and store in a sealed container. Douse a cotton ball and gently apply to affected area as needed. Do not reuse the same cotton ball.

BUG BITE RELIEF

This can be made into a vinegar liniment, poultice, or salve. If making a vinegar liniment, use apple cider vinegar.

- ¼ ounce plantain leaf
- ¼ ounce yellow dock root
- ¼ ounce yarrow flowers
- ¼ ounce chaparral powder
- ¼ ounce witch hazel bark

FUNGAL FIGHTER TINCTURE

For internal and external use

- 3 parts black walnut hull
- 3 parts pau d'arco bark
- 1 part usnea
- 1 part myrrh powder

Use 1 or 2 dropperfuls, 3 times per day, or apply liberally as needed.

LEMONGRASS TEA

To help eliminate fungal infections

- Lemongrass stalks

Use 1 or 2 teaspoons per cup, steep 10 to 12 minutes. Drink 1 to 3 cups per day.

HELPFUL TOOLS FOR TREATING SKIN ISSUES

Use lavender essential oil, which has powerful antifungal effects. Studies have shown that the oil not only stops fungi from developing, but can also kill fungal infections.

Eat foods included in the anti-inflammatory guidelines.

Take 2000 to 4000 IUs of vitamin D per day. Vitamin D deficiency is common with eczema and psoriasis.

Take vitamin A.

Apply castor oil packs to affected areas.

Take digestive enzymes and L-glutamine, the amino acid specific for healing the intestinal lining.

Stress and Adrenal Problems

Herbs are particularly helpful for the adrenal glands. They not only help regulate and return function to the adrenal system, but they nourish the body on a cellular level. As you're studying herbal formulas, remember that the cause of any disharmony in the body must always be addressed. When your adrenals have been overexerted by stress and are underfunctioning, you need to address the stress if it is still occurring, or you may need to address your body's pattern of reacting to stress. For example, if you are not happy at work and each day you are sad, angry, or tired of the idea of going to work, that stress needs to be evaluated. Or perhaps you experienced a time in your life that was particularly stressful—you were financially strapped, you had too many obligations or a tenuous relationship. In your current life those things have passed, yet each time you think about money you react as if you were in the trauma zone. That pattern needs to be addressed.

Unless noted otherwise, to make the teas in these recipes, add 4 or 5 tablespoons of herbs to 1 quart of almost boiling water. Then drink 3 cups per day or 1 quart throughout the day, hot or cold. With tinctures, for chronic complaints, take 1 dropperful 3 times per day. For acute issues, take 2 dropperfuls every 2 or 3 hours for 1 or 2 days, and then 2 dropperfuls 2 or 3 times per day for 5 days. For recipes that do not include instructions, see "An Herbalist's Laboratory" for information regarding how to create and use them.

ADRENAL REHAB TINCTURE

- 2 parts nettle leaf
- 2 parts schizandra berry
- 1½ parts rhodiola root
- 1 part skullcap herb
- 1 part wood betony herb
- ½ part black cohosh root

Take 2 dropperfuls twice per day for 12 weeks.

NERVOUS NELLY TEA

- 1 ounce skullcap herb
- 1 ounce passionflower herb
- ½ ounce burdock root
- ½ ounce chamomile flowers
- ¼ ounce rose petals
- ⅛ ounce lavender flowers
- 1/16 teaspoon cayenne powder

Use 1 or 2 teaspoons per cup, steep 8 to 10 minutes. Drink as desired.

RELAX NOW TINCTURE

- 2 parts lemon balm leaf
- 2 parts oatstraw herb
- 2 parts skullcap herb
- 1 part nettle leaf
- ½ part hops flowers
- ½ part valerian root

Take 1 or 2 dropperfuls in acute stress situations.

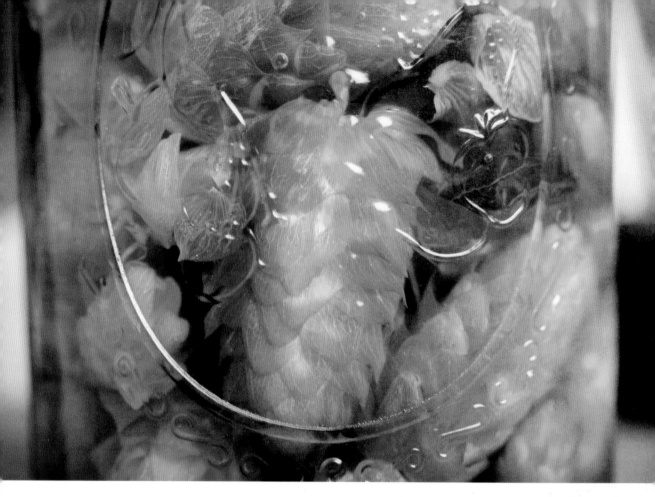

Hops

HELPFUL TOOLS FOR TREATING STRESS AND ADRENAL HEALTH

Exercise often.

Meditate daily.

Establish regular eating and sleeping patterns.

Take B vitamins, known as the stress vitamins, to help reduce the quick-fired stress response.

Take calcium and magnesium.

Use flower essences to help reduce negative habit response.

Tummy Complaints and Irritable Bowels

One of the most common bowel diseases diagnosed today, irritable bowel disease, or IBD, is a problem I often see in my office. Those who suffer IBD experience a fluctuation between constipation and diarrhea, often accompanied by abdominal cramping and pain. Patients also present with gas, bloating, and incomplete bowel movements. Often they cannot identify a pattern resulting from eating certain foods, or at least they cannot pinpoint a source of the problem. Whether it's acid reflux, burping, bloating, or gas, their gastrointestinal health seems to be challenged.

Because the health of our gastrointestinal function is vital to our well-being, we need to identify any abnormal gastrointestinal reactions that occur. Although we all may experience abdominal discomfort from time to time, particularly after eating a rich meal, we should not ignore day-to-day symptoms. Using herbs to address gastrointestinal health and stress reduction, along with diet modification, can really make a difference. I cannot tell you how many patients have experienced their first days of no abdominal bloating under my care, only to report that they had no idea they had been bloated for 20 years!

Acid reflux occurs when the stomach acid projects upward into the esophagus and mouth. Not a comfortable experience, it often results in the sensation of burning in the stomach or chest, burping, or nausea after eating. Acid reflux has many causes, but using herbs can help prevent and reduce the problem, providing relief and healing to the irritated tissues.

The symptoms of digestive imbalance often result from one or a combination of a few issues: eating under stress, inadequately preparing the body for food, chewing too quickly, and, most commonly, poor food choices. While you are investigating your own eating habits, consider taking digestive bitters before each meal. Doing so will initiate the digestive process to kick-start the production of stomach acid, and the bitter flavors let all the gastrointestinal organs know that food is on the way.

Unless noted otherwise, to make the teas in these recipes, add 4 or 5 tablespoons of herbs to 1 quart of almost boiling water. Then drink 3 cups per day or 1 quart throughout the day, hot or cold. With tinctures, for chronic complaints, take 1 dropperful 3 times per day. For acute issues, take 2 dropperfuls every 2 or 3 hours for 1 or 2 days, and then 2 dropperfuls 2 or 3 times per day for 5 days. For recipes that do not include instructions, see "An Herbalist's Laboratory" for information regarding how to create and use them.

TEA FOR ACID REFLUX

2 ounces marshmallow root

1 ounce chamomile flowers

½ ounce licorice root

½ ounce ginger root

½ ounce slippery elm bark

Use 1 or 2 teaspoons per cup, steep 5 to 8 minutes. Drink 1 cup after meals.

TINCTURE FOR ACID REFLUX

3 parts marshmallow root

2 parts chamomile flowers

1½ parts ginger root

1½ parts fennel root

Take 1 or 2 dropperfuls at first sign of acid reflux.

SLIPPERY ELM JUICE

I love this formula and recommend it often. Even young children with digestive problems will drink it to help heal their insides. It is formulated to help repair the gastrointestinal lining and reduce inflammation to tummy and intestinal mucous membranes. It is also very soothing for those who experience acid reflux and helps to heal the esophagus from chronic irritation.

- 1 ounce slippery elm
- 1 ounce comfrey leaf
- ½ ounce cinnamon chips

Simmer 15 minutes covered. Strain, and store in container in refrigerator. Take 1 or 2 tablespoons, 3 times per day on an empty stomach.

DIGESTIVE BITTERS TINCTURE

- 2½ parts angelica root
- 2½ parts gentian root
- 2 parts dandelion root
- 1 part ginger root

Take 1 dropperful, 10 minutes before each meal.

AFTER DINNER TEA

- 1 ounce fennel seed
- 1 ounce lemon peel
- ½ ounce caraway seed
- ½ ounce chamomile flowers
- ½ ounce marshmallow root

Use 1 teaspoon per cup, steep 10 minutes covered. Drink 1 cup after each meal.

TOPICAL TUMMY TREATMENT

This herbal oil is good for an upset tummy with gas and bloating.

- 4 ounces castor oil
- 1 ounce fennel seeds

Mix oil and seeds in a jar. Seal and let sit in the warm sun for 2 weeks. Strain and store in glass bottle. Apply 2 or 3 teaspoons to abdomen and relax.

PEPPERMINT OIL CAPSULES

- Peppermint oil
- Enteric-coated capsules

Take 1 or 2 capsules an hour before eating.

IBD TEA

- 1 ounce holy basil leaf
- 1 ounce catnip herb
- 1 ounce marshmallow root
- 1 ounce peppermint leaf
- ½ ounce fennel seed

Use 1 teaspoon per cup, steep 10 minutes covered. Drink 1 cup after each meal or as needed.

IBD OIL OR SALVE

- 1 ounce California poppy flowers
- 1 ounce crampbark
- 1 ounce fennel seed

Apply to abdomen freely for pain.

HELPFUL TOOLS FOR TREATING TUMMY COMPLAINTS

Take stress-reducing herbs, such as skullcap, rhodiola, and passionflower.

Take ginger or fennel essential oils internally or apply topically on abdomen.

Eat foods included in the anti-inflammatory guidelines.

Use L-glutamine amino acid powder for intestinal healing.

Take digestive enzymes with meals.

Wounds

Although cuts, burns, scrapes, and sores are quite common in little ones, adults often fall victim as well. Some of the most common wounds I see in my practice result from falls, from being confined to a bed for too long (bedsores), or from accidents in the kitchen. When wounds occur, take a moment to care for yourself. If you don't take care of wounds right away, unnecessary infections and long healing times result. Treating wounds with herbs can be extremely effective to ensure quick healing and prevent infection.

Any time a wound is bleeding, your first course of action is to stop the bleeding. This helps promote cellular functions that begin to clean and heal the wound and reduce the possibility of side effects such as dizziness or elevated pulse. To stop bleeding, apply direct pressure and elevate the injured part. In a pinch, directly applying calendula, shepherd's purse, lady's mantle, or cayenne will help.

Whenever there is damage to the skin surface, there is a threat of potential infection. You can ward off infection by using herbs both topically and internally. Using an herbal wash, salve, or oils topically can prevent infection and stimulate the cellular regeneration process. You don't need to do a harsh cleaning or debriding of a wound to prevent infection. In fact, this can often cause more inflammation to an already irritated area.

You can also use herbs to promote tissue healing. Many herbs help to pull tissues together and generate new skin formation. For deeper wounds, keep them moist with healing agents to promote continuous skin regeneration. When skin dries out, regeneration stops, which leads to pocketing of tissue or scarring. By continuing with moist treatments, such as applying salves, poultices, or other damp topical treatments, you allow the wound to heal from the inside out. My friend Ananda once nicked off the tip of her finger as she was preparing a big meal. There was no way to reattach it, and it hurt like the dickens. She kept it covered with herbal salves for weeks to help the healing process. It was a miraculous thing to witness her finger regrow to its former shape and size.

Unless noted otherwise, to make the teas in these recipes, add 4 or 5 tablespoons of herbs to 1 quart of almost boiling water. Then drink 3 cups per day or 1 quart throughout the day, hot or cold. With tinctures, for chronic complaints, take 1 dropperful 3 times per day. For acute issues, take 2 dropperfuls every 2 or 3 hours for 1 or 2 days, and then 2 dropperfuls 2 or 3 times per day for 5 days. For recipes that do not include instructions, see "An Herbalist's Laboratory" for information regarding how to create and use them.

HERBAL WASH OR TEA

To stop bleeding

Use the following formula as a topical wash or to make tea.

- 1½ ounces lemon peel
- 1 ounce agrimony herb
- 1 ounce witch hazel bark
- ¾ ounce rose petals
- ½ ounce yarrow flowers

Wash: Steep a strong infusion, 4 tablespoons per pint, for 1 hour. Then soak affected area in the infusion. Better yet, apply a cloth soaked in the infusion to the affected area with pressure. Tea: Steep 3 or 4 teaspoons in 2 cups water for at least 1 hour. Drink 4 ounces every 20 minutes or until bleeding stops; discontinue after 4 hours if no change.

INTERNAL BLEEDING TINCTURE

To stop bleeding, including heavy menstrual bleeding

- 3 parts shepherd's purse herb
- 3 parts yarrow flowers
- 2 parts rose petals

Take 2 dropperfuls every 20 minutes until bleeding subsides. If bleeding has not subsided in 3 to 4 hours, discontinue use.

Small cuts, scrapes, and burns are common injuries: I cannot tell you how many times my husband has burnt himself in the kitchen, only to shrug off my offer of a little burn salve. I often look at him perplexed, not understanding why he wouldn't accept the simple act of a quick swipe of cooling goo to soothe the stinging burn. But I pick my battles. Whether it's a burn, a cut, or a scrape, we need to be proactive. A little salve goes a long way to promote skin repair, fight infection, and cool inflammation. Most salves, including the formulas here, have antimicrobial action, meaning they fight infections of all types. Whenever I have a cut, I apply my salve 4 to 6 times per day. Bandages are rarely necessary, because the salve acts as a protective barrier, and bandages often increase unwanted heat to an injured area.

BOO BOO HERBAL WASH OR SALVE

- ½ ounce calendula flowers
- ½ ounce comfrey leaf
- ½ ounce lavender flowers

Wash: Steep a strong infusion of the formula, 4 tablespoons per pint, for 1 hour. Then soak affected part in the infusion or apply a cloth soaked in infusion for 20 minutes. Salve: Apply topically to affected area 4 to 6 times per day.

BURN HERBAL WASH OR SALVE

| 1 ounce chickweed herb
| ½ ounce plantain leaf
| ½ ounce St. John's wort herb
| ½ ounce lavender flowers

Wash: Steep a strong infusion of the formula, 4 table-spoons per pint, for 1 hour. Then soak affected part in the infusion or apply a cloth soaked in infusion for 20 minutes. Salve: Apply topically to affected area 4 to 6 times per day.

BEDSORE POWDER PACK

Painful bedsores can develop because of pressure caused by lying in a bed in one position for a long period of time, and they can be quite deep for those in the hospital or in hospice care. Some medications make the healing of bedsores extremely difficult, because the body's immune system is compromised.

I have seen great success with the use of the bedsore powder pack formula, which pulls tissues together and reduces the discharge and pain associated with infection.

| 1 ounce calendula flower powder
| 1 ounce plantain leaf powder
| 1 ounce goldenseal root powder

Mix the powders together in a bowl. Depending on the size of the bedsore, pack the wound area with 1 to 4 teaspoons of the powder mix, pouring it into the bedsore. You can also add a little warm water to make a dry paste and then apply it over the bedsore. Once the sore is filled, cover it with a bandage. Change this dressing twice per day. Store the mixture in a glass container.

HELPFUL TOOLS FOR TREATING WOUNDS

Use essential oils: Apply helichrysum directly to stop bleeding. Apply frankincense or lavender topically to prevent infection.

Use herbs rich in vitamins to help heal wounds, such as rosehips, rosemary, peppermint, coriander, and thyme. Include in your diet or drink as tea, 1 or 2 teaspoons per cup.

Use vitamins D and E and borage oil, essential for skin health and healing.

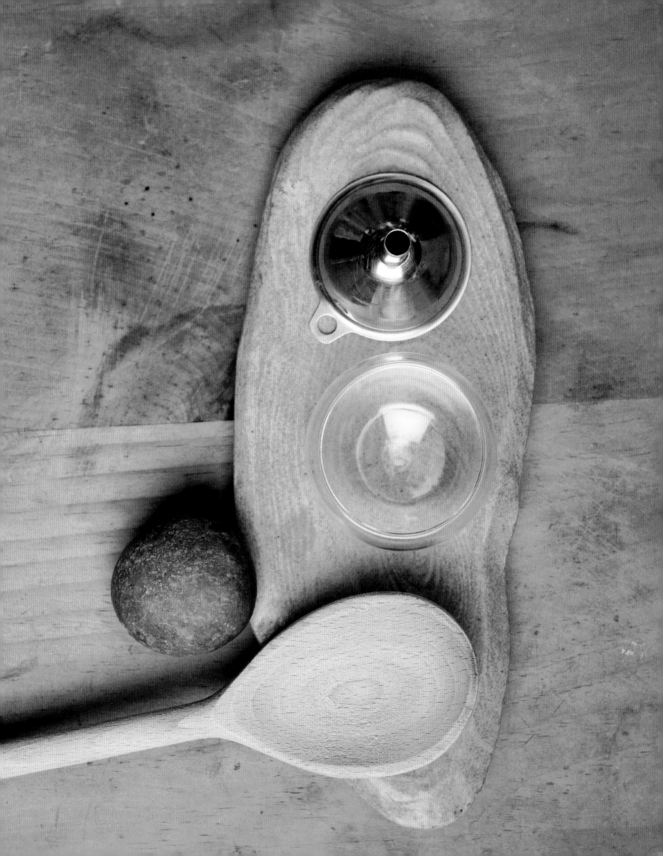

Metric Conversions

INCHES	CENTIMETERS
⅓	0.8
½	1.3
¾	1.9
1	2.5
1½	3.8
2	5.0
2½	6.4
3	7.6
4	10.0
5	12.7
6	15.2
7	17.8
8	20.3
9	22.9
10	25.4
12	30.5
14	35.5
15	38.0
18	45.7
20	50.8
24	61.0
28	71.0

FEET	METERS
1	0.3
1½	0.5
2	0.6
3	0.9
4	1.2
5	1.5
6	1.8
7	2.1
8	2.4
9	2.7
10	3.0
12	3.7
15	4.6
20	6.0
30	9.1
40	12.2
50	15.2
70	21.3
80	24.4
100	30.5
130	39.6
5000	1524.0

US VOLUME MEASURE	METRIC EQUIVALENT
¹⁄₁₆ teaspoon	0.3 milliliter
⅛ teaspoon	0.5 milliliter
¼ teaspoon	1.2 milliliters
½ teaspoon	2.5 milliliters
1 teaspoon	5.0 milliliters
1 tablespoon (3 teaspoons)	14.8 milliliters
2 tablespoons (1 fluid ounce)	29.6 milliliters
⅛ cup (2 tablespoons)	29.6 milliliters
¼ cup (4 tablespoons)	59.1 milliliters
½ cup (4 fluid ounces)	118.3 milliliters
¾ cup (6 fluid ounces)	177.4 milliliters
1 cup (16 tablespoons)	236.6 milliliters
1 pint (2 cups)	473.2 milliliters
1 quart (4 cups)	946.4 milliliters

US WEIGHT MEASURE	METRIC EQUIVALENT
¹⁄₁₆ ounce	1.8 grams
⅛ ounce	3.5 grams
¼ ounce	7.0 grams
½ ounce	14.2 grams
¾ ounce	21.3 grams
1 ounce	28.3 grams
1½ ounces	42.5 grams
2 ounces	56.7 grams
3 ounces	85.0 grams
4 ounces	113.4 grams
8 ounces	226.8 grams
10 ounces	283.5 grams
12 ounces	340.2 grams
16 ounces	453.6 grams

Herbal Suppliers

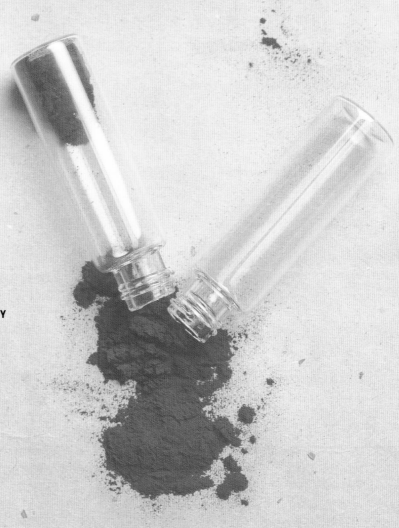

THE HERB SHOPPE—HAWTHORNE
3327 S.E. Hawthorne Boulevard
Portland, OR 97214
503-234-7801
theherbshoppe.net

THE HERB SHOPPE BROOKLYN
394 Atlantic Avenue
Brooklyn, NY 11217
718-422-7981
theherbshoppebrooklyn.com

THE HERB SHOPPE—MISSISSIPPI
3912 N. Mississippi Avenue
Portland, OR 97227
971-703-4347
Thspharmacy.com

WONDERLAND TEA AND SPICE
1305 Railroad Avenue
Bellingham, WA 98225
360-733-0517
wonderlandteanspice.com

DANDELION BOTANICAL COMPANY
dandelionbotanical.com

GAIA HERBS
gaiaherbs.com

MOUNTAIN ROSE HERBS
mountainroseherbs.com

RADIANCE HERBS
radianceherbs.com

WISE WOMAN HERBALS
wisewomenherbals.com

References

Akoachere, J. F., R. N. Ndip, E. B. Chenwi, L. M. Ndip, T. E. Njock, and D. N. Anong. 2002. Antibacterial effect of *Zingiber officinale* and *Garcinia kola* on respiratory tract pathogens. *East African Medical Journal* 79(11): 588–592.

Bode, A. Ginger is an effective inhibitor of HCT116 human colorectal carcinoma in vivo. 26 October, 2003. Paper presented at the Frontiers in Cancer Prevention Research Conference, Phoenix, AZ.

Borrelli F., R. Capasso, G. Aviello, M. H. Pittler, and A. A. Izzo. 2005. Effectiveness and safety of ginger in the treatment of pregnancy-induced nausea and vomiting. *Obstetrics & Gynecology* 105(4): 849–856.

Christopher, John. 1976. *School of Natural Healing*. Provo, Utah: BiWorld Publishers.

Culpepper, Nicholas. 1653. *The Complete Herbal*. Reprint, Hertfordshire, UK: Wordsworth, 2010.

Duke, James. 1997. *The Green Pharmacy: The Ultimate Compendium of Natural Remedies from the Word's Foremost Authority on Healing Herbs*. New York: St. Martin's Press.

Ensminger, A. H., M. E. Ensminger, J. E. Kondale, and J. R. K. Robson. 1983. *Foods & Nutrition Encyclopedia*. Clovis, CA: Pegus Press.

Ensminger, Audrey. 1986. *Food for Health: A Nutrition Encyclopedia*. Clovis, CA: Pegus Press.

Ficker, C. E., J. T. Arnason, P. S. Vindas, L. P. Alvarez, K. Akpagana, M. Gbéassor, C. DeSouza, and M. L. Smith. 2003. Inhibition of human pathogenic fungi by ethnobotanically selected plant extracts. *Mycoses* 46(1–2): 29–37.

Fischer-Rasmussen, W., S. K. Kjaer, C. Dahl, and U. Asping. 1990. Ginger treatment of hyperemesis gravidarum. *European Journal of Obstetrics & Gynecology and Reproductive Biology* 38(1990): 19–24.

Fline, Margi. 2010. *The Practicing Herbalist: Meeting with Clients, Reading the Body*. Marblehead, MA: EarthSong Press.

Fortin, Francois, and Serge D'Amico, eds. 1996. *The Visual Foods Encyclopedia*. New York: Macmillan.

Gladstar, Rosemary. 2012. *Medicinal Herbs: A Beginner's Guide*. North Adams, MA: Storey Publishing.

Green, James. 2000. *The Herbal Medicine Maker's Handbook: A Home Manual*. New York: Crossing Press.

Grieve, M. 1931. *A Modern Herbal*. New York: Harcourt, Brace & Company.

———. 1931. *A Modern Herbal*. Reprint. New York: Dover Publications, 1971.

Hoffman, David. 1996. *Holistic Herbal: A Safe and Practical Guide to Making and Using Herbal Remedies*. Rockport, MA: Element Books.

———. 2003. *Medical Herbalism: The Science and Practice of Herbal Medicine*. Rochester, VT: Healing Arts Press.

Holmes, Peter. 2007. *Energetics of Western Herbs: Treatment Strategies Integrating Western & Oriental Herbal Medicine* Volumes 1 and 2. Cotati, CA: Snow Lotus Press.

Ippoushi K., K. Azuma, H. Ito, H. Horie, and H. Higashio. 2003. [6]-Gingerol inhibits nitric oxide synthesis in activated J774.1 mouse macrophages and prevents peroxynitrite-induced oxidation and nitration reactions. *Life Sciences* 73(26): 3427–3347.

Jagetia G. C., M. S. Baliga, P. Venkatesh, and J. N. Ulloor. 2003. Influence of ginger rhizome (*Zingiber officinale* Rosc.) on survival, glutathione and lipid peroxidation in mice after whole-body exposure to gamma radiation. *Radiation Research* 160(5): 584–592.

Kiuchi F., S. Iwakami, M. Shibuya, F. Hanaoka, and U. Sankawa. 1992. Inhibition of prostaglandin and leukotriene biosynthesis by gingerols and diarylheptanoids. *Chemical & Pharmaceutical Bulletin* 40 (1992): 387–391.

Peterson, M. 2008. *Our Daily Meds: How the Pharmaceutical Companies Transformed Themselves into Slick Marketing Machines and Hooked the Nation on Prescription Drugs*. New York: Picador.

Phan P. V., A. Sohrabi, A. Polotsky, D. S. Hungerford, L. Lindmark, and C. G. Frondoza. 2005. Ginger extract components suppress induction of chemokine expression in human synoviocytes. *Journal of Alternative and Complementary Medicine* 11(1): 149–154.

Rhode, J. M., J. Huang, S. Fogoros, L. Tan, S. Zick, and J. R. Liu. 4 April, 2006. Ginger induces apoptosis and autophagocytosis in ovarian cancer cells. Abstract #4510, presented at the ninety-seventh American Association for Cancer Research Annual Meeting, Washington, DC.

Schittek, B., R. Hipfel, B. Sauer, J. Bauer, H. Kalbacher, S. Stevanovic, M. Schirle, K. Schroeder, N. Blin, F. Meier, G. Rassner, and C. Garbe. 2001. Dermcidin: a novel human antibiotic peptide secreted by sweat glands. *Nature Immunology* 2: 1133–1137.

Srivastava, K. C., and T. Mustafa. 1989. Ginger (*Zingiber officinale*) and rheumatic disorders. *Medical Hypothesis* 29(1989): 25–28.

———. 1992. Ginger (*Zingiber officinale*) in rheumatism and musculoskeletal disorders. *Medical Hypothesis* 39(1992): 342–348.

Weiner, Michael. 1990. *Weiner's Herbal: The Guide to Herb Medicine*. Mill Valley, CA: Quantum Books.

Wigler I., I. Grotto, D. Caspi, and M. Yaron. 2003. The effects of Zintona EC (a ginger extract) on symptomatic gonarthritis. *Osteoarthritis Cartilage* 11(11): 783–789.

Wood, Matthew. 2004. *The Practice of Traditional Western Herbalism: Basic Doctrine, Energetics, and Classification*. Berkeley, CA: North Atlantic Books.

———. 2008. *The Earthwise Herbal: A Complete Guide to Old World Medicinal Plants*. Berkeley, CA: North Atlantic Books.

Wood, Rebecca. 1988. *The Whole Foods Encyclopedia*. New York: Prentice-Hall Press.

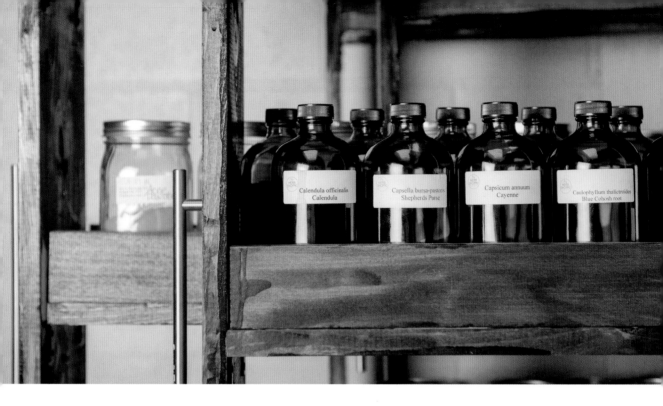

Acknowledgments

The book you hold in your hands was a gift. I'd always dreamed of having the time to return to the dedicated study of my beloved plants, but it wasn't until Timber Press reached out and asked me to do so that I was afforded the opportunity. As a teacher, I hope this book is well used and referenced by students and enthusiasts of herbal medicine. I truly believe herbal medicine is community medicine, and we all have the right to access it. So enjoy all that is contained within these pages and share it with others.

Many thanks go to my editors, Juree and Lisa, who truly taught me the beauty of what an editor does. Thank you for your patience and for helping me make my way through the initiation into authorship. To Shawn, Patrick, and the design team, for making this book come to life. I cannot fully express in words what it feels like to have someone validate your work and want to contribute to it in such a kind and loving way. Thanks Stephanie and Kecia, it was a fun photo journey! To BK and Cordelia, your patience was extraordinary, particularly in the last weeks of putting the finishing touches on my work. Your support was lifesaving. A special thank you to my dad, Don Pursell, for truly showing me the ways of the Earth, and to Linda Quintana, my herbal mentor, for taking me under your wing and then pushing me from the nest when I needed to fly.

Photo Credits

Andreas Eichler, page 93 right

Brynn, page 84 right

Christian Fischer, pages 55 below, 74, 82 left and above right, 90 below, 174 above

C T Johansson, page 106 above

Davepd19, page 131

Dietrich Krieger, page 112

Duncan R Slater, page 175 below

Ezonokuma, page 160 below

Famartin, page 145 above

Herbert Baker, page 86 above

Howcheng, page 87 below

IoannesPavlvsIII, page 87 above

Ivar Leidus, page 147

Jean-Pol GRANDMONT, page 67

Jesse Taylor, page 122

N-Baudet, pages 5, 159 above

Olivier Pichard, page 85 below

Pharaoh han, page 125 right

Schnobby, page 136 above

Teun Spaans, page 134 left

Uleli, page 106 below

Vinayaraj, page 151 above left

Vladimir Kosolapov, page 157

Vojtech Zavadil, page 66 below

Wolfgang Frisch, page 170 left

Used under a Creative Commons Attribution–Share Alike 2.5 license

böhringer friedrich, page 175 above

Marco Schmidt, page 177 below

Onderwijsgek, page 168 below

Public domain on Wikimedia Commons

Daderot, page 127 below

Javier martin, pages 85 above, 103 left

Keith Weller, pages 6 bottom, 160 above

WildBoar, page 158

All other photos are by the author.

Index

A

Abscess Poultice, 207
acid reflux, 266
acids, functions of, 47
acne, 190, 239–241
Acne Wash, 241
adaptogenics, 39, 158
Adrenal Rehab Tincture, 264
adrenals, functions of, 37, 38
adrenal support, 77–78, 124–125, 154, 158
After Dinner Tea, 267
Afternoon Pick Me Up Tea, 244
agitation, 94, 151
agrimony (Agrimonia eupatoria), 54–55
AIDS virus (HIV-1), 124
alimentary canal cleansing, 167
alkaloids, functions of, 47
allergies, 107, 137
Allergy Relief Capsules, 193
allopathic doctors in America, 23
American Association of Poison Control Centers, 24
American Botanical Council, 17–18
amylase, 34
ancient medicine, 20–22
anemia, 137

angelica (Angelica archangelica), 55–56
angina, 111–112, 126
animal bites, 159
anthraquinones, 47
anticatarrhals, and respiratory system, 32
antidepressants, 166
Anti-inflammatory Guidelines, 251–252
Anti-inflammatory Tea, 250
antimicrobial herbs, 33
antioxidants, 86, 131
Antiseptic Liniment, 204
antispasmodics, 36
antivirals, 172
anxiety, 65, 94, 111–113, 157, 217
apertifs, 34
appetite stimulants, 176
arabinogalactan, 122
arbutin, 61
arthritis, 88, 137, 148
Arvigo, Rosita, 248
asthma, 128, 135, 161, 171
astragalus, 258
astringent herbs, 36
Ayurvedic practices, 20

B

Baby Bath for Cold or Teething, 243
Baby Sleep Salve, 209
Backster, Cleve, 43
bacterial infections, 68

balsam fir (Abies balsamea), 56–57
balsam poplar (Populus balsamifera), 57–58
Barking Dogs Salve, 208
baths, 209, 243, 255, 260
bayberry (Morella cerifera, Myrica cerifera), 59–60
bearberry (Arctostaphylos uva-ursi), 60–61
Bedsore Powder Pack, 270
bedsores, 88, 166
bedwetting, 54
benefits of herb consumption, 13
Berger, Paul, 18
bile production, 90
Bird, Christopher, 42
bistort (Persicaria bistorta), 62–63
bitters, 35–36, 39, 47
blackberry (Rubus fruticosus), 63–64
black cohosh (Actaea racemosa or Cimicifuga racemosa), 64–65
black haw (Viburnum prunifolium), 66–67
black walnut (Juglans nigra), 67–68
bladder
   elimination, 58
   function support, 91, 116–118, 147

incontinence, 54, 61, 107, 144, 174
prolapsed, 162
restoratives, 83, 88, 92, 119, 173
bladder stones, 109, 174
bleeding, excessive, 62, 79, 171, 173, 269
bleeding, internal, 89
blessed thistle *(Cnicus benedictus* or *Centaurea benedicta),* 69–70
blood
    circulation, 121, 127, 180
    cleansing, 70, 80–81, 97, 140, 152, 159, 182–183
    clots, 157
    white cell production, 97, 130
blood pressure regulation, 111–112, 132, 134, 150
bloodroot *(Sanguinaria canadensis),* 70–71
blood sugar regulation, 93, 155, 167
blood vessels, cooling and constricting, 153
blue flag *(Iris versicolor),* 72–73
blue vervain *(Verbena officinalis),* 73–74
Blumenthal, Mark, 17–18
bodily fluids, balancing, 156
bodily function improvement, 129, 137

bodily systems, interconnectedness of, 27
body detoxification, 87, 100–101
body warming, 59, 129
bogbean *(Menyanthes trifoliata),* 74–75
Boil On The Bum Sitz Bath, 209
boils, 88, 164
boneset *(Eupatorium perfoliatum),* 76
Bone-up Herbal Vinegar, 235
Bonk and Boo Boo Salve, 208
Boo Boo Herbal Wash or Salve, 269
borage *(Borago officinalis),* 77–78
bowels, 146–147, 150, 170, 240, 266–267
brain function, 64, 70, 82, 120, 152, 244–245, 257
breast milk production and flow, 69, 74, 106
breath, function of, 31
breathing difficulties, 128, 135, 161, 171
bronchodilators, 33
bruises, 88
buckthorn *(Frangula alnus* or *Rhamnus frangula),* 78–79
Bug Bite Relief, 263

bugleweed *(Lycopus virginicus),* 79–80
Build My Immune Reserves Tea or Tincture Blend, 259
Bum Bum Relief Suppository, 214
Bumps and Bruises Salve, 243
burdock *(Arctium lappa),* 80–81, 230–233
Burn Herbal Wash or Salve, 270
burns, 88

C
calamus *(Acorus calamus),* 82–83
Calendula Flower Oil, 201
calendula succus, 212
California poppy flowers, 227
Calm Child Tea or Syrup, 243
Calm Tummy Salve, 208
cancer, 84, 115, 164, 168. *See also* tumors
cankers (mouth sores), 157
capsules, overview, 193–194
carbohydrates, functions of, 48
carbuncles, 164
cardiac glycosides, 27
cardiac obstructive diseases, 133

cardiactive and cardiotonic herbs, 29–30
cardiovascular system, 28–30, 111, 155, 196. *See also* heart
carminatives, 36
castor bean *(Ricinus communis)*, 202
castor oil pack, 202
cat's claw, 23–24
Causae et Curae (Hildegard von bingen), 22
Causis Plantarum, De (Theophrastus), 21
cedar *(Thuja occidentalis)*, 83–84
cellulitis, 172
centaury *(Centaurium erythraea)*, 85
central nervous system, 37, 54–55, 119, 121
Centre for Natural Healing, 18
cervical dysplasia, 70–71, 172
chaga *(Inonotus obliquus)*, 86
chaparral *(Larrea divaricata)*, 87–88
Charaka, 20
Chest Cold Tincture, 259
chickweed *(Stellaria media)*, 88–89
chicory *(Cichorium intybus)*, 90

childbirth, 133–134, 165
children, 54, 122, 242–243
Chinese herbs and herbalism, 20, 189
cholesterol reduction, 160
Christopher, John, 120, 128, 182
circulation improvement, 111–112, 132
cleavers *(Galium aparine)*, 91–92
Clymer, R. Swinburne, 153
cognitive function, 64, 70, 82, 120, 152, 244–245, 257
Cold Catcher, The, 195
colds, 154, 191, 235, 243, 259
cold uterus, 59, 134
colic, 90, 178
colon detoxification, 67–68
colorectal cancer, 115
congestion
    of lymphatic system, 60, 91, 152
    nasal, chronic, 173
    pelvic, 133
    physical, 54
    Warming Sock Treatment, 261
conical biopsies, viable options to, 71
connective tissue, 136, 138, 148
constipation, 58, 141, 150, 215

constituent, defined, 14
contraception, 174, 178
convulsions, 132
cooling, emotional and physical, 126
cordials, overview, 194–195
cortisol production and release, 37–39, 125
couch grass *(Elymus repens)*, 92–93
cough calming, 103, 114, 161, 169, 176, 217
coumarin, 24, 48, 50
cowslip *(Primula veris)*, 93–94
cranesbill *(Geranium maculatum)*, 95
Crohn's disease, 147, 150
Culpepper, Nicholas, 17, 22, 70, 114
culver's root *(Veronicastrum virginicum)*, 96–97
cure-alls, 160
cystitis, 56, 83

D

decoctions, 51, 218–219
decongestants, 83, 114
demulcent herbs, 33
depression, 77
dermatitis, 139, 262
detoxification of body, 87, 100–101
detoxification of organs, 166
diabetes mellitus, 106

diarrhea
  acute, 148, 170
  bacteria-caused, 146
  in children, 95
  sudden onset, 140–141, 165
  tough cases, 112, 165
  traveler's, 68
  with unhealthy bowels, 173
Digestif Cordial, 194
digestifs, 34
digestion
  aids, 63, 85, 102, 142, 180
  fire reduction, 183
  process optimization, 90, 140
  stimulation of, 97, 129, 179
  tonics for, 176
Digestive Bitters Tincture, 267
digestive demulcents, 36
digestive wellness, 56
discharges, excessive, 95, 167, 170
diuretics, 30
diverticulitis, 150
doctrine of signatures, 62, 82
dosing basics for adults, 238
dosing guidelines for children, 242
draughts, 195
Dreaming Syrup, 217

dry conditions in the body, 163, 168
Dry Nose Suppository, 214
dysglycemia, 155

E

ear infections, 122
EarthSong Herbals, 18
echinacea (Echinacea purpurea), 97–98, 227, 258
eczema, 118
Eczema Tincture, 262
Eczema Wash, 263
edema, 132, 174
elder (Sambucus nigra), 98–99
elderberry immune syrup, 217
Elderberry Syrup, 243
elecampane (Inula helenium), 100–101
electuaries, 196–197
elimination facilitation, 58, 78
elixirs, 194
Ellingwood, Finley, 134
emotions, holding in, 54
emunctory system support, 65
endocrine system, 37–39, 72, 77, 104
Endocrine Tea Tonic, 247
Endocrine Tincture, 247
Energy Balls, 245
Energy Now Tincture, 244

epilepsy, 132
erectile dysfunction, 115–116
essential oils, 199, 200, 243, 250, 260
Everyone's Favorite Elderberry Immune Syrup, 217
eyewashes, 165

F

false unicorn (Chamaelirium luteum), 101–102
fatigue, 37, 78, 148, 244–245
fear, 100, 144
female complaints, herbal treatment plan for, 246–248
fennel (Foeniculum vulgare), 102–103
fertility issues, 115, 165
Fertility Tea, 248
fever reduction, 76, 124, 134, 142, 144, 148
flatulence relief, 83, 174
flavonoids, functions of, 48
Flint, Margi, 18
flower essences, overview, 50
flus, 235
fomentations, overview, 204–207
food absorption, 104
formulating herbal blends, 189–191

Fresh St. John's Wort Oil, 201
Fungal Fighter Tincture, 263
fungal infections, 68, 84, 178, 181, 262

G
galactagogues, 69
Galen of Pergamon (Aelius Galenus), 21–22
gallbladder, 75, 81, 90, 96, 110
gallstones, 178
gas relief, 83, 174
gastrointestinal system
  bitters and, 35–36
  bowels, 146–147, 150, 170, 240, 266–267
  colon detoxification, 67–68
  in human anatomy, 34–36
  inflammation in, 56, 87
  intestinal lining toning, 149
  lower intestines, 58
  purgatives and laxatives, 36
  support for, 122, 178, 182
genitourinary system, 119–120
gentian (Gentiana lutea), 104–105
Get 'Er Going Suppository, 215
ginger, 14

Ginger Root or Yarrow Tea, 260
Gladstar, Rosemary, 18, 248
glucose metabolism modulation, 93
glycoside, 48
goat's rue (Galega officinalis), 106
goiter, 68
goldenrod (Solidago canadensis), 107–108
gout, 58, 148
grand cactus (Selenicereus grandiflorus), 108–109
gravel root (Eupatorium purpureum), 109–110
greater celandine (Chelidonium majus), 110–111
gum disease, 79, 157, 173

H
hair follicle stimulation, 156
hardiness zones, overview, 51
hawthorn (Crataegus laevigata), 111–112
Headache Be Gone, 194
headaches, 70, 94, 144
Head Cold or Flu Tea, 259
heart
  angina, 111–112, 126
  damp condition, 110
  support for, 108–109, 155, 195, 217

heartbeat regulation, 79, 133–134, 162, 176
hemorrhaging, 173
hemorrhoids, 88, 117, 182, 214
herbal applications, overview
  capsules, 193–194
  cordials, 194–195
  draughts, 195
  electuaries, 196–197
  essential oils, 200
  herbal oils, 198–202
  liniments, 202–204
  poultices and fomentations, 204–207
  salves, 207–209
  sitz baths, 209
  soft casts, 210–211
  succuses, 212
  suppositories, 212–215
  syrups, 216–217
  teas, 218–219
  tinctures, 219–233
  vinegars, 233–235
Herbal Bath for Cold and Flu, 260
herbal blends, getting started, 190–191
herbal education, 13, 18, 42
Herbal Inhalation, 260
herbalism, 8, 12, 14, 16–19
herbal medicine, definitions and therapeutic actions, 44–45

herbal medicine, research and regulation, 17
herbal oils, 198–202
herbal suppliers, 273
herbal treatment plans, overview, 238
Herbal Wash or Tea, 269
herbs
    blending for medicinal purposes, 190–191
    cultivation and identification, overview, 51
    drying, 53
    extractions, 220
    learning about, 13, 18
    main action, as formulation component, 190
    physiological function of, 14
    preventative use of, 16
    qualities or natures of, 14
    stimulating, as formulation component, 190
    systems affected by, overview, 44
Herb Tea for Libido, 256
herpes simplex virus (HSV), 124
Hildegard von Bingen, 22
Historia Plantarum, De (Theophrastus), 21
holism and systemic unity, 14–15
hops (Humulus lupulus), 112–113

horehound (Marrubium vulgare), 114–115
Hormone Balance Tincture, 256
hormones, 37, 64, 75, 174, 178
horny goat weed (Epimedium grandiflorum), 115–116
horse chestnut (Epimedium grandiflorum), 116–117
Hot Bath with Relaxing Bath Salts, 255
hot conditions, 74, 164
Hot Flash Tincture, 257
HPV (human papilloma virus), 172
HSV (herpes simplex virus), 124
human anatomy, basic overview, 27
    cardiovascular system, 28–30
    endocrine system, 37–39
    gastrointestinal system, 34–36
    respiratory system, 31–33
human papilloma virus (HPV), 172
humors system, 22
hydrangea (Epimedium grandiflorum), 117–118
hydration, 241
hyperactivity, 126
hypertensives, 30, 126

I
IBD (irritable bowel disease), 266–267
IBD Oil or Salve, 267
IBD Tea, 267
IC (interstitial cystitis), 92–93
identification and cultivation of herbs, overview, 51
I Like to Move It, Move It, 196
immune system
    function of, 132, 154
    reserves, building, 217, 259
    stimulation of, 86, 97, 122
    support for, 98, 101, 154, 160, 181
impotence, 115
incontinence, 54, 61, 107, 144, 174
inflammation
    bowel, 146–147, 150
    gastrointestinal system, 56, 87
    and pain, 65, 113, 137, 250–252
    prostate, 118
    reduction of, 89, 171, 176, 250
    of respiratory or lymphatic system, 87
    skin irritations and, 139, 148

inflammation (*continued*)
  sores and, 167
  of tissues, 130
infusions, 51, 218
insomnia, 37, 94, 113, 136, 158, 191, 253–255
internal bleeding, 89
Internal Bleeding Tincture, 269
interstitial cystitis (IC), 92–93
irritability relief, 178

J

Jamaican dogwood *(Piscidia piscipula)*, 118–119
jaundice, transient, 164
joint restorative, 110, 162
juniper *(Juniperus communis)*, 119–120

K

kidneys
  complaints, 61, 92, 138
  elimination, 58
  support for, 88–89, 91, 116–119, 147
Kidney Stone Relief Tincture Blend, 195
kidney stones, 54, 61, 109, 174
kitchen supplies, 187
Kloss's Herbal Liniment, 204
Knockout Tincture, 253

L

labor easing, 133, 165
lactation, 69, 74, 106
lady's slipper *(Cypripedium pubescens* or *Cypripedium parviflorum)*, 121–122
larch *(Larix occidentalis)*, 122–123
laxatives, 168
LEEP (loop electrosurgical excision procedures), viable options to, 71
lemon balm *(Melissa officinalis)*, 123–124
Lemongrass Tea, 263
libido boosters, 115, 256
licorice *(Glycyrrhiza glabra)*, 124–125
ligament restoratives, 148, 162, 211
linden *(Tilia americana)*, 126–127
liniments, 202–203
liver
  cleansing and toning, 70, 75, 80–81, 85, 96, 104, 110
  disease of, 122
  function, 54, 72
lobelia *(Lobelia inflata)*, 127–128
lochia (afterbirth) suppression, 134
Long Life Elixir, 194

loop electrosurgical excision procedures (LEEP), viable options to, 71
lovage *(Levisticum officinale)*, 129
lower back pain, 174
lower respiratory infections, 114–115
lungs, 31, 71, 75, 100, 113, 161
lungwort *(Levisticum officinale)*, 130–131
lymphatic system
  congestion, 60, 91, 152
  herbs for, 33
  inflammation, 87
  support for, 75, 101, 129
Lymphatic Tea or Tincture Blend, 240

M

maceration methods, 221, 225–227, 230, 231
macrophages, increasing, 131
Maeria Medica, De (Pedanius Dioscorides), 21
ma huang, 33
maitake *(Grifola frondosa)*, 131–132
malabsorption, 35
meadowsweet, 14–15
medicinal uses of herbs, 20–22, 50–51, 190–191
medicine, modern, limitations of, 14

medicine cabinet, overview and definitions of terms, 51
Medicines of the Earth conference (2004), 24
menopause, 64–65, 256–257
menses initiation, 141
Menstrual Cramping Tincture, 248
Menstrual Moon Cramping Sitz Bath, 209
menstrual symptoms, relief for, 66, 142, 165, 195
menstruation, lack of, 55
menstruum, defined, 51
metabolistic function, 86
metric conversions, 272
migraines, 94, 119
mineral absorption assistance, 183
miscarriage prevention, 102, 110, 178
mistletoe *(Viscum album)*, 132–133
modern medicine, limitations of, 14
mononucleosis, 153
Montezuma's Defense, 194
morning sickness, 178
motherwort *(Leonurus cardiaca)*, 133–135
mouth ulcers, 159
mucolytics, 32–33

mucous membrane support, 107, 120, 124–125, 139, 150
mullein *(Verbascum thapsus)*, 135–136
muscles, pain or cramping, 64, 65, 178, 204
musculoskeletal pain, 161
mycobacterium tuberculosis, 172

N

nasal congestion, chronic, 173
naturopathic schools, 19
nerve calming, 123–124, 155, 157, 166, 168
nerve pain, 118–119, 138–139, 166
nervines, 30, 39, 126, 139
Nervous Heart Syrup, 217
Nervous Nelly Tea, 264
nettle *(Urtica dioica)*, 136–138
Nettle Succus, 212
neuralgia, 119, 166
noses, runny, 95
Not the Souvenir I Asked For, 196
nourishing agents, in formulations, 190
nutritive tonic herbs, 137

O

oatstraw *(Avena sativa)*, 138–139
obstruction elimination, 59
Oregon grape *(Mahonia aquifolium)*, 140–141
organs. *See also names of specific organs*
    affected by herbs, 44
    detoxification and strengthening, 166
    prolapse of, 102, 162, 167
    stimulation and warming of, 71
    systems imbalance, 54.
Osteoporosis Herbal Vinegar or Tincture Blend, 257
oxygen flow, 121

P

Pain-free Tincture, 250
Papyrus Ebers (anonymous), 21
Paracelsus, 17
parasite eliminating electuary, 196
parasitic infections, 68
parasympathetic nervous system (rest-and-digest state), 37, 154
Pedanius Dioscorides, 21
pelvic congestion, 133

pennyroyal *(Mentha pulegium)*, 141–142

Peppermint Oil Capsules, 267

percolation method, 221, 228–233

perimenopause/premenopause, 74, 256–257

Peterson, Melody, 24

pharmaceuticals, 23–25

phytodynamics and the body, 50

Phytolacca (Poke Root) Oil, 201

pick, chew, and spit method, 186

plantain *(Plantago major)*, 142–144

Plantain Leaf Spot Treatment, 240

Plantar Fasciitis and Ligament Healer, 211

plant directory, overview, 44–53

plant names, Latin vs. common, 44

plants

  constituents and functions, 46–49

  families, 44

  in history of medicine, 20–22

  nature of, 46

  and pharmaceuticals, 23–25

responsiveness of, 42–43

story about, 8–9

PMS (premenstrual syndrome), 55, 66, 74

Poison Ivy Liniment, 263

Poison Oak and Ivy Relief, 235

poisonous afflictions, 142

poplar *(Populus tremuloides)*, 144–145

poultices, overview, 204–205

Practice of Traditional Western Herbalism, The (Wood), 14

Practicing Herbalist, The (Flint), 18

pregnancy

  inhibitor, 174

  miscarriage prevention, 102, 110, 178

  morning sickness, 178

  successful, 115, 165, 248

premenstrual syndrome (PMS), 55, 66, 74

Preschool Barricade Tea or Syrup, 243

prostate, 61, 118, 138

Prostate Relief Suppository, 215

protein supply and processing, 137

psoriasis, 139, 262

pulmonary infections, 56

purgatives and laxatives, 36

purple loosestrife *(Lythrum salicaria)*, 146–147

Q

queen of the meadow *(Filipendula ulmaria)*, 147–148

Quintana, Linda, 100

R

rashes, 139, 148

raspberry *(Rubus idaeus)*, 149–150

rauwolfia *(Rauvolfia serpentina)*, 150–151

Raynaud's disease, 129

red clover *(Trifolium pratense)*, 152

red root *(Trifolium pratense)*, 153

reishi *(Ganoderma applanatum)*, 154

relaxation, 66, 126–127, 139, 150, 170, 180

Relax Now Tincture, 264

reproductive health for men, 113

reproductive health for women, 55, 59, 102, 121, 182

reserpine, 150

respiratory system

  ailments, 56, 258–261

  herbs for, 32–33, 58

  in human anatomy, 31–33

inflammation in, 87
lungs, 31, 71, 75, 100, 113, 161
support for, 89, 99
throat ailments, 63–64, 82, 114–115, 157, 159
tract soothing, 77–78, 135, 142, 169
rest-and-digest state (parasympathetic mode), 34–35
rheumatic pains, 166
rheumatism, 58, 65, 148
ringworm, 161, 164
rosemary (Rosmarinus officinalis), 155–156

S

sage (Salvia officinalis), 156–157
salicylic acid, 14–15
salivation, 34
salves, overview, 207–209
saponins, functions of, 49
scalp irritations, 79
schizandra (Schisandra chinensis), 157–158
sciatica, 119, 166
Secret Life of Plants (Tompkins and Bird), 42
secretory pathways, opening of, 72
sedatives, 158
self heal (Prunella vulgaris), 159

serotonin (5-HT) receptor activation, 65
Shen Nung, Emperor of China, 20
shiitake (Lentinula edodes), 160
shingles, 75
Singh, T. C., 42
sinus infections, 68, 130
sitz baths, 209
skin
    aging, 95
    boils and carbuncles, 164
    detoxification, 70
    eruptions, 72, 81
    herbal treatment plan for, 262–263
    irritation and inflammation, 139, 148
    problems in general, 58
    spot and wrinkle reduction, 94
    tissue fortification, 138–141
    warts, ringworm, tumors, and cysts, 111
    wounds, 88
skunk cabbage (Lysichiton americanus), 161
sleep, 158, 209. See also insomnia
Sleep Capsules, 255
Sleep Pillow, 255
Sleep Salve, 255

Sleep Tea, 255
Slippery Elm Juice, 267
smoking cessation, 56
soft casts, overview, 210–211
Solomon's seal (Lysichiton americanus), 162–163
Sore Muscle Liniment, 204
sores, inflammatory, 167
sores, mouth (cankers), 157
sorrel (Rumex acetosella), 163–164
spleen, swollen, 153
Sprained Ankle Poultice, 204–207
Sprain Support Oil, 250
squaw vine (Mitchella repens), 164–165
staphylococcus, 172
Stingers Sting Away, 207
St. John's wort (Hypericum perforatum), 165–166, 201
stomach
    damp condition, 63
    purification, 128
    tissue toning, 149
    topical treatment, 208, 267
    tummy tamer capsules, 194
    upset relief, 102–103, 113, 142, 194, 243
streptococcus, 172

stress
  and adrenal problems,
    herbal treatment plan
    for, 264–265
  fatigue and, 37, 78
  hormonal imbalance and,
    246
  mental, 119
  reduction of, 123, 132
  syrup for anxiety and, 217
succuses, overview, 212
sumach *(Rhus glabra)*,
  167–168
sunburn, 94
suppliers of herbs, 273
supplies for herbal kitchen,
  187
supplies for wild harvesting,
  52
suppositories, overview,
  212–215
Sushruta, 20
sweating inducers, 182
sweet violet *(Viola odorata)*,
  168–169
swelling reduction, 168
sympathetic nervous system
  (fight-or-flight state),
  37, 134, 144
syrups, overview, 215–217

T
tannins, functions of, 49
T-cells, increasing, 131
Tea Blend for Zinc

Deficiency, 240
Tea For Acid Reflux, 266
Tea for Keeping Things
  Cool, 257
Tea for Memory and Cere-
  bral Circulation, 257
Tea or Tincture Blend for
  Acne, 239–240
Tea or Tincture Blend for
  Bowel Toxicity, 240
teas, overview, 218–219
teeth, 117, 159, 173
tendons, 156, 162
Tenney, Louise, 136
tension, 54, 73–74, 94,
  118–119, 121
Theophrastus, 21
therapeutic actions of herbal
  medicines, overview
  and definitions, 44–45
Thomson, Samuel, 128
throat ailments, 63–64, 82,
  114–115, 157, 159
Throat Soother, 196
thyme *(Thymus vulgaris)*, 43,
  169–170
thyroid, 68, 79, 124, 138
Tincture For Acid Reflux,
  266
tinctures, overview, 219–223
tissues
  connective, 136, 138, 148
  function of, 170
  inflammation reduction,
    130

rebuilding, 88
  sedating and cooling, 176
  states concept, 14
  toning, 149, 170
  vaginal, healing of, 256
Tompkins, Peter, 42
tonics, 30, 32, 247
tonsillitis, 159
Topical Tummy Treatment,
  267
tormentil *(Potentilla erecta)*,
  170–171
toxic mineral buildup, 110
toxin release, 59, 148
tremors, 157
tribal cultures' use of healing
  plants, 16
Tummy Tamer (capsule),
  194
Tummy Tea, 243
tumors, 120, 122, 160, 168

U
ulcers, 150, 167
United Plant Savers, 18
urinary tract, 118, 174
urination, painful, 174
usnea *(Usnea barbata)*,
  171–172
Uterine Fibroids Tea or
  Tincture Blend, 247
uterine prolapse, 102, 162
uteruses, 59, 83, 133–134,
  149, 165

V

vaginal discharges, excessive, 95
vaginal dryness, 257
Vaginal Tissue Healer, 256
Varicose Vein Soft Cast, 211
vascular tonics, 30
vasodilators, 30
vein health, 117
Vinegar of the Four Thieves, 235
vinegars, 16, 233–235
viral rashes, 139
Virchow, Rudolf, 22
vision, 147
Vogel, Marcel, 42–43
voice, 82, 114, 169
volatile oil, 45, 46, 49, 199, 258

W

Wake Up Tea, 244
Warming Sock Treatment, 261
Warrior Heart (cordial), 195
warts, 79, 84
water brash, 83
Weed, Susun, 134
well-being, sense of, 65
wellness, in general, 104
white oak *(Quercus alba)*, 173
whooping cough, 169
wild carrot *(Daucus carota)*, 174–175

wild cherry *(Prunus serotina)*, 175–177
Wild Cherry Cough Syrup, 217
wildcrafting, 52
wild yam *(Dioscorea villosa)*, 177–178
women. *See also* pregnancy
childbirth, 133–134, 165
reproductive health, 55, 59, 102, 121, 182, 246–248
Women's Moon Magic Tincture Blend, 195
Wood, Matthew, 14
wood betony *(Stachys officinalis)*, 178–179
wormwood *(Stachys officinalis)*, 179–180
wounds, 88, 142, 144, 159, 166, 176, 268–270

Y

Yance, Donnie, 18
yarrow *(Achillea millefolium)*, 181–182
yellow dock *(Rumex crispus)*, 182–183

Z

zinc deficiency, 240

Dr. JJ Pursell is a board certified naturopathic physician and licensed acupuncturist and has worked with medicinal herbs for more than 20 years. Having spent many hours on her father's flower farm, her love of plants began at an early age. She began working at herb farms and herb shoppes, which inspired her to enroll in graduate studies in health and medicine. While in school, having returned to the urban life, she missed the plants and the community that an herb shoppe offers. During school she decided to open The Herb Shoppe while finishing her degree in Portland, Oregon. She has taught and trained with herbalists all over the world but prefers the practice of close-to-home grown western herbs.

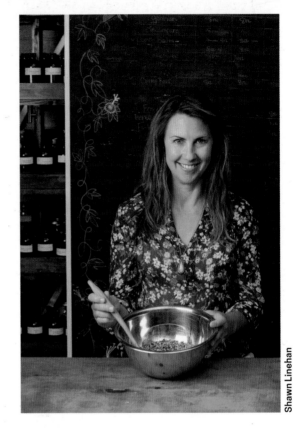

Shawn Linehan

The Herb Shoppe focuses on offering the most vital organic herbs available, while sustaining local growers. Over the years, The Herb Shoppe has received countless words of thanks for all it has to offer and has been asked by many patrons to open shoppes in other parts of the country. The Herb Shoppe's second location is in Brooklyn, New York. With the continued success of both businesses, The Herb Shoppe is now available for franchise for those who are passionate about community and herbal medicine.

The Herb Shoppe was voted "the best apothecary in Portland" by *Willamette Week* and was written up in *Portland Monthly* magazine and *The L Magazine* in New York City. JJ and her shoppe have been featured in several blogs and Tumblr sites, including Gardenista, White & Warren Inspired, Kale and Coriander, Portland Healing Project, PoppySwap, and Girl Gift Gather. JJ appeared on "Green Living," a BCAT television show in Brooklyn; the "Bread and Roses" radio show on Portland's KBOO; and "Wise Woman Radio" with Susun Weed. She is also included in the book *Curing Canine Cancer* and contributed to the new edition of *Hot Pants: A Do It Yourself Gynecology and Herbal Remedies*. She has her own YouTube channel for those who want to learn more about making herbal medicine.